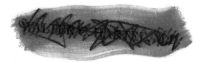

THE EYE AND ORBIT IN THYROID DISEASE

The Eye and Orbit in Thyroid Disease

Editors

Colum A. Gorman, M.D.

Division of Endocrinology and
Department of Internal Medicine
Mayo Clinic
and
Professor of Medicine
Mayo Graduate School of Medicine
Rochester, Minnesota

Robert R. Waller, M.D

Department of Ophthalmology
Mayo Clinic
and
Professor of Medicine
Mayo Graduate School of Medicine
Rochester, Minnesota

John A. Dyer, M.D.

Department of Ophthalmology
Mayo Clinic
and
Professor of Medicine
Mayo Graduate School of Medicine
Rochester, Minnesota

Raven Press ■ New York

Raven Press, 1140 Avenue of the Americas, New York, New York 10036

Made in the United States of America

Library of Congress Cataloging in Publication Data
Main entry under title:

The Eye and orbit in thyroid disease.

　Includes bibliographies and index.
　1. Grave's disease.　I. Gorman, Colum A.
II. Waller, Robert R.　III. Dyer, John A.
(John Allen)
RC657.5.G7E94　1984　　　616.4′42　　　84–18124
ISBN 0–88167–036–7

Preface

It sometimes seems that back to back in their academic tower, the endocrinologist, ophthalmologist, and immunologist gaze at the scene of Graves' ophthalmopathy through different windows. Each sees a part of the landscape but shares the view of his or her colleague to only a limited extent.

This book is intended to broaden the perspective of those interested in Graves' ophthalmopathy by collecting, in one volume, a compendium of current information ranging from theories of etiology to detailed advice regarding practical clinical management.

The reader will find detailed information on orbital embryology, soft tissue anatomy, and pathology. The multifaceted clinical expression of Graves' ophthalmopathy is presented and the role of autoimmunity in its production is discussed. Advances in diagnosis of Graves' ophthalmopathy are reviewed, ranging from ultrasound to computerized tomography and nuclear magnetic resonance. Also covered are the relationships among Graves' disease, Hashimoto's thyroiditis, and myasthenia gravis, concluding with a review of current treatment methods, their successes and limitations.

We have endeavored throughout the book to present information from different disciplines in a manner readily understandable to the reader not well versed in that discipline. With regard to therapy, while not neglecting medical forms of treatment, we have devoted most attention to surgical management, which we believe is the most effective treatment available for the patient with severe ophthalmopathy. Throughout the treatment section runs the consistent thread of planned, coordinated, multidisciplinary medical and surgical management.

The fundamental cause of Graves' ophthalmopathy remains unknown. The best management is controversial. If we manage to stimulate a few readers to test and discard some of the hypotheses and approaches discussed herein, we shall be well rewarded.

This volume will be of interest to endocrinologists, ophthalmologists, and ophthalmic surgeons.

COLUM A. GORMAN
JOHN A. DYER
ROBERT R. WALLER

Acknowledgment

The editors wish to gratefully acknowledge the invaluable secretarial assistance of Ms. Claudia Pietsch, Mrs. Shirley Richardson, and Mrs. Maree Kraft.

Contents

The Eye and Orbit

Thyroid and Autoimmunity

Patient Evaluation

Treatment

Contributors

L. Bartalena, M.D.
Cattedra di Patologia Medica II
University of Pisa
Via Roma 67
56100 Pisa, Italy

Michael D. Brennan, M.D.
Division of Endocrinology and Department
of Internal Medicine
Mayo Clinic
Rochester, Minnesota 55905

R. Jean Campbell, M.B., Ch.B.
Department of Ophthalmology and Section
of Surgical Pathology
Mayo Clinic
Rochester, Minnesota 55905

L. Chiovato, M.D.
Cattedra di Endocrinologia e Medicina
Costituzionale
University of Pisa
Via Roma 67
56100 Pisa, Italy

Roger L. Dawkins, M.D.,
F.R.A.C.P., F.R.C.P.A.
Department of Clinical Immunology
Royal Perth Hospital
G.P.O. Box X2213
Perth, Western Australia 6001

Lawrence W. DeSanto, M.D.
Department of Otorhinolaryngology
Mayo Clinic
Rochester, Minnesota 55905

John A. Dyer, M.D.
Department of Ophthalmology
Mayo Clinic
Rochester, Minnesota 55905

Charles Eil, M.D., Ph.D.
Department of Endocrinology
Box 396
Bethesda Naval Hospital
Bethesda, Maryland 20814

Glenn Forbes, M.D.
Department of Diagnostic Radiology
Mayo Clinic
Rochester, Minnesota 55905

Paul G. Galentine III, M.D.
Department of Ophthalmology
Bethesda Naval Hospital
Bethesda, Maryland 20814

George T. Gamblin, M.D.
Hypertension Clinic, Building 123
Naval Regional Medical Center
Portsmouth, Virginia 23708

Michael J. Garlepp, Ph.D.
Department of Clinical Immunology
University of Western Australia
Perth, Western Australia 6001

Colum A. Gorman, M.D.
Division of Endocrinology and Department
of Internal Medicine
Mayo Clinic
Rochester, Minnesota 55905

Stephen G. Harner, M.D.
Department of Otorhinolaryngology
Mayo Clinic
Rochester, Minnesota 55905

Ian D. Hay, M.B., Ph.D.,
M.R.C.P.(UK), F.A.C.P.
Division of Endocrinology and Department
of Internal Medicine
Mayo Clinic
Rochester, Minnesota 55905

David H. Jacobson, M.D.
4555 N. Shallowford Road
Suite 203
Atlanta, Georgia 30338

Leo Koornneef, M.D.
Wilhelmina Gasthius
Koopvaardijstraat 52
Amsterdam, The Netherlands

C. Marcocci, M.D.
*Cattedra di Endocrinologia e Medicina
  Costituzionale
University of Pisa
Via Roma 67
56100 Pisa, Italy*

William M. McConahey, M.D.
*Division of Endocrinology and Department
  of Internal Medicine
Mayo Clinic
Rochester, Minnesota 55905*

Henry S. Metz, M.D.
*Department of Ophthalmology
University of Rochester Medical Center
601 Elmwood Avenue, Box 659
Rochester, New York 14642*

John F. O'Brien, Ph.D.
*Section of Clinical Chemistry
210 Hinton Building
Mayo Clinic
Rochester, Minnesota 55905*

Karl C. Ossoinig, M.D.
*Department of Ophthalmology
University of Iowa Hospitals and Clinics
Iowa City, Iowa 52242*

A. Pinchera, M.D.
*Cattedra di Endocrinologia e Medicina
  Costituzionale
University of Pisa
Via Roma 67
56100 Pisa, Italy*

John R. Samples, M.D.
*Department of Ophthalmology
Mayo Clinic
Rochester, Minnesota 55905*

David Sevel, M.D., Ph.D.
*Division of Ophthalmology
Scripps Clinic
10666 North Torrey Pines Road
La Jolla, California 92037*

**Robert Volpé, M.D., F.R.C.P.(C),
  F.A.C.P.**
*Department of Medicine
Room 109, E. K. Jones Building
The Wellesley Hospital
160 Wellesley Street East
Toronto, Ontario M4Y 1J3, Canada*

J. R. Wall, M.D.
*The Montreal General Hospital Research
  Institute
1650 Avenue Cedar
Montreal, Quebec H3G 1A4, Canada*

Robert R. Waller, M.D.
*Department of Ophthalmology
Mayo Clinic
Rochester, Minnesota 55905*

R. Patrick Yeatts
*Department of Ophthalmology
Mayo Clinic
Rochester, Minnesota 55905*

Brian R. Younge, M.D.
*Department of Ophthalmology
Mayo Clinic
Rochester, Minnesota 55905*

The Eye and Orbit in Thyroid Disease, edited by
C. A. Gorman et al. Raven Press, New York 1984.

Graves' Disease: An Overview

Colum A. Gorman

*Division of Endocrinology and Department of Internal Medicine, Mayo Clinic,
Rochester, Minnesota 55905*

The association of eye disease and goiter has apparently been recognized as early as the twelfth century (7), but modern focus on the triad of hyperthyroidism, diffuse nonnodular goiter, and ophthalmopathy developed after publication of the works of Caleb Parry (6), Robert Graves (4), and Carl von Basedow (4). Graves' name is predominantly associated with the syndrome for Parry's observations were published posthumously by his son and von Basedow published his findings a few years after Graves.

In patients with fully developed Graves' disease the constellation of clinical findings may include not only diffuse goiter, ophthalmopathy, and hyperthyroidism but also pretibial dermopathy and thyroid acropachy (Fig. 1). Pretibial dermopathy is characterized by the accumulation of acid mucopolysaccharides beneath the skin of the anterior tibial region. Thyroid acropachy is recognized radiologically as a lacy subperiosteal pattern on the metacarpal bones.

Not all patients with Graves' disease exhibit the full spectrum of manifestations. Hyperthyroidism is by far the most common overt manifestation. Clinically obvious infiltrative ophthalmopathy is seen in 3 to 5% of the hyperthyroid group (5), but, by careful study, evidence of subtle ophthalmopathy has been found in most if not all patients with diffuse toxic goiter (1,2,8). Pretibial dermopathy is rarely seen in the absence of overt ophthalmopathy. Thyroid acropachy, the rarest expression of Graves' disease, is, so far as I am aware, found only in patients who also have had the thyroid, eye, and skin manifestations of Graves' disease.

Normally the function of the thyroid gland is regulated by thyroid-stimulating hormone (TSH) released from the pituitary. The TSH attaches to a specific receptor on the surface of thyroid follicular cells and induces production of cyclic nucleotides. These in turn promote the production and release of thyroid hormone (see Brennan, *this volume*). When thyroid hormone levels in the blood rise, the production of pituitary TSH is inhibited and thyroid hormone production and release decline. When serum thyroid hormone concentrations fall, the levels of serum TSH rise and thyroid hormone is released into the circulation. In Graves' disease, this finely regulated balance between serum thyroxine and TSH is disrupted by a new participant in the regulation of thyroid function—the thyroid-stimulating immunoglobulins.

The fundamental cause of Graves' disease remains unknown; however, there is general agreement that the hyperthyroidism of Graves' disease is caused by a family of thyroid-stimulating immunoglobulins which are stimulatory antibodies directed toward the TSH receptor. Whether these or related antibodies are also responsible for Graves' ophthalmopathy is addressed by the chapters by Volpé and by Wall (*this volume*). What evokes the production of antibodies in the first instance remains a mystery. Volpe favors the forbidden

1

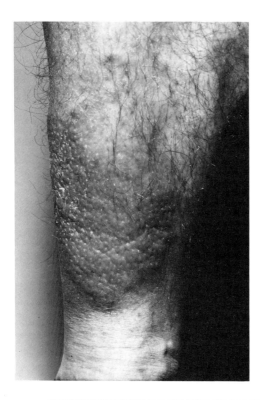

FIG. 1. Top: Pretibial dermopathy is characteristically a raised reddened indurated dermal plaque. Biopsy reveals extensive cutaneous mucopolysaccharide infiltration. **Bottom:** Thyroid acropachy. Note the irregular margin along the radial surface of the 1st metacarpal bone.

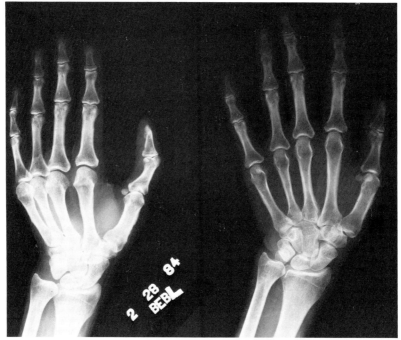

clone hypothesis in which, due to defective immunologic surveillance, a "forbidden" clone of lymphocytes produces self-directed antibodies, in this case against the TSH receptor. The recent discovery of TSH receptors in several types of bacteria gives rise to the intriguing alternative possibility that infection with an organism carrying the TSH receptor is the first event in the genesis of Graves' disease. One may speculate that as part of the body's reaction to the infection, antibodies might be developed against multiple antigenic determinants on the surface of the bacteria, including antibodies to the TSH receptor which could cross-react with the TSH receptor on thyroid cells and thereby stimulate them into overactivity.

Not all patients with eye changes characteristic of Graves' disease are hyperthyroid. Careful study of ostensibly euthyroid patients with thyroid eye disease reveals that, in most, a subtle disorder of thyroid function or regulation can be recognized. This is a very important point because if hyperthyroidism and thyroid eye disease are caused by the same process, one would expect an invariable association. If they are caused by different processes which just happen to be frequently associated, then a much wider degree of variance in their occurrence is to be expected. Certainly strong temporal correlations exist between the onset of ophthalmopathy and the diagnosis of hyperthyroidism (3).

The treatment of Graves' disease remains unsatisfactory. Treatment of hyperthyroidism is directed toward reduction or elimination of the bulk of functioning thyroid tissue by radioiodine or surgery. Alternatively, the chemical synthesis of thyroid hormones in the gland is blocked by antithyroid drugs. Yet in Graves' disease the thyroid, toward which all these treatments are directed, is almost an innocent bystander responding passively to the inappropriate presence of the thyroid-stimulating immunoglobulins. Our hopes for better therapy of the hyperthyroidism of Graves' disease must rest on finding the means to prevent or inhibit this abnormal autoimmune stimulus to thyroid hyperfunction.

Treatment of pretibial dermopathy is symptomatic and consists of local steroid applications under occlusive dressings. It is protracted and not very effective. There is no treatment for thyroid acropachy.

Treatment of the eye changes of Graves' disease is dealt with in detail in the following chapters. It is also unsatisfactory. Our efforts are aimed, imprecisely and with limited success, at suppression of the immune response by using steroids and other immunosuppressive drugs or by radiotherapy to the orbits. Surgery either creates more space for swollen muscles by the various decompression procedures or corrects the late ravages of the diseases by rehabilitative operations directed toward realigning extraocular muscles and repositioning eyelids. We must learn more about effective prevention of ophthalmopathy through improving our understanding of the basic mechanics underlying the eye changes of Graves' disease.

REFERENCES

1. Amino, N., Yuasa, T., Yabu, Y., Miyai, K., and Kumahara, Y. (1980): Exophthalmos in autoimmune thyroid disease. *J. Clin. Endocrinol. Metab.*, 51:1232.
2. Gamblin, G. T., Harper, D. G., Galentine, P., Buck, D. R., Chernow, B., and Eil, C. (1983): Prevalence of increased intraocular pressure in Graves' disease: evidence of frequent subclinical ophthalmopathy. *N. Engl. J. Med.*, 308:420.
3. Gorman, C. A. (1983): Temporal relationship between onset of Graves' ophthalmopathy and diagnosis of thyrotoxicosis. *Mayo Clin. Proc.*, 58:515.
4. Graves, R. J. (1835): *London Med. Surg. J.*, 7:516.
5. Hamilton, H. E., Schultz, R. O., and De Gowin, E. L. (1960): The endocrine eye lesion in hyperthyroidism: its incidence and course in 165 patients treated for thyrotoxicosis with iodine. *Arch. Intern. Med.*, 105:675.

6. Parry, C. H. (1825): *Collections from Unpublished Medical Writings of the Late Caleb Hillier Parry*, Vol. 2. Underwoods, London.
7. Rolleston, H. D. (1936): *The Endocrine Organs in Health and Disease with an Historical Review*. Oxford University Press, London.
8. Tamai, H., Nakagawa, T., Ohsako, N., Fukino, O., Takahashi, H., Matsuzuka, F., Kuma, K., and Nagataki, S. (1980): Changes in thyroid functions in patients with euthyroid Graves' disease. *J. Clin. Endocrinol. Metab.*, 50:108.

The Eye and Orbit in Thyroid Disease, edited by
C. A. Gorman et al. Raven Press, New York 1984.

Orbital Bony and Soft Tissue Anatomy

Leo Koornneef

*Orbital Center Amsterdam, University Eye Hospital, Academic Medical Center,
1105 AZ Amsterdam, The Netherlands*

The human orbit is encaged by the areas of various specialties: above by the neurosurgeons, laterally by maxillofacial, ear, nose, and throat, and plastic surgeons, and below again by maxillofacial and ENT surgeons. Medially the nasal and ethmoidal area is mainly dealt with by ENT surgeons. Orbital surgeons should have a detailed anatomical knowledge of these areas when dealing with orbital disease.

SPATIAL AND SYSTEMATIC APPROACH

Bony Structures

The orbital cavity is pear-shaped; its base is the orbital opening on the face, its long axis directed backward and medially (Fig. 1). The orbital roof and rim are mainly formed by the frontal bone which separates the orbital contents from the anterior cranial fossa. Within this frontal bone the frontal sinus lies medially near the orbital rim. The orbital roof, which is thin, is frequently pierced by various emissary vessels to the dura mater of the frontal lobe. The supraorbital foramen or notch contains the supraorbital artery, the supraorbital nerve, and the superior branch of the superior ophthalmic vein. Laterally the orbital roof bulges upward behind the orbital rim, forming the lacrimal fossa in which the lacrimal gland lies. Posteriorly the frontal bone meets the lesser and greater sphenoidal wings.

Two large openings (i.e., the optic canal, which transmits the optic nerve and ophthalmic artery, and the superior orbital fissure) dominate the sphenoidal bone. Through the fissure run the oculomotor, trochlear, and abducent nerves and the terminal branches of the ophthalmic nerve, together with the ophthalmic veins. The lateral orbital wall is relatively thick posteriorly in the area of the spongy part of the greater wing of the sphenoid bone which separates the orbit from the middle cranial fossa, but it becomes thinner anteriorly where the posterior part of the zygomatic bone meets the greater wing. Outside these bony boundaries, the temporal fossa containing the temporal muscle surrounds the orbit.

This part of the zygomatic bone is generally pierced by two holes through which the zygomaticofacial and zygomaticotemporal arteries and nerves emerge. Anteriorly the zygomatic bone forms the strong lateroinferior orbital margin.

The orbital floor is thick laterally near the inferior orbital fissure, where the zygomatic bone is built-up spongy and compact bone. Following it medially, the floor becomes thinner, finally reaching the maxilla, where the latter forms the roof of the maxillary sinus. In this thin lamella the infraorbital canal is present, containing the infraorbital artery and nerve, the continuation of the maxillary artery and nerve.

Anteriorly the maxilla forms the relatively thick and strong medial inferior orbital margin. The upper part of the maxilla in this area, the frontal process, meets the lacrimal bone

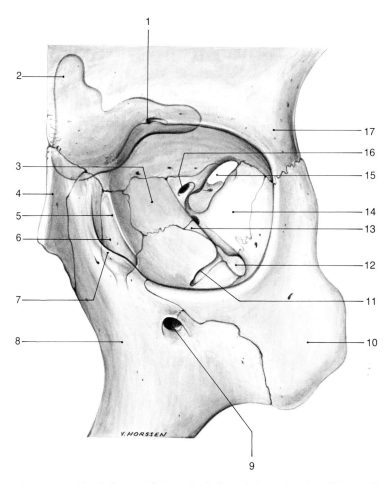

FIG. 1. Left human orbit. *1*: Supraorbital notch, *2*: frontal sinus, *3*: ethmoid bone, *4*: nasal bone, *5*: posterior lacrimal crest, *6*: lacrimal fossa, *7*: anterior lacrimal crest, *8*: maxilla, *9*: infraorbital foramen, *10*: zygomatic bone, *11*: infraorbital sulcus or canal, *12*: infraorbital fissure, *13*: palatine bone, *14*: greater wing of sphenoid bone, *15*: supraorbital fissure, *16*: optic canal, *17*: frontal bone.

inside the orbit, forming the anterior lacrimal crest. Behind this crest lies the lacrimal fossa, the area of the lacrimal sac. Downward, this fossa is continuous with the nasolacrimal canal in the maxilla containing the nasolacrimal duct. The posterior border of the lacrimal bone, the posterior lacrimal crest, meets the ethmoid bone, containing the ethmoidal air cells. The upper border of the ethmoid bone joins the frontal bone. In this area, the anterior and posterior ethmoidal arteries generally leave the orbit. Below, the ethmoid bone meets the maxilla and posteriorly it meets the orbital process of the palatine bone.

Muscles for the Globe

The orbit contains 7 muscles, 6 of which are involved in eye movements (Fig. 2). The seventh muscle, the levator muscle, governs the movements of the upper eyelid. Except for one, the inferior oblique eye muscle, which originates from the area below the lacrimal fossa, all these muscles emerge from a common tendinous ring (Zinn's annulus) in the

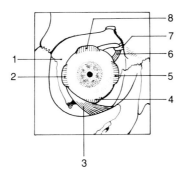

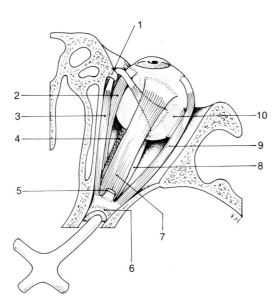

FIG. 2. Schematic drawing muscles for the globe. **Top:** Anterior view right orbit. *1*: Orbit, *2*: lateral rectus muscle, *3*: inferior oblique muscle, *4*: inferior rectus muscle, *5*: medial rectus muscle, *6*: superior oblique muscle, *7*: trochlea (pulley superior oblique), *8*: superior rectus muscle. **Bottom:** Cranial axial view same orbit after orbital roof has been removed. *1*: Trochlea, *2*: medial rectus muscle, *3*: superior oblique muscle, *4*: inferior rectus muscle, *5*: levator palpebrae muscle, *6*: common tendinous ring (Zinn's), *7*: superior rectus muscle, *8*: optic nerve, *9*: lateral rectus muscle, *10*: inferior oblique muscle.

orbital apex. The superior rectus muscle and the levator muscle are closely related throughout their course to the anterior. All straight eye muscles—the superior, the medial, the inferior, and the lateral rectus muscles—insert to the globe anterior from its equator about 6 mm from the margin of the cornea. The superior oblique muscle follows the medial orbital wall up to the trochlea (a pulley) where it turns obliquely backward passing below the superior rectus muscle and attaches behind the equator to the lateral superior surface of the globe, between the superior rectus and lateral rectus muscles. The inferior oblique muscle, unlike the superior oblique muscle, passes below the inferior rectus muscle before attaching behind

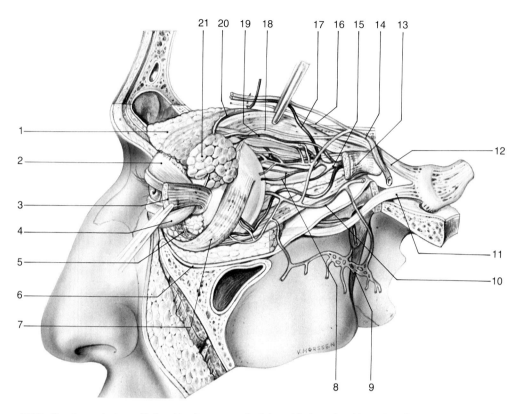

FIG. 3. Lateral view of left orbit after removal of the orbital roof and lateral wall. *1*: Preaponeurotic fat pad, *2*: superior tarsal plate, *3*: lateral rectus muscle (cut), *4*: inferior tarsal plate, *5*: capsulopalpebral ligament, *6*: periorbita, *7*: inferior oblique muscle, *8*: posterior ciliary arteries, *9*: pterygoid venous network, *10*: inferior ophthalmic vein, *11*: maxillary nerve, *12*: ophthalmic nerve, *13*: lateral rectus muscle (cut), *14*: superior ophthalmic vein, *15*: ophthalmic artery, *16*: frontal nerve, *17*: supraorbital artery, *18*: lacrimal nerve, *19*: dorsal nasal artery, *20*: levator muscle, *21*: lacrimal gland.

the eyeball equator to the posterior inferior surface, again between the lateral and superior rectus muscles.

Five of the 7 orbital muscles are innervated by the oculomotor nerve. The superior oblique muscle is innervated by the trochlear nerve; the lateral rectus muscle, by the abducent nerve.

Orbital Vessels and Nerves, Muscles for the Eyelids

The ophthalmic artery originates from the internal carotid artery and enters the orbital cavity through the optic canal, below and lateral to the optic nerve (Fig. 3). In the orbit, it runs for a short distance medial to the oculomotor and abducent nerves, the ciliary ganglion, and the lateral rectus muscle. Then it crosses, in ~85% of the cases, obliquely above the optic nerve and below the superior rectus muscle to reach the medial wall of the orbit.

Running anteriorly between the superior oblique and the medial rectus muscles, the ophthalmic artery divides into two branches: the supratrochlear and dorsal nasal arteries. Other branches of the ophthalmic artery are the central artery of the retina, the lacrimal artery, the muscular branches for the eye muscles, the long and short posterior ciliary arteries for the globe, the supraorbital artery, and the posterior and anterior ethmoidal arteries.

The two ophthalmic veins, the superior and inferior, are devoid of valves. The superior ophthalmic vein begins behind the medial angle of the upper eyelid by union of the supraorbital vein and the angular vein, which communicates with the facial vein. It runs along the medial orbital wall near the orbital roof backward for a short distance and then crosses between the superior rectus muscle and the optic nerve lying inside a connective tissue band: the superior ophthalmic vein hammock. Along its trajectory in the orbit, it receives tributaries of the lacrimal gland, the globe, and medial, lateral, and superior eye muscles, and the ethmoidal veins. Finally it passes through the medial part of the superior orbital fissure and ends in the cavernous sinus.

The inferior ophthalmic vein is far less prominent and begins anteriorly in a venous network; it receives branches from the inferior rectus muscle, the inferior oblique muscle, the lacrimal sac, and the eyelids, and runs backward above the inferior rectus muscle. It frequently joins the superior ophthalmic vein before entering the cavernous sinus, and communicates with the pterygoid venous plexus via a small vein that passes through the inferior orbital fissure.

Aside from the optic nerve and the nerves innervating the orbital muscles, mentioned already, the orbit contains the first division of the trigeminal nerve, called the ophthalmic nerve, a sensory nerve. It supplies branches to the globe, the lacrimal gland, the conjunctiva; to a part of the mucous membrane of the nose; and to the skin of the nose, eyelids, forehead, and scalp. It divides into three branches: the lacrimal, frontal and nasociliary nerves.

Three muscles, i.e., the levator palpebrae, the orbicularis oculi, and Müller's smooth muscle, are involved in the movements of the eyelid. The levator palpebrae aponeurosis splits into two lamellae (Fig. 4) before inserting to the superior eyelid. The anterior lamella interweaves with fibers of the pretarsal part of the orbicularis muscle and attaches to the skin of the upper eyelid forming the upper lid crease. The posterior lamella (Müller's smooth muscle) attaches to the upper border of the tarsal plate. Anterior from the anterior lamella, the preaponeurotic fat pad is present, which in turn is bordered anteriorly from the preseptal part of the orbicularis muscle by the orbital septum. In the lower lid a similar architecture is conceivable. From the inferior rectus muscle, connective tissue septa run anteriorly (the capsulopalpebral ligament) with smooth muscle cells (Müller's muscle) and attach to the inferior border of the tarsal plate, conjunctiva, and pretarsal part of the orbicularis muscle. The medial and lateral inferior orbital fat pads are again separated from the preseptal orbicularis muscle by the far less prominent orbital septum.

The Lacrimal Apparatus

The lacrimal apparatus consists of three units: the tear production part, the conductive part (blinking of eyelids) for moistening of the cornea, and a drainage system to the nose (Fig. 4). Aqueous production forming the middle layer of the tear film mainly occurs in the lacrimal gland, lying in the lacrimal fossa. The gland itself is partly divided into two portions—orbital and palpebral—by the lateral levator aponeurosis. The tear ducts of the gland drain into the lateral part of the superior conjunctival fornix. Additional aqueous production takes place in accessory lacrimal glands (Krause's and Wolfring's glands) lying in the upper eyelid. The mucous layer of the tear film covering the corneal epithelium is formed in other accessory lacrimal glands, those of Manz and Henle. The top lipid layer of the tear film is produced by the meibomian glands, the glands of Moll and Zeis, roughly located in the lid margin area. The tears flowing into the lacrimal lake near the lacrimal puncta are conducted via a superior and inferior canaliculus to the common canaliculus

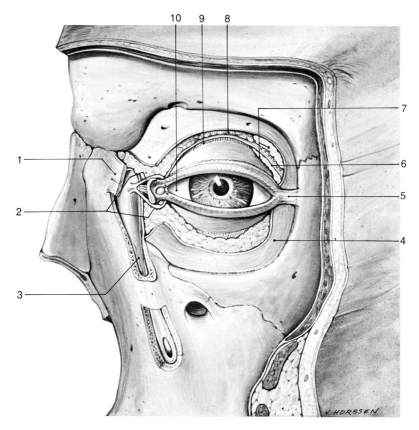

FIG. 4. Lacrimal apparatus of left orbit after skin, orbicularis muscle, and orbital septum have been partially removed. *1*: Medial canthal tendon (landmark in dacryocystorhinostomies), *2*: superior and inferior canaliculus, *3*: nasolacrimal duct, *4*: remnant of orbital septum, *5*: lateral canthal tendon, *6*: levator palpebrae aponeurosis, *7*: lacrimal gland palpebral and orbital parts, *8*: preaponeurotic fat pad (below it the anterior lamella of the levator), *9*: posterior lamella levator muscle (Müller's muscle), *10*: lacrimal lake.

draining into the lacrimal sac. This sac, ~10 mm long, drains into the nose below the inferior nasal concha via the nasolacrimal duct, which in turn is twice the length of the sac.

Orbital Connective and Adipose Tissue

Apart from the eye muscles governing the eye movements, an additional supportive system is present in the orbit and best developed at eyeball level. This system is definitely involved in orbital fractures, which accounts for the bizarre motility disturbances in these cases. Probably it is also involved in patients with Graves' ophthalmopathy because again the severe motility disturbances in these patients cannot be explained by eye muscle involvement only. That this connective tissue is more conspicuous on CT scans of these patients lends support to this assumption.

Orbital Connective Tissue Medially and Inferiorly

The medial rectus muscle connective tissue has a predominantly craniocaudal direction (Fig. 5). The muscle appears to have a large area of attachment to both the orbital roof and

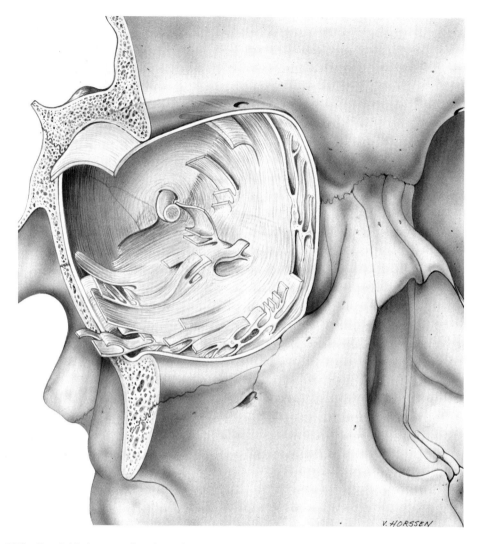

FIG. 5. Orbital connective tissue in medial and inferior orbital areas (right orbit). The medial rectus, the inferior oblique, and the inferior rectus are invisible because they are completely enveloped by this connective tissue system (see text).

floor. In a trajectory of 16 mm from the orbital apex to the anterior, the inferior border of the muscle has connections with the periorbita covering Müller's muscle in the inferior orbital fissure. There, cranial connections with the orbital roof start, and septal connections are established with the optic nerve and the hind surface of the globe.

At a distance of 2.6 cm from the apex, the connective tissue systems of the medial rectus muscle and the superior oblique muscle tendon join. Other septa from the medial rectus muscle contribute to the formation of the superior ophthalmic vein hammock. The connections with the orbital roof and floor are still maintained. Some of the caudal septa change their direction laterally and reach the connective tissue of the inferior oblique and rectus muscles.

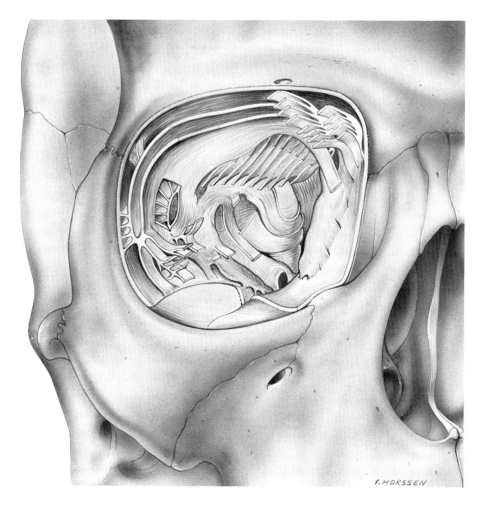

FIG. 6. The orbital connective tissue systems of the superior oblique, the superior rectus, the levator, and the lateral rectus muscles (see text).

The inferior oblique muscle connective tissue is generally parallel to the orbital floor and intermingles extensively with the inferior rectus muscle connective tissue. Medially, near the lacrimal sac fossa, the septa of the inferior oblique muscle are connected to the caudal attachments of the medial rectus muscle septa. The lateral part of the inferior oblique muscle connective tissue, on the other hand, is connected with caudal septa of the lateral rectus muscle (Lockwood's ligament).

The inferior rectus muscle near the apex is connected to Müller's smooth muscle by a number of connective tissue septa. At a distance of ~ 1.5 cm from the apex, this connection is lost. Nevertheless, other septa now connect the medial aspect of the muscle with the medial rectus muscle. Anteriorly lateral septal extensions attach the muscle to the periorbita, which covers the inferior orbital fissure. At a distance of 2 cm from the orbital apex, relationships with the connective tissue system of the lateral rectus muscle are established. The muscle is closely adherent to the orbital floor. This close relationship is maintained anteriorly, and archlike septa surround the muscle and several fingerlike offshoots reach the

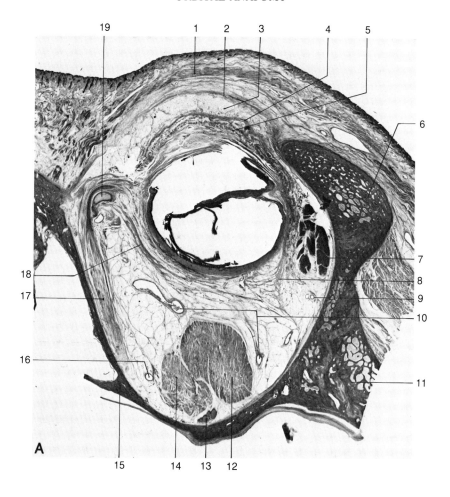

A

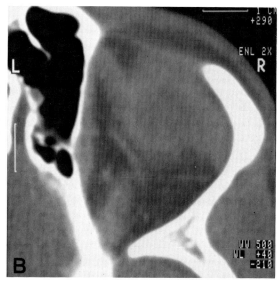

B

FIG. 7. A: Axial section through the upper one-third of a right orbit (see text). *1*: Preseptal part of orbicularis muscle, *2*: orbital septum, *3*: preaponeurotic fat pad, *4*: anterior lamella levator muscle, *5*: posterior lamella levator (Müller's muscle), *6*: zygomatic bone, *7*: lacrimal gland, *8*: lateral levator aponeurosis, *9*: lacrimal artery, *10*: superior ophthalmic vein cut twice, *11*: sphenoid bone, *12*: superior rectus muscle, *13*: frontal nerve, *14*: superior levator muscle, *15*: frontal bone, *16*: ophthalmic artery, *17*: superior oblique muscle, *18*: superior oblique muscle connective tissue (tendon), *19*: trochlea. **B:** CT scan of same area.

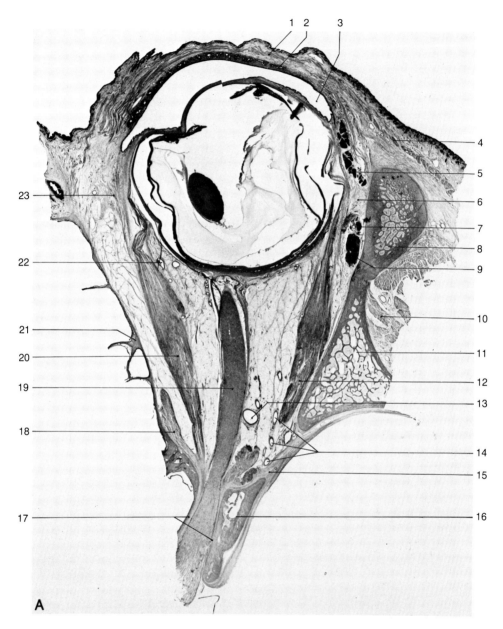

FIG. 8. A: Midaxial section, right orbit. *1:* Pretarsal part of orbicularis muscle, *2:* tarsal plate, *3:* conjunctival fornix, *4:* orbital part of orbicularis muscle, *5:* lacrimal gland, palpebral part, *6:* lateral check ligament, *7:* lacrimal artery, *8:* zygomatic bone, *9:* lacrimal gland, orbital part, *10:* temporalis muscle, *11:* sphenoid bone, *12:* lateral rectus muscle, *13:* ophthalmic artery, *14:* superior ophthalmic vein, *15:* supraorbital fissure, *16:* sphenoid bone, lesser wing, *17:* optic canal, *18:* superior oblique muscle, *19:* optic nerve, *20:* medial rectus muscle, *21:* ethmoid bone, *22:* superior ophthalmic vein, *23:* medial check ligament, **B:** CT scan of same area.

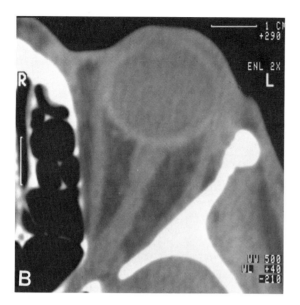

FIG. 8. *(Continued).*

inferolateral orbital wall, fixing the muscle in its position. The close relationship with the orbital floor is abruptly lost at the moment the floor bulges out into the maxillary sinus. The muscle fails to conform to this bulge, but passes straight on, leaving room for the inferior oblique muscle and its connective tissue septa.

Orbital Connective Tissue Superiorly and Laterally

At a distance of 1 cm from the apex, connective tissue septa of the superior rectus muscle reach the superior ophthalmic vein, forming the caudal prolongation of the medial part of the superior ophthalmic vein hammock (Fig. 6). Anteriorly the vein gradually becomes embedded in the connective tissue septa of the medial rectus muscle.

From the lateral end of the muscle, fingerlike connective tissue septa run laterally and attach it to the adjacent periorbita. More to the anterior these fingerlike connections are gradually replaced by a single thick septum, the lateral aponeurosis of the levator muscle. Further, a second septum is added cranially which attaches the levator to Whitnall's tubercle and envelopes the palpebral part of the lacrimal gland. This septum finally attaches together with the orbital septum to the superior border of the tarsal plate containing smooth muscle fibers (posterior lamella). The medial aponeurosis, because it is interfered with by the superior oblique muscle connective tissue, is far less well developed.

The superior oblique muscle belly, running along the medial orbital wall, has connective tissue septa enveloping it. Thus, the muscle lies in its own adipose tissue compartment until it reaches the trochlea. After passing the trochlea, the superior oblique muscle tendon has extensive septal connections over a long distance to the medial upper and posterior surface of the globe.

Going back to the orbital apex, now more laterally, connective tissue septa of the inferior border of the lateral rectus muscle reach the periorbita covering Müller's muscle in the inferior orbital fissure. Immediately anterior to this area, fingerlike offshoots reach the lateral orbital wall and attach the muscle to the adjacent periorbita over a large area anteriorly.

This area includes the whole lateral orbital wall. The muscle is thus firmly anchored to the lateral wall on its whole journey through the orbit. At a distance of 1.5 cm anterior from the apex, the lateral rectus muscle connective tissue joins the connective tissue septa originating from the lateral border of the inferior rectus muscle. These connections are maintained over an area of ~1 cm. Further to the anterior, the lateral rectus muscle connective tissue system becomes continuous with the inferior oblique muscle connective tissue system. Like the superior and medial rectus muscles, the lateral rectus muscle also contributes to the formation of the superior ophthalmic vein hammock. At a distance of 2.2 cm from the apex, septa running from the medial part of the lateral rectus muscle reach the optic nerve and the posterior part of Tenon's capsule. At the area of Whitnall's tubercle, cranial extensions of the lateral rectus muscle connective tissue blend with the lateral aponeurosis of the levator.

SECTIONAL ANATOMY OF THE ORBIT IN THREE PLANES

Axial Sections

In these sections the orientation is as follows: above is anterior, left is nasal, below is posterior, and right is temporal (Fig. 7). The first section lies in a plane through the lacrimal gland on the right and the trochlea on the left. The orbital walls are formed, from medial to lateral, by the frontal bone, a small part of the sphenoid bone (greater wing) and the zygomatic process of the frontal bone. Anteriorly the orbital contents are separated from the skin and orbicularis muscle by the orbital septum and the preaponeurotic fat pad. Below this fat pad, the anterior and posterior lamellae of the levator muscle are visible. Medially the superior oblique muscle lies close to the bone, and passes through the trochlea becoming tendinous. The tendon cannot be seen in Fig. 7, but the connective tissue of the muscle swings backwards and intermingles with the lateral aponeurosis of the levator muscle. Posteriorly, Fig. 7 shows the superior ophthalmic vein sectioned twice, the ophthalmic artery, the lacrimal artery, the bellies of the levator, and the superior rectus muscle and divisions of the supraorbital nerve. Laterally the orbital part of the lacrimal gland lying in the lacrimal fossa is present.

In the midaxial section (Fig. 8), the orbital walls are formed by the zygomatic bone, the lesser and greater wings of the sphenoid and ethmoid bones. In the upper eyelid, the pretarsal part of the orbicularis muscle is seen, as well as the tarsal plate with the meibomian glands. The optic nerve running through the optic canal is flanked medially by the medial rectus muscle and laterally, in part, by the lateral rectus muscle. Between the latter and the nerve, the ophthalmic artery and branches of the superior ophthalmic vein near the superior orbital fissure are visible. Lateral from the lateral rectus muscle and more anteriorly the orbital and palpebral part of the lacrimal gland is present. As illustrated in this section, the orbital connective tissue should be considered a continuous network. Thus, the palpebral and orbital parts of the lacrimal gland are separated in appearance only by the lateral check ligament, since it is actually continuous with the lateral levator aponeurosis.

Coronal Sections

In these sections right is medial and left is lateral (Fig. 9). This first coronal section goes approximately through the orbital aperture, which consists of the frontal bone, zygomatic bone, maxilla, and lacrimal bone. The lacrimal bone is absent however, because the plane of sectioning has not yet reached it. In its place, medially the orbicularis muscle is visible.

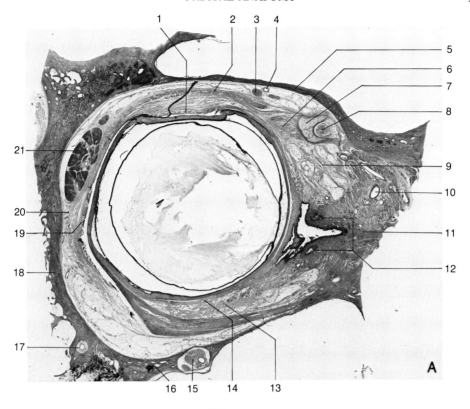

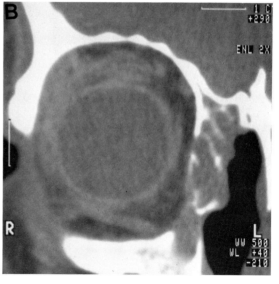

FIG. 9. A: Coronal section, right orbit. *1*: Superior rectus muscle, *2*: levator muscle, *3*: frontal nerve, *4*: supraorbital artery, *5*: frontal bone, *6*: superior oblique muscle tendon, *7*: trochlea, *8*: superior oblique muscle, *9*: medial levator aponeurosis, *10*: angular vein, *11*: medial canthal tendon, *12*: superior and inferior canaliculi, *13*: capsulopalpebral ligament, *14*: inferior oblique muscle, *15*: infraorbital nerve and artery, *16*: maxilla, *17*: zygomaticofacial canal, *18*: zygomatic bone, *19*: lateral rectus muscle, *20*: lateral check ligament, *21*: lacrimal gland. **B:** CT scan of same area.

Below the trochlea is the medial extension of the superior levator aponeurosis. The tendon and connective tissue of the superior oblique muscle are continuous with the levator aponeurosis. The muscle belly of the latter is broad and flat. The lateral aponeurosis passing below the lacrimal gland is continuous with the lateral check ligament. Medially below the ligament, the inferior oblique muscle attaches to the globe. Above this muscle is the

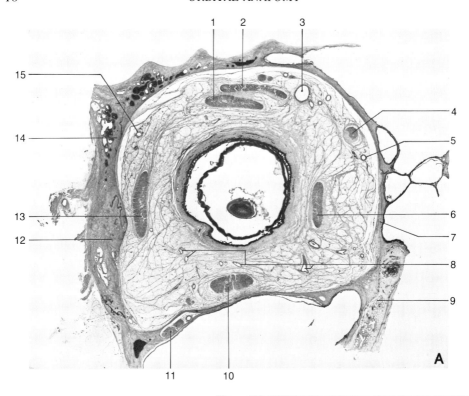

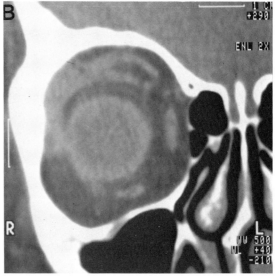

FIG. 10. **A:** Coronal section, half-way equator and the posterior pole of the globe. *1*: Superior rectus muscle, *2*: levator muscle, *3*: superior ophthalmic vein, *4*: superior oblique muscle, *5*: dorsal nasal artery, *6*: medial rectus muscle, *7*: ethmoid bone, *8*: inferior ophthalmic vein, *9*: nasolacrimal duct, *10*: inferior rectus muscle, *11*: infraorbital nerve and artery in their canal, *12*: zygomatic bone, *13*: lateral rectus muscle, *14*: greater wing of sphenoid bone, *15*: lacrimal artery. **B:** CT scan of same area.

capsulopalpebral ligament and the inferior rectus muscle. Medially there is the T-forked conjunctival formix, with the lacrimal canaliculi which are present in the striated muscle fibers of the orbicularis muscle

In the section illustrated by Fig. 10, which goes approximately halfway through the equator and posterior pole of the eye, the orbital walls are built up by the frontal, sphenoid, zygomatic, and ethmoid bones and the maxilla. Orbital connective tissue is best developed

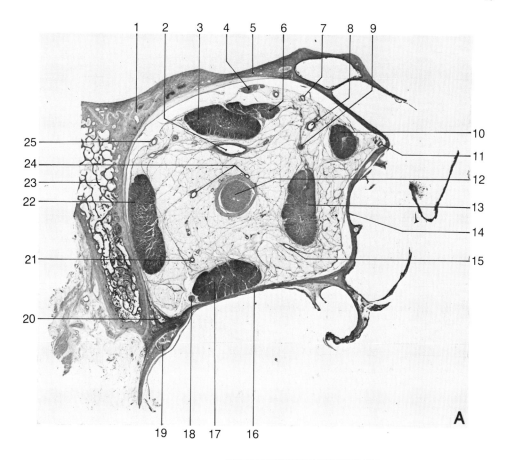

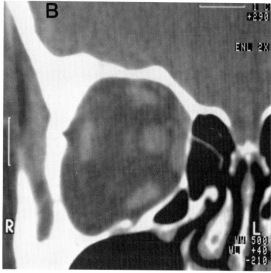

FIG. 11. A: Coronal section through the anterior one-third of the retrobulbar space. *1*: Zygomatic bone, *2*: superior ophthalmic vein, *3*: superior rectus muscle, *4*: frontal nerve, *5*: frontal bone, *6*: levator muscle, *7*: dorsal nasal artery, *8*: ophthalmic artery, *9*: nasociliary nerve, *10*: superior oblique muscle, *11*: supratrochlear artery, *12*: optic nerve, *13*: medial rectus muscle, *14*: ethmoid bone, *15*: inferior ophthalmic vein, *16*: maxilla, *17*: inferior rectus muscle, *18*: oculomotor nerve branch to inferior oblique muscle, *19*: intraorbital nerve, *20*: infraorbital fissure, *21*: muscular branch inferior oblique muscle, *22*: lateral rectus muscle, *23*: greater wing of sphenoid bone, *24*: posterior ciliary arteries, *25*: lacrimal artery. **B:** CT scan same area.

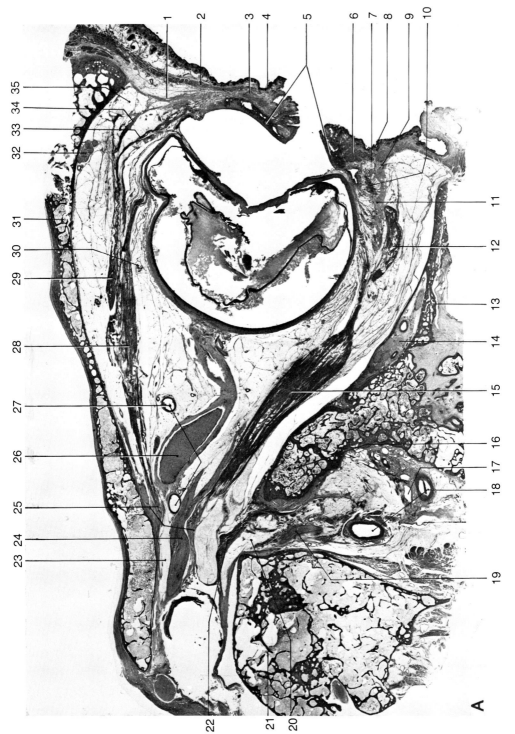

FIG. 12A *(legend on p. 21).*

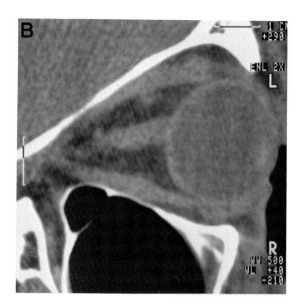

FIG. 12. A: Midsagittal section through right orbit. *1*: Orbital septum, *2*: orbicularis muscle, *3*: pretarsal part of orbicularis muscle, *4*: superior eyelid skin crease, *5*: tarsal plates, *6*: orbicularis muscle, *7*: orbital septum, *8*: lower lid skin crease, *9*: capsulopalpebral ligament, *10*: Müller's muscle, *11*: Lockwood's ligament, *12*: inferior oblique muscle, *13*: maxilla, *14*: infraorbital canal, *15*: inferior rectus muscle, *16*: palatine bone, *17*: pterygoid venous network, *18*: maxillary artery, *19*: maxillary nerve, *20*: infraorbital fissure, *21*: sphenoid bone, *22*: Müller's muscle, *23*: supraorbital fissure, *24*: oculomotor nerve, *25*: common tendinous ring (Zinn's), *26*: optic nerve, *27*: ophthalmic artery, *28*: superior rectus muscle, *29*: levator muscle, *30*: superior ophthalmic vein, *31*: frontal bone, *32*: frontal nerve, *33*: posterior levator lamella, *34*: anterior levator lamella, *35*: preaponeurotic fat pad. **B:** sagittal CT scan same area.

in this area. Laterally from the supraorbital vein, the superior rectus muscle and levator have septal connections to the orbital roof.

A thick septum (intermuscular membrane) connects the superior rectus muscle to the lateral rectus muscle. Below the lateral rectus muscle, radial septa are present, gradually intermingling with the archlike septa surrounding the inferior rectus muscle. Many branches of the inferior ophthalmic vein are present in this area. The medial rectus muscle, anteriorly completely enveloped by the medial check ligament connective tissue, now makes craniocaudal connections with the orbital roof and floor. The superior oblique muscle belly lies in its own fat compartment.

The section illustrated by Fig. 11 covers the anterior one-third of the retrobulbar space. The zygomatic bone, lying between the greater wing of the sphenoid and the frontal bone, makes up only a small part of the lateral orbital wall.

The inferior orbital fissure lies between the greater sphenoid wing and the maxilla, closed off by Müller's smooth muscle. Below the latter is the infraorbital nerve. The orbital floor is extremely thin in this area. Equally thin is the medial orbital wall, which consists of the frontal and ethmoid bones. Unfortunately, the orbital contents in this section are artificially separated from the orbital walls by shrinkage in lateral superior and medial areas. Below the superior rectus muscle, which lies in close relation to the levator muscle, the superior ophthalmic vein, lying in its hammock, is visible. The connective tissue system is far less developed as compared to the previous section. Craniocaudal connections of the medial rectus are still discernible. The inferior rectus muscle lies close to the orbital floor in this section. The ophthalmic artery lies above the nasociliary nerve. In this area the main arterial trunk has divided into muscular branches, posterior ciliary arteries, the lacrimal artery, and supra- and infratrochlear arteries.

Midsagittal Section

The midsagittal section passes through the orbital apex (left of section) and the superior and inferior orbital fissures (Fig. 12). The orbital walls consist of the frontal bone, the greater wing of the sphenoid bone, the palatine bone, and the maxilla. Anteriorly on the right are the eyelids. In the upper eyelid below the skin, the orbicularis muscle, the subcutaneous fat, and the orbital septum are present. Also present are the preaponeurotic fat pad and the anterior and posterior levator (Müller's muscle) lamellae. The posterior lamella attaches to the tarsal plate; the anterior lamella interweaves with the orbicularis muscle and attaches to the skin forming the upper lid crease. In the lower eyelid the tarsal plate is smaller, the suborbicularis fat pad is absent, and the orbital septum lies immediately posterior to the orbicularis muscle. The inferior oblique and inferior rectus muscles are closely adherent and enveloped by connective tissue (Lockwood's ligament). Anteriorly this tissue is continuous with the capsulopalpebral ligament. This ligament in turn divides into two lamellae: the posterior one (Müller's muscle) attaches to the inferior border of the tarsal plate; the anterior to the orbicularis muscle and to the skin forming the lower eyelid skin crease. The anatomy of the upper and lower eyelids are comparable. Below the orbital roof several fasciculi of the frontal nerve are present, and the bellies of the superior levator muscle and the superior rectus muscle are adherent. Between the globe and the superior rectus muscle, the superior ophthalmic vein lies inside its hammock. The ophthalmic artery is sectioned twice because it partially encircles the optic nerve. Below the posterior division of the artery is the oculomotor nerve. The inferior rectus muscle originates from Zinn's common annulus. In the inferior orbital fissure lies Müller's muscle; below it, the pterygopalatine fossa with the maxillary artery and nerve are visible.

CLINICAL BEARINGS

Detailed anatomical knowledge is of paramount importance for surgeons dealing with orbital disease. In progressive malignant Graves' ophthalmopathy, when steroids and/or supervoltage irradiation fail, orbital decompression can halt visual acuity decrease. The medial and inferior orbital walls are easiest to remove because they are thinnest and also yield the most volume effect. However, it is advised to start the decompression procedure with a lateral orbitotomy and removal of the lateral orbital wall, because this is a relatively low-risk first approach and yields preliminary relief to the tensed orbital structures. In this way, visibility of the apex is better and chance of damage to the infraorbital nerve is lessened. Additional volume effect can be created permanently by removing the anterior one-third of the temporalis muscle. Taking away the orbital walls alone, however, is not enough; one should always incise the periorbita. This should be done posteriorly parallel to the connective tissue system which runs from apex to aperture and anteriorly, approximately at eyeball level parallel to the connective tissue systems of the oblique muscles that encircle the globe. A decompression procedure performed in this manner minimizes chances of a further increase in motility disturbances and even proves to have a beneficial effect on motility in some cases.

Knowledge of the orbital sectional anatomy presented above can be helpful with regard to eyelid surgery. The various layers of the eyelids and the comparable architecture of the upper and lower eyelids are clarified by the various sections in different planes. Additional information is provided by the sections for the interpretation of CT scans and for decisions about the direction in which a scan should be made. With Graves' disease, for instance, the coronal scanning direction or, even better, the one parallel to the orbital aperture per orbit seem best, because the straight eye muscles are sectioned perpendiclar to their axes, and volume increase can be compared in one section. Furthermore, compression of the optic nerve in the apex can be evaluated.

ACKNOWLEDGMENTS

The author wishes to thank Frans Zonneveld for providing the CT scans, Ad van Horssen for his drawings, Pem Goldsmidt for assisting with the English, and Jeanine Haages-Manck for editing the manuscript. The basis for this chapter was formed while the author worked in the reconstructive morphology group (head, Prof. dr. J. A. Los) of the Department of Anatomy, University of Amsterdam.

The Eye and Orbit in Thyroid Disease, edited by
C. A. Gorman et al. Raven Press, New York 1984.

Pathology of Graves' Ophthalmopathy

R. Jean Campbell

*Department of Ophthalmology and Section of Surgical Pathology, Mayo Clinic,
Rochester, Minnesota 55905*

The pathologic changes that occur in Graves' disease may be widespread, and the changes that occur within the orbit are merely part of a generalized pathologic process that also affects the thyroid, thymus, heart, skeletal muscles, and subcutaneous tissues. Within these structures the pathologic changes are similar with respect to cellular infiltrate and edema but differ in degree and from patient to patient.

NATURE OF ORBITAL TISSUE

Over the years, authors have debated and presented conflicting evidence as to the precise nature of the increased volume of tissue within the orbit above its average volume of 26 ml. In 1840 von Basedow (4) described what he called "hypertrophy of the orbital tissue," especially orbital fat. Many other authors (1,22,23) have also emphasized the increased amount of fibrofatty tissue. Dobyns (8) demonstrated an increase in the fat content of the orbit in animals treated with thyrotropic hormone. Smelser (30) considered both water and fat to be responsible for the increased amount of retrobulbar tissue in experimental animals. Other authors (1,9,17) emphasized the muscle changes and reported enlargement up to eight (17) or 10 (5) times normal. Computed tomography scanning and pathology (7,32) and ultrasound (11,33) studies have shown that the extraocular muscles are responsible for the proptosis and are the primary focus of the disease process.

It is interesting that in 1944 Rundle and Pochin (23) performed quantitative analysis studies of the orbital contents of 17 autopsy cases with thyrotoxicosis, with and without eye signs, and found an increase in the amount of "muscle fat." The content of fat within the muscle was more than double that of tissue from control subjects. This increase in fat was found to be proportional to the contents of the muscle; that is, the levator superioris muscle showed the greatest increase in fat, and the medial rectus muscle showed the least. In a normal control patient, fat formed approximately half of the total weight of the tissue. Because the fat content of muscles is not increased in obesity, this finding may suggest an abnormal regeneration of fat.

To the surgeon and the pathologist, the orbital contents appear glistening and edematous. The muscles are tan in color and firm or rubbery in consistency. The microscopic picture of the tissues that is responsible for the gross appearance is a combination of edema, accumulation of mucin, cellular infiltrate, and fibrosis of varying degrees. These changes are seen predominantly within the extraocular muscles and the lacrimal gland. They are present in the fibrofatty tissue to a lesser degree. How do such changes occur, and what are the pathways for production of the edema and the cellular infiltrate?

In normal persons, 70% of the orbital content is occupied by retrobulbar and peribulbar structures and is comprised chiefly of muscle, fat, nerves, and vessels. The vessels include

25

arterial and venous channels as well as lymphatics (24). The eye is an extension of the central nervous system and is therefore without lymphatics; but it is important to recognize that lymphatic channels *are* present within the fat and muscle of orbital tissue. Because fibrofatty tissue elsewhere in the body contains lymphatic channels, there is no reason to presume that the fibrofatty tissue within the orbit should differ. The popular misconception that lymphatic channels do not exist within the orbit was fostered in part by the experiments of Patek and Bernick (19), who failed to demonstrate the channels. Other investigators (10) have ligated the lymphatic ducts within the necks of dogs and cats as well as the submandibular and deep cervical lymph glands. At autopsy they demonstrated the presence, both grossly and microscopically, of edema of the superficial and deep orbital fascia, fibrofatty tissues, extraocular muscles, and lacrimal gland. Some of the animals had exophthalmos due to the retro-orbital edema. Kozma and Gellért (14) demonstrated that skeletal muscles contain lymphatics; thus by analogy, extraocular muscles, also striated, contain similar channels. These authors were able to demonstrate experimentally the presence of lymphatic pathways within the extraocular muscles. They ligated the ducts within the necks of dogs as well as the submandibular and deep cervical lymph glands. Evans blue dye was simultaneously injected into the vitreous body, and 3 days later at autopsy the dye was found in the epimysium and perimysium of the extraocular muscles and within the retrobulbar connective tissues. Also supporting the concept that lymphatic channels are present within the orbit is the fact that lymphangiomas occur at this site (12). Thus a body of evidence supports the presence of orbital lymphatic channels and hence a pathway for the development of orbital edema and the infiltration of mononuclear cells in Graves' disease.

PATHOLOGIC TISSUE CHANGES

Wybar (34) considered five pathologic changes within the orbital tissues: increase in fat content, increase in mucin content, increase in water content, fibrosis, and lymphocytic infiltration. To what extent any or all of these factors contribute to the production of exophthalmos has been debated over the years, but many studies (7,11,21,31,32; R. J. Campbell, *personal observation*) agree that the extraocular muscles are predominantly affected. The seven extraocular muscles are striated and easily recognizable microscopically by the abundance of nerve fibers within the interstitium (Fig. 1). The seven extraocular muscles are not equally affected by the pathologic process, although all of the muscles show histopathologic changes to some degree. These changes are most marked in the inferior and medial rectus muscles (4; *personal observation*). In specimens obtained during decompression procedures, the inferior rectus muscle shows the earliest exudate and the earliest fibroblastic proliferation.

In Graves' disease the interstitium of the extraocular muscles shows an infiltration with mononuclear cells and fibroblasts with an admixture of edema fluid and an accumulation of mucin. These changes are present in the endomysium and perimysium and to a lesser extent in the epimysium. The fibrofatty tissue that surrounds the muscle is involved to a lesser extent, and the tendon is not involved at all.

The cellular infiltrate is composed predominantly of mature lymphocytes with some plasma cells and a few macrophages. The histologic picture depends on the stage of the disease. In the early stages the cellular infiltrate is sparse and is both focal and diffuse within the endomysium (Fig. 2). Mast cells may be present but are few in number; they are found in a perivascular distribution (22). As the lymphocytes and plasma cells increase in number (Fig. 3), the fibroblasts within the interstitium enlarge and proliferate, and in so doing produce collagen and mucopolysaccharide material.

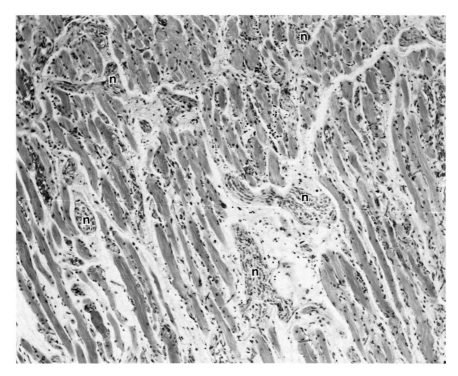

FIG. 1. Numerous nerve fibers *(n)* characteristic of extraocular muscles. Diffuse interstitial mononuclear infiltrate in patient with Graves' disease. Hematoxylin and eosin. × 100.

Ludwig et al. (16) likened the orbital changes to those of localized myxedema occurring in human skin (13) and demonstrated an increased amount of hexosamine content in the orbit of guinea pigs treated with thyroid-stimulating hormone. In humans (26) the localized myxedema of Graves' disease contains 16 times the normal skin concentration of acid mucopolysaccharides. Accumulation of glycosaminoglycans is a characteristic feature of the orbital tissues in humans and most experimental animals with exophthalmos. Normal human retrobulbar connective tissue contains hexosamine in the glycoprotein fraction, and one-third is in the glycosaminoglycan fraction. These substances were formerly considered to be produced by mast cells (2,3,31), but morphologic and experimental evidence shows that these substances are actually produced by fibroblasts. The fibroblasts are stimulated to proliferate and to secrete hyaluronic acid by lymphocytes and lymphocytic products. Sisson et al. (27–29) demonstrated the enhanced synthesis of hyaluronic acid in retrobulbar fibroblasts in response to dibutyryl cyclic $3',5'$-adenosine monophosphate and theophylline and to an increase in intracellular cyclic $3',5'$-adenosine monophosphate after exposure to lymphocytes and their products. Cell cultures of human fibroblasts also show secretion of hyaluronic acid after exposure to lymphocytes and lymphocytic products (28,29). We have demonstrated such mucinous materials in tissue that was removed during orbital decompression procedures, fixed in cetylpyridinium chloride for 1 week, and stained with 0.025% Alcian blue in 0.025 M acetate buffer, pH 5.8, with 0.4 M magnesium chloride. This tissue stained more strongly than did control tissue from autopsy cases with normal orbits. Increased mucin content of the tissue leads to an increased water-holding property and hence edema.

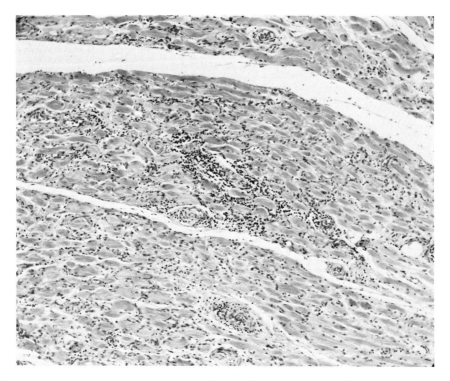

FIG. 2. Sparse interstitial inflammatory cellular infiltrate, focal and diffuse. Hematoxylin and eosin. × 100.

As the fibroblasts proliferate within the perimysium, bundles of fibers are compressed and atrophy. Fibrous strands within the epimysium may extend into the adjacent sector of the orbital fat. Dense orbital scarring is the end stage and is associated with severe muscle atrophy and loss of function.

The histopathologic changes described above are also observed within the connective tissue of the lacrimal gland. Fibrosis occurs to a lesser degree than within the extraocular muscles and results in only a mild atrophy of the glandular elements.

Early reports stated that muscle fibers show definite degenerative changes with loss of striation (1,6,17,20,23). Giant fibers were described, and staining was noted to be irregular and unequal. These findings were probably artifactual and resulted from poor sampling procedures and poor fixation. In the older literature the terms "degeneration" and "atrophy" are often used interchangeably. Electron microscopic studies of tissues obtained during orbital decompression procedures at the Mayo Clinic (21; R. J. Campbell, *personal observation*) support the studies of others (15) in that they fail to show early degenerative features of the muscle fibers. Thus one can conclude that any muscle changes that do occur are secondary to fibrosis. Most of the collagen fibers in the early stages have a diameter of 400 to 500 μm, which is a feature of active collagen synthesis (21). These fibers are separated by a finely amorphous material with a diameter of 100 to 120 μm, and this material has been suggested to be mucopolysaccharide (22).

The pathologic changes that may occur to the globe are secondary and are by no means specific to Graves' disease. The two important complications are keratitis and papilledema.

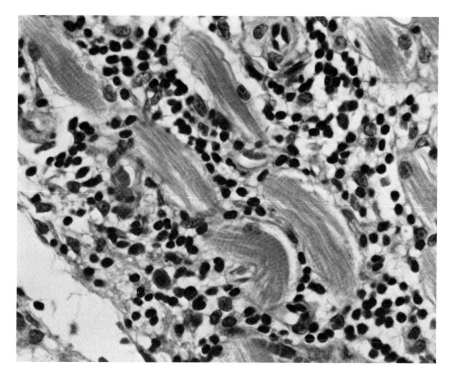

FIG. 3. Mononuclear cells (lymphocytes or plasma cells) in close association with striated extraocular muscle. Hematoxylin and eosin. ×640.

The keratitis is caused by exposure and is secondary to the proptosis and nonprotection of the cornea by the lids. The tear film quickly evaporates, the cornea dries, and in the most severe cases of proptosis the corneal epithelium changes from the normal five-layer epithelium to one that is keratinized, stratified, and squamous. Ulceration may occur. Inflammatory cells are present within the corneal stroma and may be acute or chronic. New vessels may grow into the corneal stroma from the limbal area. If the patient is not treated, panophthalmitis may occur in ~1 to 2% of patients (18), and orbital cellulitis may result.

Papilledema results from compression of the vessels to and within the optic nerve by the increased orbital bulk. On histologic examination the disc head varies in its degree of swelling and shows separation of nerve fibers by edema fluid. Subretinal fluid may accumulate and is first seen adjacent to the optic disc. However, the histopathologic appearance of the optic disc in Graves' disease in no way differs from that of papilledema produced from other causes.

SUMMARY

Morphologic and experimental evidence shows that the fibroblast is responsible for the production of collagen and a mucopolysaccharide material, and that the lymphocyte and lymphocytic products stimulate the fibroblast to produce these substances. Exactly how and why the lymphocyte and its products trigger this production is an enigma at this time. Many aspects of the disease suggest an autoimmune disorder. It is interesting that the lymphocytes accumulate within the interstitium of the extraocular muscles but without the production of primary muscle degeneration. This finding suggests that surface membrane antigens of the muscles are *not* involved, and one might speculate that the surface antigens of the fibroblasts may be of importance. One might also speculate that surface antigens of Schwann cells of the numerous nerve fibers of the interstitium attract the lymphocyte or that the neuromuscular junction is the focus of the attack. Abnormalities in circulating T lymphocytes have been demonstrated in Graves' ophthalmopathy by Sergott and Glaser (25), but more detailed studies on the exact site of action are required.

REFERENCES

1. Aird, R. B. (1940): Experimental exophthalmos and associated myopathy induced by the thyrotropic extract. *Arch. Ophthalmol.*, 24:1167–1178.
2. Asboe-Hansen, G. (1952): The mast cell: cortisone action on connective tissue. *Proc. Soc. Exp. Biol. Med.*, 80:677–679.
3. Asboe-Hansen, G., and Iversen, K. (1951): Influence of thyrotrophic hormone on connective tissue: pathogenetic significance of mucopolysaccharides in experimental exophthalmos. *Acta Endocrinol. (Copenh.)*, 8:90–96.
4. Basedow, C. A. von (1840): Exophthalmos durch Hypertrophie des Zellgewebes in der Augenhöhle. *Wissensch. Ann. Ges. Heilk. Berl.*, 6:198–205; 220–228.
5. Bouzas, A. G. (1980): The Montgomery lecture, 1980: endocrine ophthalmopathy. *Trans. Ophthalmol. Soc. U.K.*, 100:511–520.
6. Burch, F. E. (1929): The exophthalmos of Graves' disease. *Minn. Med.*, 12:668–675.
7. Daicker, B. (1979): Das gewebliche Substrat der verdickten äuberen Augenmuskeln bei der endokrinen orbitopathie. *Klin. Monatsbl. Augenheilkd.*, 174:843–847.
8. Dobyns, B. M. (1946): Studies on exophthalmos produced by thyrotropic hormone. II. Changes induced in various tissues and organs (including the orbit) by thyrotropic hormone and their relationship to exophthalmos. *Surg. Gynecol. Obstet.*, 82:609–617.
9. Dobyns, B. M. (1950): Present concepts of the pathologic physiology of exophthalmos. *J. Clin. Endocrinol.*, 10:1202–1230.
10. Földi, M., Kukán, F., Szeghy, G., Gellért, A., Kozma, M., Poberai, M., Zoltán, O. T., and Vanga, L. (1963): Anatomical, histological and experimental data on fluid circulation of the eye. *Acta Anat. (Basel)*, 53:333–345.
11. Hodes, B. L., and Shoch, D. E. (1979): Thyroid ocular myopathy. *Trans. Am. Ophthalmol. Soc.*, 77:80–103.
12. Jones, I. S. (1961): Lymphangiomas of the ocular adnexa: an analysis of sixty-two cases. *Am. J. Ophthalmol.*, 51:481–509.
13. Kobayasi, T., Danielsen, L., and Asboe-Hansen, G. (1976): Ultrastructure of localized myxedema. *Acta Derm. Venereol. (Stockh.)*, 56:173–185.
14. Kozma, M., and Gellért, A. (1958): Mikroskopische beiträge zur frage der lymphgefässe in der skelettmuskulatur. *Acta Morphol. Acad. Sci. Hung.*, 8:15–20.
15. Kroll, A. J., and Kuwabara, T. (1966): Dysthyroid ocular myopathy: anatomy, histology, and electron microscopy. *Arch. Ophthalmol.*, 76:244–257.
16. Ludwig, A. W., Boas, N. F., and Soffer, L. J. (1950): Role of mucopolysaccharides in pathogenesis of experimental exophthalmos. *Proc. Soc. Exp. Biol. Med.*, 73:137–140.
17. Naffziger, H. C. (1933): Pathologic changes in the orbit in progressive exophthalmos: with special reference to alterations in the extra-ocular muscles and the optic disks. *Arch. Ophthalmol.*, 9:1–12.
18. Ogura, J., Wessler, S., and Avioli, L. V. (1971): Surgical approach to the ophthalmopathy of Graves' disease. *JAMA*, 216:1627–1631.
19. Patek, P. R., and Bernick, S. (1960): Extravascular pathways of the eye and orbit. *Am. J. Ophthalmol.*, 49:135–141.
20. Paulson, D. L. (1939): Experimental exophthalmos and muscle degeneration induced by thyrotropic hormone. *Proc. Staff Meet. Mayo Clin.*, 14:828–832.
21. Riley, F. C. (1972): Orbital pathology in Graves' disease. *Mayo Clin. Proc.*, 47:975–979.
22. Rundle, F. F., Finlay-Jones, L. R., and Noad, K. B. (1953): Malignant exophthalmos: a quantitative analysis of the orbital tissues. *Australas. Ann. Med.*, 2:128–135.
23. Rundle, F. F., and Pochin, E. E. (1944): The orbital tissues in thyrotoxicosis: a quantitative analysis relating to exophthalmos. *Clin. Sci.*, 5:51–74.
24. Rusznyák, I., Földi, M., and Szabó, G. (1967): *Lymphatics and Lymph Circulation: Physiology and Pathology*, 2nd ed., edited by L. Youlten, pp. 187–194. Pergamon Press, New York.
25. Sergott, R. C., and Glaser, J. S. (1981): Graves' ophthalmopathy: a clinical and immunologic review. *Surv. Ophthalmol.*, 26:1–21.
26. Sisson, J. C. (1968): Hyaluronic acid in localized myxedema. *J. Clin. Endocrinol. Metab.*, 28:433–436.
27. Sisson, J. C. (1977): Mechanisms by which retrobulbar fibroblasts are stimulated by lymphocytes: role of cyclic nucleotide. *Proc. Soc. Exp. Biol. Med.*, 154:386–390.

28. Sisson, J. C., Kothary, P., and Kirchick, H. (1973): The effects of lymphocytes, sera and long-acting thyroid stimulator from patients with Graves' disease on retrobulbar fibroblasts. *J. Clin. Endocrinol. Metab.*, 37:17–24.

29. Sisson, J. C., and Vanderburg, J. A. (1972): Lymphocyte-retrobulbar fibroblast interaction: mechanisms by which stimulation occurs and inhibition of stimulation. *Invest. Ophthalmol.*, 11:15–20.

30. Smelser, G. K. (1937): A comparative study of experimental and clinical exophthalmos. *Am. J. Ophthalmol.*, 20:1189–1203.

31. Tengroth, B. (1964): Histological studies of orbital tissues in a case of endocrine exophthalmos before and after remission. *Acta Ophthalmol. (Copenh.)*, 42:588–591.

32. Trokel, S. L., and Jakobiec, F. A. (1981): Correlation of CT scanning and pathologic features of ophthalmic Graves' disease. *Ophthalmologica*, 88:553–564.

33. Werner, S. C., Coleman, D. J., and Franzen, L. A. (1974): Ultrasonographic evidence of a consistent orbital involvement in Graves's disease. *N. Engl. J. Med.*, 290:1447–1450.

34. Wybar, K. C. (1957): The nature of endocrine exophthalmos. *Bibl. Ophthalmol.*, 49:119–220.

The Eye and Orbit in Thyroid Disease, edited by
C. A. Gorman et al. Raven Press, New York 1984.

Extraocular Muscles: Their Development and Peculiarities

David Sevel

Division of Ophthalmology, Scripps Clinic, La Jolla, California 92037

The extraocular muscles (12 in all), although one of the most highly organized, systemized, and coordinated group of muscles in the body, have certain morphological and functional peculiarities. Each muscle is surrounded by a capsule formed by Tenon's capsule. The capsules of the rectus muscles are connected by intervening septae, thus dividing the orbit into an extra- and an intraconal compartment. Within the latter two compartments is fat, so the extraocular muscles are indeed surrounded by a milieu of fatty tissue.

Early in development, the extraocular muscles, Tenon's capsule, and the orbital fat are derived from the same mesenchymal tissue, and it is therefore not surprising that thyroid eye disease may involve either the extraocular muscles or the orbital fat. The concept of the development of the extraocular muscles has recently been reappraised, not only from the origin of these muscles but from the standpoint of cellular morphogenesis.

It has been suggested (17,23) that the anlage of extraocular muscles commence adjacent to the head cavities and then "grow" into the orbit, dragging their respective nerves in the process. However, investigations by Sevel (28–30) indicate that the extraocular muscles develop from a condensation of mesenchymal tissue in the orbit and do not commence development in the posterior aspect of the orbit and then grow forward.

A "trail" or connection of mesenchymal cells is not observed to extend from the cranial cavities to the orbit. The origin, belly, and insertion of the muscles develop contemporaneously. Furthermore, individual extraocular muscles develop at the same time.

The extraocular muscles arise basically from a superior and an inferior mesodermal complex (Fig. 1). The superior rectus, levator palpebrae superioris, and superior oblique muscles develop from the superior complex, whereas the inferior rectus and inferior oblique muscles develop from the inferior complex. The medial and the lateral rectus muscles arise from both complexes (Figs. 2 and 3). The cellular morphogenesis of the extraocular muscles develops in six stages. These stages are not distinct, but merge into one another.

STAGES OF MUSCLE DEVELOPMENT

Muscle develops in six cellular stages: (a) mesenchymal cells; (b) early myoblasts; (c) myoblasts; (d) fusion of myoblasts; (e) myotube cells; and (f) mature muscle cells. Cells at successive stages of development can be seen in a single muscle fiber.

Mesenchymal Cell Stage

Mesenchymal tissue (in up to 36.0-mm embryos) is composed of a spongy meshwork of cells situated in ground substance. These cells are widely separated from one another. Their

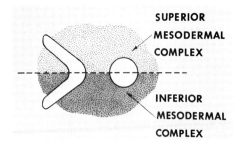

FIG. 1. The extraocular muscles are derived from a superior mesodermal complex and an inferior mesodermal complex (section through superior orbital fissure and optic foramen at apex of orbit).

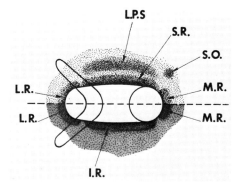

FIG. 2. Section through the apex of the orbit showing the superior orbital fissure and optic foramen. Muscles derived from the superior mesodermal complex are the levator palpebrae superioris *(L.P.S.)*, superior rectus *(S.R.)*, and superior oblique muscle *(S.O.)*. Muscle derived from the inferior mesodermal complex is the inferior rectus muscle *(I.R.)*. Muscles derived from both superior and inferior mesodermal complexes are the lateral rectus *(L.R.)* and the medial rectus *(M.R.)*.

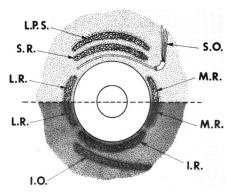

FIG. 3. Section through the anterior aspect of the orbit demonstrating muscles derived from the superior and inferior mesodermal complexes. Note the trochlea of the superior oblique *(S.O.)* muscle and its tendon derived from superior mesodermal complex, and the inferior oblique muscle *(I.O.)* derived from the inferior mesodermal complex. See Fig. 2 for other abbreviations.

nuclei are large and vesicular, and are surrounded by a fine rim of cytoplasm. The cells taper and have long wavy processes that are arranged in a stellate fashion about the nucleus. These cytoplasmic "arms" touch and join those of adjacent cells (7,19,21).

Early Myoblast Cell Stage

The term "early myoblast" (seen in 13.6-mm embryos) is preferred to "premyoblast." Premyoblast implies a distinct, well-defined cell with specific features that can be recognized, whereas early myoblasts are transitional cells—ongoing developing cells. These cells have features akin to both myoblasts and mesenchymal cells.

Early myoblasts are located at the site of the future extraocular muscles. At these sites the processes of the mesenchymal cells retract. The nuclei of these cells become round to oval and are located centrally. The cytoplasm becomes basophilic.

An individual cell considered in isolation cannot be differentiated from a fibroblast using light microscopy. The features of the early myoblast are considered together with those

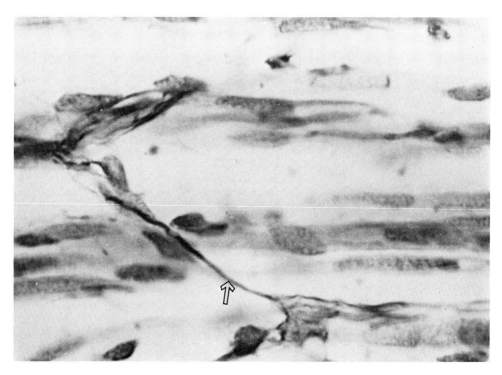

FIG. 4. Fusion of myoblasts is noted with fine nerve fibers present *(arrow)*. The nucleoli are eccentric, and the cytoplasm is granular. Silver stain. ×507.

features of adjacent cells. Furthermore, their cell morphology is compared with cells at the sites of other extraocular muscles and with cells found at deeper sections of the same muscle.

Myoblast Stage

Unless well-developed cross-striations are observed, it is not possible, except in muscle culture, to identify positively myoblasts (from 38.2-mm embryos) with the light microscope. However, the situation and orientation of the cells, as observed in a serial section, are features in favor of a specific cell being labeled a myoblast.

Myoblasts are fusiform mononucleated spindle-shaped cells. The round, centrally positioned nuclei are large. Nuclear chromatin is dispersed but mainly concentrated at the periphery of the nucleus. One or two prominent nucleoli are present. Furthermore, wavy fine filaments are noted within the basophilic cytoplasm. The myoblast cell becomes mature when there is loss of cytoplasmic basophilia, migration of the nuclei from the center to the periphery of the cell, and accumulation of myofibrils with cross-striations.

Fusion of Myoblasts

A syncytium of multinucleated myoblasts develops (54.0-mm embryos). The nuclei are round and the nucleoli eccentric. The cytoplasm is basophilic and granular (Fig. 4).

Myotube Cell

The sarcolemmal layers of the myotubes are parallel to one another (54.0-mm embryos). The oval nuclei, which have eccentric nucleoli, become centrally situated in the cell and

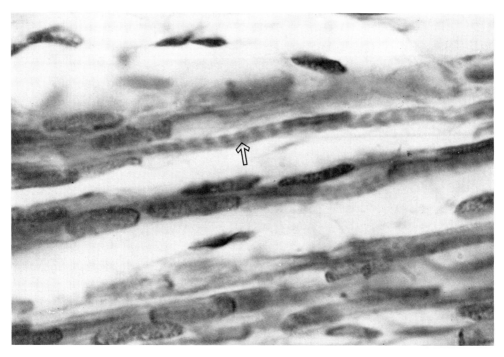

FIG. 5. Cross-striations *(arrow)* are noted in the muscle fibers in the mature muscle stage. In the adjacent area, there is evidence of the fusion of the myoblasts. Hematoxylin and eosin. ×488.

are arranged in tandem throughout the length of the cell. The cytoplasm loses its basophilia and stains more lightly in the center of the cell. This clear region stains with periodic acid-Schiff stain. Longitudinal and cross-striations are present in the periphery of the cytoplasm.

Mature Muscle

The mature muscle (Fig. 5) is a syncytium of elongated cells (80.0-mm fetuses). The nuclear membrane can be distinguished, and the fine chromatin is mainly related to this membrane. Four to eight nuclei are present in a muscle cell.

The nuclei, which are oval and are situated in a subsarcolemmal position, lie parallel to the long axis of the muscle fiber. The nuclei are granular and contain eccentrically placed nucleoli. The cytoplasm, which contains longitudinal striations and cross-striation, has less basophilic staining. Occasional internal nuclei are also seen in the mature muscle cell.

As the fetus develops and matures, the mature muscle fibers increase in length and width. At this stage of development, myoblasts, multinucleated myoblasts, and myotubes are not observed.

PECULIARITIES OF EXTRAOCULAR MUSCLE

The reason for extraocular muscle involvement in thyroid disease cannot be explained by morphological or embryological reasons. However, there are certain anatomical and embryological peculiarities of extraocular muscles which distinguish them from other muscles.

Extraocular muscles differ in certain respects from the skeletal muscles of the extremities. These differences are considered under morphological and stimulatory responses, embryological features, nerve fibers, spindles, nuclei, muscle fiber size.

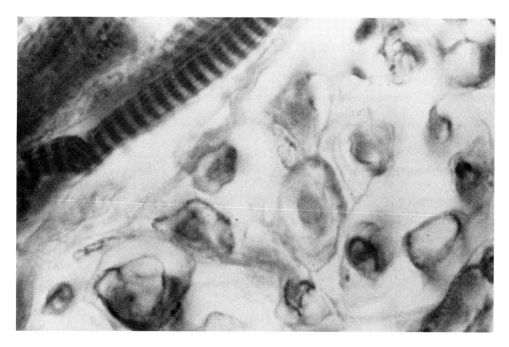

FIG. 6. There are cross-striations in the mature muscle, and adjacent to this is a spindle. Phospho-tungstic acid hematoxylin. ×624.

Morphological and Stimulatory Responses

The average muscle fiber diameter is small, ∼18 μm (1). Two types of muscle fibers are described in extraocular muscles: twitch fibers and slow fibers. The twitch muscle fibers are 25 to 50 μm in diameter and have much sarcoplasm and abundant mitochondria. The sarcoplasmic reticulum and T systems are well marked. The slow fibers are smaller (9 to 15 μm in diameter) and contain less sarcoplasm and fewer mitochondria. The sarcoplasmic reticulum and T system are not well marked.

There is great rapidity, fine grading, and accuracy of extraocular muscle contraction (13). The duration of the twitch is short (9), and the muscle has a high frequency of stimulation for tetanic fusion (26). Peachey (25) noted that in the inferior oblique muscle of the cat both "slow" and "fast" fibers were morphologically similar to twitch fibers of other mammalian muscles. The amplitude of the action potentials of the extraocular muscles is greatly reduced (9), the frequencies of contraction of individual muscles are high, and their recruitment is rapid (9).

Embryological Features

Extraocular muscles have features which are observed in embryological mammalian muscle: A large number of spindles are present in the extraocular muscles which may represent modified embryological skeletal muscle (Fig. 6). Central muscle nuclei commonly observed in mammalian embryological muscle are seen in extraocular muscle.

A further embryological feature of the extraocular muscles is the short duration of the twitch response and the high frequency of stimulation for tetanic fusion. This characteristic is noted in frog muscle but not in other mature mammalian muscle.

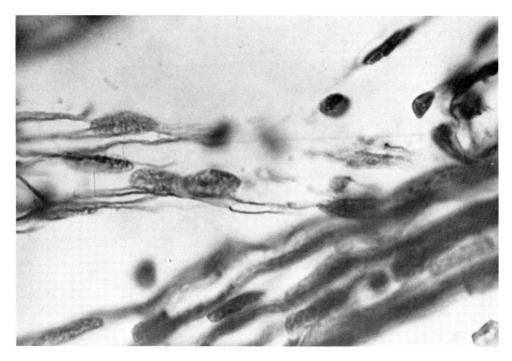

FIG. 7. Numerous nerve fibers are seen within the extraocular muscles. Silver. ×488.

The response of intact extraocular muscle to the application of acetylcholine is characteristic of the muscle of submammalian species. Without previous denervation, the extraocular muscles have a prolonged tonic contraction following the application of acetylcholine (16,18,37).

Nerve Fibers

There is a strikingly high ratio of nerve to muscle fibers in extraocular muscles (11,30) (Figs. 7 and 8). The nerve/muscle ratio in extraocular muscle is 1:5–6, whereas in semitendinosus muscle it is 1:50 (8). Stibbe (33) noted in the human fetus that the abducent nerve is as large as the inferior gluteal nerve, although the gluteus maximus muscle is 74 times as heavy as the lateral rectus muscle.

Spindles

Spindles are not found in extraocular muscles of the cat, the dog, the rabbit, and the horse (10–12,32). Sunderland (34) examined the levator palpebrae superioris, superior rectus, and superior oblique muscles in man and concluded that spindles were present in all. There were approximately 12 in each muscle and were widely distributed. The human extrinsic eye muscles are richly endowed with a degree of sensibility that bears comparison with the lumbrical muscles of the human hand (10,11). The spindles are probably under the influence of the retina and the periorbital tissue in much the same way as the intrafusal muscle fibers of the muscle spindle of the extensor muscles of the limbs are affected by the skin and movements of the joints.

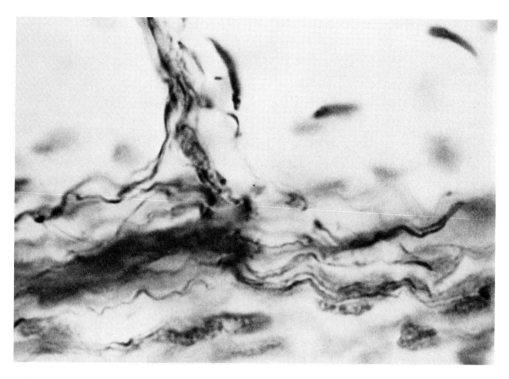

FIG. 8. The nerve fibers divide extensively within the extraocular muscles. They have a tortuous course between the muscle fibers and vary in thickness throughout their course. Silver. × 520.

Cooper and Daniel (11) found that the spindles in extraocular muscles of man were shorter than in limb muscles, and that their capsules were thinner. The spindles of extraocular muscles were not evenly distributed in the muscle and were mainly observed either near the origin or near the insertion. The extrafusal fibers in these regions were small.

Cooper et al. (12) noted that in each human extrinsic eye muscle there were ~50 muscle spindles. A comparable number were found in the lumbrical muscles of the human hand. In the inferior rectus muscle approximately 45 of the muscle spindles were found to be situated near the origin of the muscle; the remaining five were scattered between the origin and the insertion. There were approximately 130 spindles per gram of muscle, which was more than the number of spindles in most other human muscles (27,35).

Kupfer (22) assessed cholinesterase localization of the motor nerves in human extraocular muscles. He found multiple motor end-plates on extrafusal fibers as well as small areas of cholinesterase activity near these end-plates. It was suggested that these sites represented postganglionic parasympathetic efferent nerve endings. Furthermore, cholinesterase cuffing at the ends of extrafusal fibers was also noted at the musculotendinous junction. On the basis of cholinesterase localization in the muscle spindle, there seemed to be two types of motor nerve ending in extraocular muscle. It was concluded that both alpha and gamma efferent nerve fibers could innervate some intrafusal fibers, whereas others were innervated only by gamma efferent nerves.

The extrinsic eye muscles also have close connections with the cerebellum and the brainstem so that supraspinal influences may also be of importance in controlling the discharge to the gamma efferent fibers.

The motor innervation of spindles is from the collaterals of the motor supply to the extrafusal muscles. Extraocular muscles do not have a specific gamma efferent innervation (2–6). Numerous zebra bodies are present close to the plasma membrane of extraocular muscles.

Central Connections of the Spindles

The intracranial connections of the spindles remains uncertain (12,24). Whitteridge (36) suggested that, in the goat, proprioceptive fibers from the superior oblique muscle passed into the brainstem via the trigeminal nerve. Also in the goat there are obvious connections between the oculomotor nerve and the branches of the trigeminal nerve.

Nuclei

Subsarcolemmal Nuclei

Approximately two to six nuclei are found in extraocular muscle cells. The nuclei are ~8 μm in length and 4 to 5 μm in width; they do not significantly differ from the nuclei of skeletal muscle elsewhere in the body. They are flattened and elongated in the long axis of muscle. Usually one, but occasionally two, nucleoli are present. Scattered throughout the nucleoplasm are clumps of chromatin. The finer details of the nucleoli and the chromatin cannot be distinguished with light microscopy. A nuclear membrane is observed which stains with hematoxylin.

Internal Nuclei

Internal nuclei are said to occur if they are in excess of three to six of the number of muscle fibers (15,20). In fetal life the nuclei of skeletal muscle are centrally placed (internal nucleus) within the muscle cell. Internal nuclei are present in at least 10% of the muscle cells of extraocular muscles. Approximately two or three internal nuclei are present in these muscle cells. The nuclei are less flattened than the subsarcolemmal nuclei but in all other respects are structurally similar. Internal nuclei are also observed at the myotendinous junction at both the insertion and the origin.

Muscle Fiber Size

Denny-Brown (14) suggested that, in the cat, muscle fibers which produced similar speed of contraction formed a group, and that these fibers were probably the same diameter. Normal adult extraocular muscles contain uniform small fibers of ~20 μm, the largest being rarely >25 μm.

Cellular limits in muscle are best assessed if muscle fibers are stained for types I and II fibers. It is possible to compare the fiber size of all extraocular muscles except for the inferior oblique muscle, which has basically a horizontal course and therefore is sectioned only in the coronal plane. The remaining extraocular muscles have a general anteroposterior course.

It is found that the diameter of muscle fibers of all the extraocular muscles is similar. Furthermore, the fibers of the respective muscles develop at the same rate throughout their maturation to term and then on to adulthood.

It is not possible to measure the diameters of myoblasts with any accuracy because the cytoplasmic membranes of these cells are ill-defined and merge with the surrounding mesenchymal tissue. Furthermore, the cell membranes in multinucleated myoblasts (first seen in 54.0-mm embryos) are not accurately discernible.

Myotubes can be measured because their cell membranes are reasonably well defined. Myotubes (first seen in the 54.0-mm embryos) are found to be an average of 15 μm. The diameter of mature (adult) muscle fibers (first seen in the 80.0-mm fetus) is 25 μm.

REFERENCES

1. Adams, R. D., Denny-Brown, D., and Pearson, C. M. (1962): Embryology and histology of skeletal muscle. In: *Diseases of Muscle*, 2nd ed., pp. 3–15. Harper Brothers, New York.
2. Barker, D. (1948): The innervation of the muscle spindle. *Q. J. Microsc. Sci.*, 89:143–186.
3. Barker, D. (1967): The innervation of mammalian skeletal muscle. In: *Myotatic, Kinesthetic and Vestibular Mechanisms*, edited by A. V. S. De Reuck and J. Knight, pp. 3–19. Churchill, London.
4. Barker, D., and Gidumal, J. L. (1961): The morphology of intrafusal muscle fibres in the cat. *J. Physiol. (Lond.)*, 157:513–528.
5. Barker, D., and Ip, M. C. (1965): The motor innervation of cat and rabbit muscle spindles. *J. Physiol. (Lond.)*, 177:27P.
6. Barker, D., Stacey, M. D., and Adal, M. N. (1970): Fusimotor innervation in the cat. *Philos. Trans. R. Soc. Lond. [Biol.]* 258:315–346.
7. Bloom, W., and Fawcett, D. W. (1964): *Textbook of Histology*, 8th ed., pp. 90–209. Saunders, Philadelphia.
8. Bors, E. (1925): Uber das Zahlenverhaltnis Zwischen Nerven—und Muskelfasern. *Anat. Anz.*, 60:415.
9. Bjork, A., and Kugelberg, E. (1953): Motor unit activity in the human extraocular muscles. *Electroencephalogr. Clin. Neurophysiol.*, 5:271–278.
10. Cilimbaris, P. A. (1910): Histologische Untersuchungen Uber die Muskelspindeln der Augenmuskeln. *Arch. Mikrosc. Anat. EntwMech.*, 75:692–747.
11. Cooper, S., and Daniel, P. M. (1949): Muscle spindles in human extrinsic eye muscles. *Brain*, 72:1–24.
12. Cooper, S., Daniel, P. M., and Whitteridge, D. (1955): Muscle spindles and other sensory endings in the extrinsic eye muscles; the physiology and anatomy of these receptors and of their connections with the brainstem. *Brain*, 78:564–583.
13. Cooper, S., and Eccles, J. C. (1930): The isometric responses of mammalian muscles. *J. Physiol. (Lond.)*, 69:377–385.
14. Denny-Brown, D. E. (1929): The histological features of striped muscle in relation to its functional activity. *Proc. R. Soc. Lond. [Biol.]*, 104:371–411.
15. Dubowitz, V., Brooke, M. H., and Neville, H. E. (1973): *Muscle Biopsy: A Modern Approach, Vol. 2: Major Problems in Neurology*, edited by J. N. Walton, pp. 98–101. Saunders, Philadelphia.
16. Duke-Elder, W. S. (1930): New observations on the physiology of the extra-ocular muscles. *Trans. Ophthalmol. Soc. U.K.*, 50:181–200.
17. Duke-Elder, W. S. (1963): *System of Ophthalmology, Normal and Abnormal Development*, Vol. III, Part I. Mosby, St. Louis.
18. Duke-Elder, W. S., and Duke-Elder, P. M. (1930–1931): The contraction of the extrinsic muscles of the eye by choline and nicotine. *Proc. R. Soc. Lond. [Biol.]*, 107:332–343.
19. Garven, H. S. D. (1965): *A Student's Histology*, 2nd ed. Livingstone, Edinburgh.
20. Greenfield, J. G., Shy, G. M., and Ellsworth, C. A. (1957): *Neuromuscular Disease*. Livingstone, Edinburgh.
21. Ham, A. W. (1974): *Histology*, 7th ed. Pitman, London.
22. Kupfer, C. (1960): Motor innervation of extraocular muscle. *J. Physiol. (Lond.)*, 153:522–526.
23. Mann, I. (1950): *The Development of the Human Eye*. Grune & Stratton, New York.
24. Manni, E., Descole, C., and Palmieri, G. (1970): On whether eye muscle spindles are innervated by ganglion cells located along the oculomotor nerves. *Exp. Neurol.*, 28:333–343.
25. Peachey, L. D. (1966): Fine structure of two fiber types in cat extra-ocular muscles. *J. Cell Biol.*, 31:84A.
26. Reid, G. (1949): The rate of discharge of the extraocular motorneurones. *J. Physiol. (Lond.)*, 110:217–225.
27. Schulze, M. L. (1955): Die absolute und relative zahl der Muskel-spindeln in den Kurzen Daumenmuskeln des Menschen. *Anat. Anz.*, 102:290–291.
28. Sevel, D. (1981): A reappraisal of the origin of the human extraocular muscles. *Ophthalmology*, 88:1330–1338.
29. Sevel, D. (1981): Brown's syndrome—a possible etiology explained embryologically. *J. Pediatr. Ophthalmol. Strabismus*, 18:26–31.
30. Sevel, D. (1982): Development of the Nerves of the Extraocular Muscles. Presented at the ISA-AAPO&S Meeting, Asilomar, CA.
31. Sevel, D. (1982): Discussion on the trochlea: a study of the anatomy and physiology. *Ophthalmology*, 89:124–133.
32. Sherrington, C. S. (1897): Further note on the sensory nerves of muscles. *Proc. R. Soc.*, 61:247–249.
33. Stibbe, E. P. (1929): Sensory components of the motor nerves of the eye. *J. Anat.*, 64:112–113.

34. Sunderland, S. (1949): A preliminary note on the presence of neuromuscular spindles in the extrinsic ocular muscles in man. *Anat. Rec.*, 103:561–562.

35. Voss, H. (1937): Untersuchungen Uber Zahl, Anordnung und Lange der Muskelspindeln in den Lumbrical-muskeln des Menschen und einiger Tiere. *S. Mikrosk. Anat. Forsch.*, 42:509–542.

36. Whitteridge, D. (1955): A separate afferent nerve supply from the extraocular muscles of goats. *Q. J. Exp. Physiol.*, 40:331–336.

37. Woollard, H. H. (1930–1931): The innervation of the ocular muscle. *J. Anat.*, 65:215–223.

The Eye and Orbit in Thyroid Disease, edited by
C. A. Gorman et al. Raven Press, New York 1984.

Glycosaminoglycans and Exophthalmos

John F. O'Brien

Section of Clinical Chemistry, Mayo Clinic, Rochester, Minnesota 55905

Glycosaminoglycan (GAG) is a relatively new term for what formerly was termed mucopolysaccharide. GAG refers to a polysaccharide chain which consists of repeating disaccharide units, usually one uronic acid and one *N*-acetylhexosamine. The major structural variations between GAGs are due to substitutions of either the *N*-acetylhexosamine or the glycuronic acid moieties, which are the components in repeating disaccharide units of GAGs. Further heterogeneity in structure results from the site and extent to which a GAG is sulfated. Heparan sulfate is unique in this respect as sulfate groups are substituted for some *N*-acetyl groups and, as with dermatan sulfate, it contains periodic 2-*O*-sulfate groups on constituent iduronic acid. Hyaluronic acid is exceptional in that it is probably not covalently bound to a protein backbone (i.e., does not occur naturally as a *proteoglycan*, which is the rule for the other GAGs), and it is not sulfated. The GAGs are found in most abundance, but not exclusively, in connective tissues. Fibroblasts synthesize large amounts of GAGs; the mast cell is noted for its granular stores of heparin; and heparan sulfate is associated with the hepatocyte surface. The structures of three representative GAGs are shown in Fig. 1. Glycosaminoglycans and their proteoglycan forms have been thoroughly reviewed by Roden (12).

The localization of glycosaminoglycans in tissue matrices and the surface of cells suggests that these complex molecules may function in regulating cell associations and in contributing to the ground substance in all tissues, particularly in the connective tissues of the body. Briefly, timing of the biosynthesis of specific glycosaminoglycans during ontogeny has led to the conclusion that hyaluronic acid accumulation precedes that of other GAGs and affords migrating cells a hydrated milieu through which to move. The matrix at this point is not yet occupied by sulfated GAGs and matrix proteins, e.g., collagen. Subsequently, hyaluronate is digested by hyaluronidase, the tissue loses water, and cells and their matrix differentiate (18). This differentiation occurs concomitantly with rapid synthesis of sulfated GAGs; and the remaining hyaluronic acid, which is no longer the predominant GAG, associates with sulfated proteoglycans (GAGs with a protein "backbone") to form part of the bulk of connective tissue matrix. This intriguing association has been in large measure elucidated by Hascall and his associates, who reviewed this phenomenon elsewhere (6). Thus there is evidence that GAGs function by influencing cell association and providing the ground substance of differentiated tissues.

The volumes which hydrated forms of hyaluronate and cartilage proteoglycan occupy are as much as 100 and 1,000 times larger than the volume of the dry molecules, respectively (3). Thus their domains in solution are very large relative to other biological polymers. The retention of H_2O by the polysaccharide confers a resistance to compression. Gels formed by dissolving hyaluronate in water can be shrunk by the action of hyaluronidase. If the hydration and compressibility, and therefore the volume of a tissue, depend qualitatively and

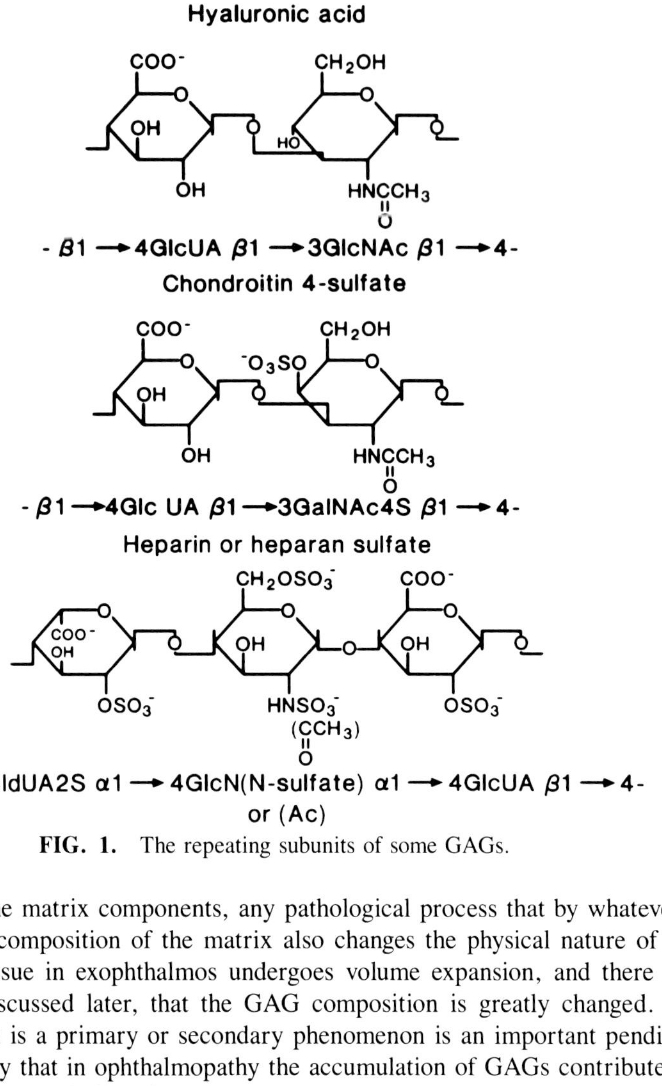

FIG. 1. The repeating subunits of some GAGs.

quantitatively on the matrix components, any pathological process that by whatever means changes the GAG composition of the matrix also changes the physical nature of a tissue. The retrobulbar tissue in exophthalmos undergoes volume expansion, and there is ample evidence, to be discussed later, that the GAG composition is greatly changed. Whether GAG accumulation is a primary or secondary phenomenon is an important pending issue. However, it is likely that in ophthalmopathy the accumulation of GAGs contributes greatly to the volume of the retrobulbar tissues.

EVIDENCE FOR GAG IN RETROBULBAR TISSUE

The finding of increased GAGs and water in exophthalmos occurred nearly 50 years ago and was aided by the guinea pig model for exophthalmos (17). The guinea pig model may not be a valid replica of human exophthalmos because presumably the exophthalmic response to thyroid-stimulating hormone (TSH) resides in the harderian gland, which is not found in humans. Nevertheless, some of the histochemical findings, particularly relative to GAGs, seem remarkably similar to those in humans and are of value. Ludwig et al. (11) reported that exophthalmos was induced with TSH in guinea pigs regardless of whether they had undergone prior thyroidectomy. The thyroidectomized group showed the most dramatic exophthalmos. The histological findings were of large deposits of metachromatic material, presumably GAGs, in the connective tissue, adipose tissue, extraocular muscles, and capsules of the harderian and lacrimal glands. This phenomenon occurred in the absence of lympho-cytic infiltration, which is an important component of more recent exophthalmic mechanisms discussed below. Furthermore, the water content, particularly that of the muscle–fat fraction, increased in proportion to the metachromatic material. The identity of the anionic staining matrix component and GAGs was further supported by showing that the increase in staining was paralleled with an increase in tissue hexosamine. Ludwig et al. (11) concluded that this phenomenon consists mainly of expansion of "interfibrillar ground substance," which is further defined as hyaluronic acid. This observation was confirmed in Graves' patients, and samples including ocular muscle and the tibialis anterior muscle showed metachromatic staining (21). Localized myxedema, particularly pretibial myxedema, occasionally accom-panies Graves' exophthalmos. The occurrence of elevated GAGs in affected skin in patients with pretibial myxedema has been reported (19). Because this phenomenon was present even in clinically uninvolved dermal areas, it seems reasonable that the GAG accumulation is enough to be translated to the two- to three-fold increase in urinary excretion of GAGs in patients with exophthalmos (22). The increased urinary GAGs were composed of sulfated GAG, although hyaluronic acid could be missed because of hyaluronidase digestion prior to isolation. Serum GAGs were also elevated, and this elevation is unrelated to thyroid function or plasma long-acting thyroid stimulator (LATS) in the patients studied by Winand (22).

From the preceding, there is strong evidence that accumulation of GAG in retro-orbital tissue occurs in ophthalmopathy. Furthermore, there is reason to believe that such an accumulation would result in volume expansion, which could cause proptosis. This must be weighed against the possibility that a primary effect on muscle is the underlying cause of the proptosis. The accumulation of excessive GAGs in retro-orbital tissue still remains to be explained mechanistically.

One simplistic mechanism that might be hypothesized is that in Graves' disease the existence of high circulating thyroxine (T_4) levels stimulates GAG synthesis. Thyroxine does, in fact, stimulate GAG synthesis in certain experimental animal models. These systems include the metamorphosing tadpole backskin (10), the skin of hypothyroid rats (13), and in synergism with somatomedins the chick sternum (16). However, thyrotoxicosis is not a constant feature in Graves' patients with attendant ophthalmopathy. Moreover, the common occurrence and mechanistic similarity of the infiltrative process in ophthalmopathy and myxedema is remarkable. The occurrence of pretibial myxedema in both hypo- and hyper-thyroid patients strongly suggests that neither circulating thyroid hormone nor "TSH-like" activity is the stimulator of GAG production in ophthalmopathy.

The role of TSH or TSH fragments in the pathogenesis of ophthalmopathy requires further study. It has been shown that TSH and proteolytic fragments thereof which induce exophthal-mos in guinea pig also induce $^{35}SO_4$ incorporation into GAGs in retro-orbital tissue (23). Again, this effect is not confined to the harderian gland but is also found in perirenal fat tissue, nonglandular retro-orbital tissue, and small intestine. Because adipocytes are target cells for TSH or thyroid-stimulating immunoglobulins (TSI) (4,5,8), it could be postulated that it is the adipose component in retro-orbital tissue that is stimulated to overproduce GAGs. The variability in the expression of exophthalmos with Graves' disease may be explained by the fact that TSI interaction with adipocytes is variable (7). This mechanism is in some doubt because Abe (1) raised the question as to whether human retro-orbital adipose tissue has the same TSH response as guinea pig epididymal fat.

Lymphocytes which commonly infiltrate orbital tissues in ophthalmopathy induce GAG synthesis by fibroblasts derived from retro-orbital tissue of Graves' patients (14,15). Whether this induction is sufficient to cause the massive deposition of GAGs one would expect from the histology and the extent of the proptosis is speculative. This response of fibroblasts may, in fact, be an early component of fibrosis evoked by muscle cell loss due to the cytotoxicity of Graves' lymphocytes toward orbital muscle, recently demonstrated by Blau et al. (2). The increased synthesis may not depend on lymphocytes but may be a constitutive property of Graves' fibroblasts, according to our laboratory's limited data.

Although GAGs have been amply demonstrated in retro-orbital tissues, as alluded to earlier, and a few studies on the dynamic *in vitro* systems have shown induction of GAG synthesis, current investigations have not been concerned with ground substance expansion as a primary mechanistic explanation. From this, one may arrive at the conclusion with justification that the role of GAGs, though physically important in the process of ophthalmopathy, is secondary to some autoimmune process, such as that recently reported by Kodama et al. (9). This concept is supported by the beneficial effect of immunosuppression with steroids or cyclosporin (20) on patients with Graves' ophthalmopathy.

REFERENCES

1. Abe, Y. (1980): Studies on the thyrotropin receptor and adenylate cyclase activity in various thyroid diseases. I. The properties of TSH receptor and adenylate cyclase in Graves' thyroid and retro-orbital adipose tissues. *Folia Endocrinol. Jpn.*, 56:739–753.
2. Blau, H. M., Kaplan, I., Tao, T., and Kriss, J. P. (1983): Thyroglobulin-independent, cell-mediated cytotoxicity of human eye muscle cells in tissue culture by lymphocytes of a patient with Graves' ophthalmopathy. *Life Sci.*, 32:45–53.
3. Comper, W. D., and Laurent, T. C. (1978): Physiological function of connective tissue polysaccharides. *Physiol. Rev.*, 58:255–315.
4. Endo, K., Amir, S. M., and Ingbar, S. H. (1981): Development and evaluation of a method for the partial purification of immunoglobulins specific for Graves' disease. *J. Clin. Endocrinol. Metab.*, 52:1113–1123.
5. Gill, D. L., Marshall, N. J., and Ekins, R. P. (1978): Binding of thyrotropin to receptors in fat tissue. *Mol. Cell. Endocrinol.*, 10:89–102.
6. Hascall, V. C., and Hascall, G. K. (1981): Proteoglycans. In: *Cell Biology of Extracellular Matrix*, edited by E. D. Hay, pp. 39–63. Plenum Press, New York.
7. Hearn, M. T. W. (1980): Graves' disease and the thyrotrophin receptor. *TIBS*, 5:75–79.
8. Kishihara, M., Nakao, Y., Baba, Y., Kobayashi, N., Matsukura, S., Kuma, K., and Fujita, T. (1981): Interaction between thyrotropin (TSH) binding inhibitor immunoglobulins (TBII) and soluble TSH receptors in fat cells. *J. Clin. Endocrinol. Metab.*, 52:665–670.
9. Kodama, K., Sikorska, H., Bandy-Dafoe, P., Bayly, R., and Wall, J. R. (1982): Demonstration of a circulating autoantibody against a soluble eye-muscle antigen in Graves' ophthalmopathy. *Lancet*, 2:1353–1356.
10. Lipson, M. J., Cerskus, R. A., and Silbert, J. E. (1971): Glycosaminoglycans and glycosaminoglycan-degrading enzyme of Rana catesbeiana back skin during late stages of metamorphosis. *Dev. Biol.*, 25:198–208.
11. Ludwig, A. W., Boas, N. F., and Soffer, L. J. (1950): Role of mucopolysaccharides in pathogenesis of experimental exophthalmos. *Proc. Soc. Exp. Biol. Med.*, 73:137–140.
12. Roden, L. (1981): Structure and metabolism of connective tissue proteoglycans. In: *The Biochemistry of Glycoproteins and Proteoglycans*, edited by W. J. Lennarz, pp. 267–371. Plenum Press, New York.
13. Schiller, S., Slover, G. A., and Dorfman, A. (1962): Effect of the thyroid gland on metabolism of acid mucopolysaccharides in skin. *Biochim. Biophys. Acta*, 58:27–33.
14. Sisson, J. C. (1971): Stimulation of glucose utilization and glycosaminoglycan production by fibroblasts derived from retrobulbar tissue. *Exp. Eye Res.*, 12:285–292.
15. Sisson, J. C., and Vanderburg, J. A. (1972): Lymphocyte-retrobulbar fibroblast interaction: mechanisms by which stimulation occurs and inhibition of stimulation. *Invest. Ophthalmol.*, 11:15–20.
16. Sissons, H. A. (1971): The growth of bone. In: *The Biochemistry and Physiology of Bone*, edited by G. H. Bourne, pp. 145–180. Academic Press, New York.
17. Smelser, G. K. (1936): Experimental production of exophthalmos resembling that found in Graves' disease. *Proc. Soc. Exp. Biol. Med.*, 35:128–130.
18. Toole, B. P. (1981): Glycosaminoglycans in morphogenesis. In: *Cell Biology of Extracellular Matrix*, edited by E. D. Hay, pp. 259–294. Plenum Press, New York.
19. Watson, A. M., and Pearce, R. H. (1947): The mucopolysaccharide content of the skin in localized pretibial myxoedema. *Am. J. Clin. Pathol.*, 17:507–512.
20. Weetman, A. P., McGregor, A. M., Ludgate, M., Beck, L., Mills, P. V., Lazarus, J. H., and Hall, R. (1983): Cyclosporin improves Graves' ophthalmopathy. *Lancet*, 2:486–489.

21. Wegelius, O., Asboe-Hansen, G., and Lamberg, B. A. (1957): Retrobulbar connective tissue changes in malignant exophthalmos. *Acta Endocrinol. (Copenh.)*, 25:452–456.
22. Winand, R. J. (1968): Increased urinary excretion of acidic mucopolysaccharides in exophthalmos. *J. Clin. Invest.*, 47:2563–2568.
23. Winand, R. J., and Kohn, L. D. (1973): Retrobulbar modifications in experimental exophthalmos: the effect of thyrotropin and an exophthalmos-producing substance derived from thyrotropin on the [35]SO$_4$ incorporation and glycosaminoglycan content of harderian glands. *Endocrinology*, 93:670–680.

The Eye and Orbit in Thyroid Disease, edited by
C. A. Gorman et al. Raven Press, New York 1984.

Thyroid Dysfunction and Ophthalmopathy

Michael D. Brennan and Colum A. Gorman

*Division of Endocrinology and Department of Internal Medicine, Mayo Clinic,
Rochester, Minnesota 55905*

Although the cause of Graves' ophthalmopathy remains unknown, it is widely agreed that thyroid-stimulating immunoglobulins cause the hyperthyroidism of Graves' disease (29). Here we intend to discuss for our ophthalmologist readers the recognition of thyroid dysfunction and the relationships between thyroid overactivity and ophthalmopathy.

THYROID PHYSIOLOGY

Dietary iodine is absorbed all along the intestinal tract. It acts to regulate the thyroid and to serve as a substrate for thyroid hormone synthesis. The thyroid concentrates the iodine 30-fold, oxidizes it, and attaches it to tyrosine molecules on thyroglobulin in the thyroid follicle (14) (Fig. 1). One iodine atom per molecule of tyrosine produces monoiodotyrosine (MIT), and two iodine atoms give diiodotyrosine (DIT). The coupling of MIT with DIT produces triiodothyronine (T_3) (Table 1). When two diiodotyrosine molecules couple, the product is tetraiodothyronine (thyroxine; T_4) (Fig. 2). Antithyroid drugs, e.g., methimazole and propylthiouracil, act by inhibiting the oxidation, iodination, and coupling steps. In addition, propylthiouracil acts peripherally to impair T_4 to T_3 conversion.

THYROID HORMONE TRANSPORT AND METABOLISM

T_4 and T_3 in the circulation are almost entirely bound to transport proteins, which serve to control their volume of distribution (17,20,24,25). In order of diminishing importance, these transport proteins are thyroxine-binding globulin (TBG), thyroxine-binding prealbumin (TBPA), and albumin (Fig. 3). The amount of thyroid hormone bound to a transport protein

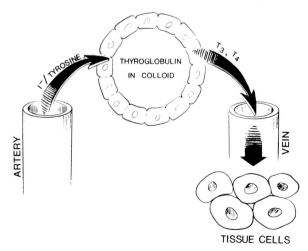

FIG. 1. Iodine trapped by the thyroid is incorporated into tyrosine in thyroglobulin at the luminal surface of the follicular cell.

49

TABLE 1. *Characteristics of thyroxine and triiodothyronine*

Characteristic	Triiodothyronine	L-Thyroxine
Production/24 hr (μg)	≈ 30	≈ 80
Fractional turnover rate/24 hr (%)	50–70	10
Volume of distribution (liters)	35–45	10–12
Thyroid-binding globulin affinity	1	30
Unbound to proteins— "free" (%)	0.18–0.46	0.03
Thyroid content (μg/tissue)	15	200

IODIDE (I^-) is trapped by the thyroid gland and oxidized—becomes IODINE (I_2)...

one or two molecules of IODINE are incorporated into TYROSINE...

to form MIT (Monoiodotyrosine) or DIT (Diiodotyrosine)...

one molecule each of MIT and DIT couple to form TRIIODOTHYRONINE (T_3)...

OR

two molecules of DIT couple to form TETRAIODOTHYRONINE (Thyroxine or T_4).

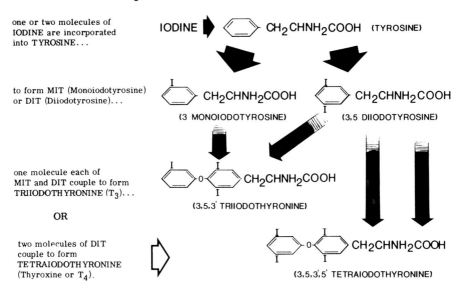

IODINE ➤ CH$_2$CHNH$_2$COOH (TYROSINE)

CH$_2$CHNH$_2$COOH (3 MONOIODOTYROSINE)

CH$_2$CHNH$_2$COOH (3,5 DIIODOTYROSINE)

CH$_2$CHNH$_2$COOH (3,5,3' TRIIODOTHYRONINE)

CH$_2$CHNH$_2$COOH (3,5,3,5' TETRAIODOTHYRONINE)

Thyroxin is then stored as part of a molecule of THYROGLOBULIN (contained as colloid in thyroid follicles) until released by proteolysis.

FIG. 2. Synthesis of thyroid hormones.

is determined by the capacity of the protein for T_4 or T_3 and the affinity with which T_4 and/or T_3 bind to the protein. TBG has high affinity and relatively low capacity (20 μg/dl). Albumin has almost unlimited capacity but very low affinity. TBG is the major T_4- and T_3-binding protein. Remember that only free thyroid hormones enter the peripheral cells to exert the effects noted in Fig. 4. Free hormones constitute <0.1% of the total, yet they are critically important (30). On the other hand, large variations can occur in the amount of thyroid hormones attached to the binding proteins without any change in the patient's metabolic status. TBG can be measured in blood by radioimmunoassay, or the binding capacity of TBG for T_4 can be tested. Results are reported as micrograms of T_4 bound by TBG per 100 ml of serum. The number of unoccupied binding sites on thyroxine-binding

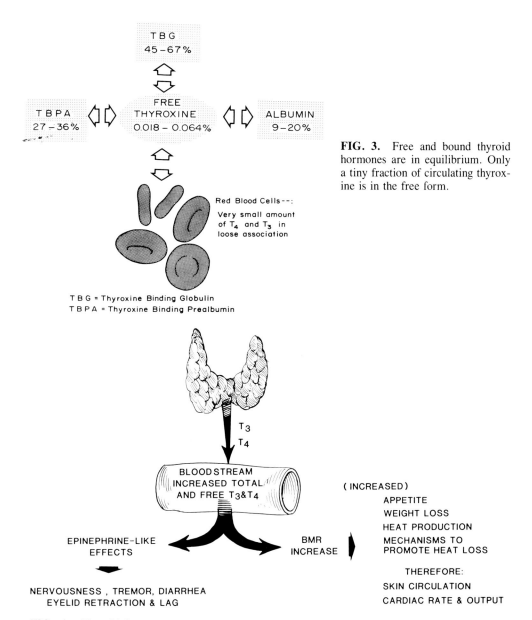

FIG. 3. Free and bound thyroid hormones are in equilibrium. Only a tiny fraction of circulating thyroxine is in the free form.

FIG. 4. Thyroid hormones exert sympathomimetic and colorigenic effects. Adaptive responses which serve to dispose of the increased heat generated include tachycardia and increased skin blood flow.

proteins is indirectly assessed by the T_3 resin uptake test (33). Do not confuse this test with the direct measurement of T_3 in serum as performed by the T_3 radioimmunoassay (31,32).

In the peripheral tissues, much of the T_4 secreted by the thyroid is monodeiodinated to T_3 (26), which is the more physiologically active thyroid hormone (Table 1). The rate of deiodination is influenced by illness and by certain drugs (16). Thyroid hormone effects are brought about, at least in part, by binding of T_3 to nuclear receptors in tissue cells (19). The consequences of excessive free T_4 and free T_3 levels are shown in Fig. 4.

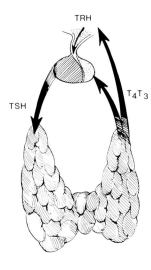

FIG. 5. In patients with Graves' disease, pituitary TSH-mediated control of thyroid function is superseded by TSIs, which induce excessive and unregulated production of thyroid hormones.

THYROID GLAND REGULATION

The pituitary gland produces thyroid-stimulating hormone (TSH), which interacts with receptors on the surface of the thyroid cell to induce growth and increased function of the cell. In consequence, more T_4 and T_3 are manufactured and released into the circulation; T_4 and T_3 feed back to the pituitary and hypothalamus and inhibit the production of TSH when their concentration in serum exceeds a preset level.

The operation of this system is precisely analogous to the operation of a thermostatically controlled furnace (Fig. 5). In addition to T_4 and T_3, another factor modifies TSH release. Thyrotropin-releasing hormone (TRH) from the hypothalamus is a tripeptide which is commercially available. When given by injection in a dose of 200 to 400 μg i.v., this substance induces a burst of TSH secretion which can readily be measured in blood (21–23,27,35). When serum T_4 and T_3 levels are even slightly raised above the physiological set point, the pituitary does not respond to TRH stimulation and no TSH is secreted into the circulation. This is the basis for a very sensitive test for early hyperthyroidism called the TRH stimulation test. A few patients who become thyrotoxic disproportionately increase T_3 in their blood. When the serum T_4 is normal and the T_3 is high, the condition is referred to as T_3 toxicosis. It occurs in about 5% of Graves' patients (11,13).

THYROID REGULATION IN GRAVES' DISEASE

In Graves' disease and other autoimmune thyroid diseases a variety of autoantibodies are directed against membrane and colloid thyroid antigens (see the chapter by Volpé, *this volume*). Among these are a group of autoantibodies termed thyroid-stimulating immuno-globulins which have in common the property of binding to or near the TSH receptor and initiating the series of stimulatory steps normally set in motion by TSH (Fig. 6). Although TSH production is tightly regulated by the level of thyroid hormone in the circulation, this is not true for TSI. In thyrotoxic Graves' disease, the unregulated continuing production of a potent thyroid stimulator results in inappropriately high levels of T_4 and T_3 in blood and peripheral tissues, consequences of excess thyroid hormone (Fig. 4). Because the thyroid is no longer driven by TSH (28,34,36,37), serum TSH levels are usually undetectable. If one were to administer T_4 or T_3 in supraphysiological doses (37), the thyroid, acting independently of TSH, would continue to trap iodine and to release T_4 and T_3 into the circulation. The normal thyroid faced with a high serum concentration of T_3 inhibits iodine uptake completely.

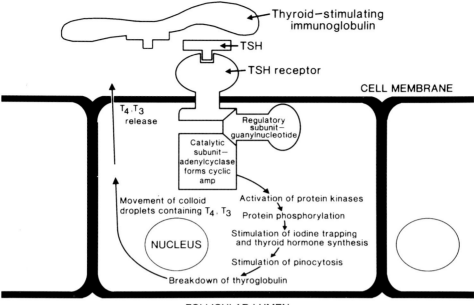

FOLLICULAR LUMEN

FIG. 6. The TSH receptor consists of a catalytic subunit, which actually initiates a chain of intracellular events, and a guanylnucleotide regulatory subunit, which couples the catalytic unit to the membrane-bound receptor. Intracellular proteins are phosphorylated by activated protein kinases. Iodine trapping and thyroxine synthesis are accelerated. Pinocytotic ingestion of thyroglobulin and thyroglobulin breakdown are accelerated, and colloid droplets containing thyroid hormones move through the cell. T_4 and T_3 are released into the perifollicular capillary. TSI binds to or near the TSH receptor and initiates the same series of events.

TABLE 2. *T_3 suppression test in euthyroid Graves' ophthalmopathy*

Daily T_3 dose (µg)	No. of days	Timing of uptake (hr)	No. studied	Nonsuppressible	%	Ref.
75	8	24	10	10	100	36
120	6	4	16	15	94	12
75	8	24	8	4	50	7
120	6	4	12	11	92	2
75	5	24	6	5	83	38
120	6	4	23	15	65	3
100	7	6	26	13	50	10
100	5	24	56	45	80	15
100	5	24	20	9	45	18
75	8	24	10	6	60	8
75	8	24	16	8	50	28
75	8	24	57	41	72	34
Total:			260	182	70	

This principle underlies the T_3 suppression test, which is a test for abnormal thyroid regulation in Graves' disease (37) (Table 2). The procedure is as follows. Radioiodine uptake by the thyroid gland is measured 24 hr after an oral tracer dose is administered. The patient is then given triiodothyronine 25 µg t.i.d. daily for 7 days, and the radioiodine uptake test is repeated. In normal patients thyroid radioiodine uptake declines to <50% and usually

TABLE 3. *TRH/T_3 suppression tests in euthyroid Graves'*
ophthalmopathy[a]

No. studied	Dose (μg i.v.)	S−/T−	S−	S−/T+	S+/T−	S+/T+	Ref.
2	200	1	1	—	—	—	?1
10	200	4	—	2	0	4	8
57	500	35	—	6	1	15	34

[a]From Tamai et al. (34); S−, T_3-nonsuppressible; S+, T_3-suppressible; T−, TRH-nonstimulable; T+, TSH-stimulable.

TABLE 4. *Levels at which thyroid function or regulation can be tested*

Parameter	Test
Hypothalamic pituitary function	TRH stimulation
Pituitary thyroid function	TSH radioimmunoassay
Thyroid iodine trap	Radioiodine uptake
Distribution of function across thyroid	Thyroid scan
Circulating thyroid hormone levels	Total and free T_4 and T_3 assays
Thyroid-binding proteins	Serum TBG; TBG binding capacity (indirectly assessed by tests such as T_3 resin uptake, normalized thyroxine, T_7
Abnormal thyroid stimulators	TSI assays (see text); T_3 suppression; TRH stimulation
Impact of thyroid hormone on peripheral tissues	Basal metabolic rate; serum cholesterol; reflex relaxation time; systolic time intervals

$<10\%$ of the administered dose. In patients with Graves' disease, due to persistent stimulation from immunoglobulins, suppression to this degree does not occur (28,34,35,38) (Table 2).

Note that the TRH stimulation test described earlier is a test for subtle degrees of thyroid hyperfunction (1,8). The T_3 suppression test is a test for the presence of abnormal thyroid stimulators (i.e., TSI) and still gives positive results when thyroid hormone levels are normal or low. One must have sufficiently high uptake of radioiodine by the thyroid gland, however, to permit a decline to be recognized (2,7) (Table 2). Neither test is absolutely consistently abnormal in patients with Graves' ophthalmopathy (28,34,38). The frequency with which abnormal results are encountered is displayed in Tables 2 and 3.

GRAVES' DISEASE AND LYMPHOCYTIC THYROIDITIS

Both Graves' disease and lymphocytic thyroiditis are thought of as autoimmune thyroid diseases. The main point of distinction between them may be the population of antibodies directed toward the thyroid. If the family of antibodies produced are predominantly stimulatory, hyperthyroidism may result, whereas if the antibodies are mainly inhibitory or cytotoxic in type lymphocytic thyroiditis may result. Some patients have both stimulatory and inhibitory antibodies, and thyroid function may be hypothyroid or balanced in the normal range but is characteristically nonsuppressible (3,4,38). Such patients may histologically exhibit lymphocytic (Hashimoto's) thyroiditis, whereas their eye findings are characteristic of Graves' disease.

TABLE 5. *Thyroid function tests commonly used to assess ophthalmopathy*

Test	Method	Normal range	Comment
Serum total thyroxine (total T_4)	Radioimmunoassay	5–12.5 μg/dl	Preferred screening test. Results are influenced by altered thyroxine binding, and it is sometimes increased after radiographic contrast administration or during therapy with thyroxine. Do not use for patients receiving estrogens, androgens, diphenylhydantoin, or salicylates
Serum free thyroxine (total T_3)	Radioimmunoassay	0.8–1.8 ng/dl	Usually reliable indicator of thyroid function when total thyroxine results are modified due to altered thyroxine binding
Total serum triiodothyronine (total T_3)	Radioimmunoassay	80–180 ng/dl	This test is abnormal in ~5% of thyrotoxic patients in whom total T_4 is normal. This condition is colloquially referred to as T_3 thyrotoxicosis
TBG binding capacity	Electrophoresis	16–24 μg/dl	A direct check on the normality of thyroxine-binding proteins. Use this test if results of total thyroxine are modified by estrogen, androgen, salicylate, pregnancy, or diphenylhydantoin
TRH stimulation test	Intravenous injection of 200–400 μg TRH	Serum TSH level increases by 100% or 6 MIU/ml	Use this test when serum total T_4 and T_3 are in the normal range but subtle hyperthyroidism is suspected, e.g., "euthyroid Graves' disease." No TSH response to TRH is consistent with early hyperthyroidism
Radioiodine uptake	^{131}I 3 mCi orally; measure percent of dose in thyroid at 24 hr	8–29% (varies regionally)	This test distinguishes Graves' hyperthyroidism from other causes of increased serum thyroxine
T_3 suppression test	Baseline radioiodine uptake (24 hr), T_3 25 μg t.i.d. for 7 days, repeat radioiodine uptake	Reduction of 50% or more in radioiodine uptake	This test can be thought of as a bioassay for circulating non-TSH stimulators of thyroid function. Because of the T_3 dose, it is contraindicated in elderly or cardiac patients
TSI in serum	Various methods (see text)	None present	This test is positive in >90% of patients with thyrotoxic Graves' disease and in a smaller percentage of those who have "euthyroid Graves' disease"

DETECTION OF TSI IN BLOOD

There exists no direct radioimmunoassay for TSI in blood. One can infer its presence from an abnormal TRH stimulation test, but *any* cause of high thyroid hormone levels gives positive results on this test so it is not specific for Graves' disease. The T_3 suppression test is not specific either, as it is abnormal in patients with toxic nodular goiters which function autonomously. It is also time-consuming, the doses of T_3 used may be risky for elderly or cardiac patients, and it requires two (albeit small) doses of radioiodine. It is not surprising that the search for more direct assays for TSI has been so assiduously pursued. No absolutely specific technique has yet been developed, and existing assays named in accordance with the specific effect of TSI that is examined (Fig. 6). Thus assays exist which are based on the ability of TSI to displace ^{125}I-labeled TSH from its receptor on thyroid cells (TSH

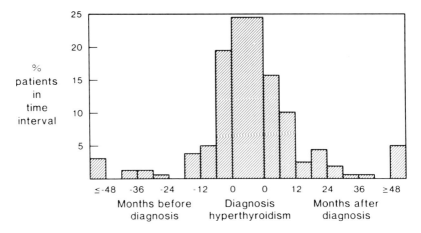

FIG. 7. Onset of eye symptoms in relation to date of diagnosis of hyperthyroidism. Among patients who required transantral orbital decompression for Graves' ophthalmopathy, 83% experienced their first eye symptom within 18 months of the date when hyperthyroidism was diagnosed. (From ref. 9.)

displacement assay). Other assays assess the amount of cyclic AMP generated in thyroid cell monolayers or thyroid slices when they are exposed to serum containing TSI (cyclic AMP generation assays). Yet others reveal the presence of TSI by detecting the stimulation of movement in colloid droplets bearing thyroid hormones from the follicular lumen toward the apex of the cell (colloid droplet assay) or by measuring the tiny quantities of T_3 and T_4 released into the medium by TSI-stimulated thyroid slices (iodothyronine release assays). Sometimes the results of these assays are presented as an index or ratio which relates the performance of the test serum to the effects of control serum, which contains no TSI. Measurement of TSI is discussed further in chapters by Volpé and by Wall, *this volume*.

LEVELS AT WHICH THYROID FUNCTION OR CONTROL CAN BE TESTED

It should now be clear that one can select from a wide variety of thyroid tests, each of which is specific to a given purpose (Tables 4 and 5). From among this extensive pool of tests, which should the ophthalmologist order? Assuming that the eye specialist will be working with an internist or endocrinologist, the first-line tests to order are measurements of serum T_4 and T_3, a check for abnormal binding (e.g., serum TBG or T_3 resin test), and a radioiodine uptake test. Radiographic contrast material and amiodarone invalidate the uptake test (5,6). If thyroid hormone levels and ^{131}I uptake are high, the problem is solved. If one or both are normal, TSI assays, T_3 suppression testing, or TRH stimulation testing may be selected before the diagnosis of Graves' disease is excluded. Remember too that a few patients who have normal levels of thyroid hormone in their blood and the histologic change of lymphocytic thyroiditis in their thyroid glands may show the typical eye findings of Graves' ophthalmopathy.

TEMPORAL RELATIONSHIPS BETWEEN GRAVES' OPHTHALMOPATHY AND HYPERTHYROIDISM

One may reasonably inquire why a patient who has circulating TSI (which is the hallmark of Graves' disease) is not necessarily hyperthyroid (10,18). The answer may be that there was previous therapy with surgery or radioiodine. A thyroid reduced to a fraction of its usual functional mass is probably incapable of producing hyperthyroidism no matter how vigorously it is stimulated by TSI. A second explanation may lie in the presence of competing antibodies, some of which may act to block the action of TSI. Lastly, it may be simply a matter of timing (9,15,34) (Fig. 7). Most patients with severe ophthalmopathy experience altered thyroid function and ophthalmopathy concurrently, but this is not invariably true. In many instances repeat thyroid function testing confirms the presence of a regulatory abnormality (34). In these circumstances consultation with an endocrinologist is advised.

REFERENCES

1. Arizi, F., Vagenakis, A. G., Portnay, G. I., Rapoport, B., Ingbar, S. H., and Braverman, L. E. (1975): Pituitary thyroid responsiveness to intramuscular thyrotrophin-releasing hormone based on analyses of serum thyroxine, triiodothyronine and thyrotrophin concentration. *N. Engl. J. Med.*, 292:273–277.
2. Bayliss, R. I. S. (1967): Stimulation and suppression tests of thyroid function. *Proc. R. Soc. Med.*, 60:303–306.
3. Bowden, A. N., and Rose, F. C. (1969): Dysthyroid exophthalmos. *Proc. R. Soc. Med.*, 62:13–15.
4. Broumlee, B. E. W., Newton, O. A. G., and Singh, S. P. (1975): Ophthalmopathy associated with primary hypothyroidism. *Acta Endocrinol. (Copenh.)*, 79:691–699.
5. Burger, A., Dinichert, D., Nicod, P., Jenny, M., Lemarchand-Beraud, T., and Vallottow, M. B. (1976): Effect of amiodarone on serum triiodothyronine, reverse triiodothyronine, thyroxine and thyrotrophin: a drug influencing peripheral metabolism of thyroid hormones. *J. Clin. Invest.*, 58:255–259.
6. Burgi, H., Wimpfheimer, C., Burger, A., Zaunbaucr, W., Rosler, H., and Lemarchand-Beraud, T. (1976): Changes of circulating thyroxine, triiodothyronine and reverse triiodothyronine after radiographic contrast agents. *J. Clin. Endocrinol. Metab.*, 43:1203–1210.
7. Burke, G. (1967): The triiodothyronine suppression test. *Am. J. Med.*, 42:600–608.
8. Chopra, I. J., Chopra, U., and Orgiazzi, J. (1973): Abnormalities of hypothalamo-hypophyseal-thyroid axis in patients with Graves' ophthalmopathy. *J. Clin. Endocrinol. Metab.*, 37:955–967.
9. Gorman, C. A. (1983): Temporal relationship between onset of Graves' ophthalmopathy and diagnosis of thyrotoxicosis. *Mayo Clin. Proc.*, 58:515–519.
10. Hall, R., Domach, D., Kirkham, K., and El Kabir, D. (1970): Ophthalmic Graves' disease. *Lancet*, 1:375–378.
11. Hesch, R. D., Huefner, M., Von Zur Muhlen, A., and Emrich, D. (1974): Triiodothyronine levels in patients with euthyroid endocrine exophthalmos and during treatment of thyrotoxicosis. *Acta Endocrinol. (Copenh.)*, 75:514–522.
12. Hobbs, J. R. (1963): M.D. thesis, University of London.
13. Hollander, C. S., Stevenson, C., Mitsuma, T., Peneda, G., Shenkman, L., and Silva, E. (1972): T_3 toxicosis in an iodine deficient area. *Lancet*, 2:1276–1278.
14. Ingbar, S. H. (1972): Autoregulation of the thyroid; response to iodide excess and depletion. *Mayo Clin. Proc.*, 47:814–823.
15. Ivy, H. K. (1972): Medical approach to ophthalmopathy of Graves' disease. *Mayo Clin. Proc.*, 47:980–985.
16. Kristensen, B. O., and Weeke, J. (1977): Propranolol induced increments in total and free serum thyroxine in patients with essential hypertension. *Clin. Pharmacol. Ther.*, 22:864–867.
17. Lutz, H. J., Gregorman, R. I., Spaulding, S. W., Hornack, R. B., and Dankins, A. I. (1972): Thyroxine binding proteins, free thyroxine and thyroxine turnover inter-relationships during acute infectious illness in man. *J. Clin. Endocrinol. Metab.*, 35:230–249.
18. Mornex, R., Fournier, G., and Berthezene, F. (1975): Ophthalmic Graves' disease. *Mod. Probl. Ophthalmol.*, 14:426–431.
19. Oppenheimer, J. H., Schwartz, H. L., Surks, M. I., Koerner, D., and Dillman, W. H. (1976): Nuclear receptors and the initiation of thyroid hormone action. *Recent Prog. Horm. Res.*, 32:529–558.
20. Oppenheimer, J. H., Squef, R., Surks, M. J., and Hauer, H. (1963): Binding of thyroxine by serum proteins evaluated by equilibrium dialysis of electrophoretic techniques: alterations in thyroidal illness. *J. Clin. Invest.*, 42:1769–1782.
21. Patel, Y. C., and Burger, H. G. (1972): Effect of synthetic thyrotrophin releasing hormone (TRH) in man. *Aust. N. Z. J. Med.*, 4:366–375.
22. Pokroy, H., Epstein, S., Hendricks, S., and Pimstone, B. (1974): Thyrotrophin response to intravenous thyrotrophin releasing hormone in patients with hepatic and renal disease. *Horm. Metab. Res.*, 6:132–136.
23. Re, R. N., Kourides, I. A., Ridgway, E. C., Weintraub, B. D., and Maloof, F. (1976): The effect of glucocorticoid administration on human pituitary secretion of thyrotropin and prolactin. *J. Clin. Endocrinol. Metab.*, 43:338–346.

24. Refetoff, S. (1979): Thyroid hormone transport. In: *Endocrinology*, edited by L. J. DeGroot, pp. 347–356. Grune & Stratton, New York.

25. Roberts, R. C., and Nicolai, T. F. (1969): Determination of thyroxine binding globulin; a simplified procedure utilizing dextran coated charcoal. *Clin. Chem.*, 15:1132–1140.

26. Schimmel, M., and Utiger, R. D. (1977): Thyroidal and peripheral production of thyroid hormones: review of recent findings and their clinical implications. *Ann. Intern. Med.*, 87:760–768.

27. Snyder, P. J., and Utiger, R. D. (1972): Response to thyrotrophin releasing hormone (TRH) in man. *J. Clin. Endocrinol. Metab.*, 34:380–385.

28. Solomon, D. H., Chopra, I. J., Chopra, U., and Smith, F. J. (1977): Identification of subgroups of euthyroid Graves' ophthalmopathy. *N. Engl. J. Med.*, 296:181–186.

29. Spaulding, S. W., and Utiger, R. D. (1981): The thyroid; physiology, hyperthyroidism, hypothyroidism and the painful thyroid. In: *Endocrinology and Metabolism*, edited by P. Felig, J. D. Baxter, A. E. Broadus, and L. A. Frohman, pp. 281–350. McGraw-Hill, New York.

30. Sterling, K., and Brenner, M. A. (1966): Free thyroxine in human serum; simplified measurement with the aid of magnesium precipitation. *J. Clin. Invest.*, 45:153–163.

31. Sterling, K., Brenner, M. A., Newman, E. S., Odell, W. D., and Bellalarla, D. (1971): The significance of triiodothyronine (T_3) in maintenance of euthyroid status after treatment of hyperthyroidism. *J. Clin. Endocrinol. Metab.*, 33:729–731.

32. Sterling, K., Refetoff, S., and Selenkow, H. A. (1970): T_3 toxicosis: thyrotoxicosis due to elevated serum triiodothyronine levels. *JAMA*, 213:571–575.

33. Sterling, K., and Talachnick, M. (1961): Resin uptake of I^{131} triiodothyronine as a test of thyroid function. *J. Clin. Endocrinol. Metab.*, 21:456–464.

34. Tamai, H., Nagagawa, T., Ohsako, N., Fukino, O., Takahashi, H., Matsuzuka, F., Kuma, K., and Nagataki, S. (1980): Changes in thyroid function in patients with euthyroid Graves' disease. *J. Clin. Endocrinol. Metab.*, 50:108–112.

35. Weintraub, B. D., Gershengorn, M. C., Kounides, I. A., and Fein, H. (1981): Inappropriate secretion of thyroid stimulating hormone. *Ann. Intern. Med.*, 95:339–351.

36. Werner, S. C. (1955): Euthyroid patients with early eye signs of Graves' disease: their responses to L-triiodothyronine and thyrotrophin. *Am. J. Med.*, 16:608–612.

37. Werner, S. C., and Spooner, M. (1955): A new and simple test for hyperthyroidism employing L-triiodothyronine and the 24-hour I^{131} uptake method. *Bull. N.Y. Acad. Med.*, 31:137–145.

38. Wyse, E. P., McConahey, W. M., Woolner, L. B., Scholz, D. A., and Kearns, T. P. (1968): Ophthalmopathy without hyperthyroidism in patients with histologic Hashimoto's thyroiditis. *J. Clin. Endocrinol. Metab.*, 28:1623–1629.

The Eye and Orbit in Thyroid Disease, edited by
C. A. Gorman et al. Raven Press, New York 1984.

Autoimmunity in Graves' and Hashimoto's Diseases

Robert Volpé

*Department of Medicine, University of Toronto; and The Wellesley Hospital,
Toronto, Ontario M4Y 1J3, Canada*

In 1897 Ehrlich coined the term "horror autotoxicus" to describe his idea that the body appeared to be "unwilling" to mount an immune assault on its own tissues (1). During the early part of the twentieth century it was hypothesized that the hyperplastic thymus, in some obscure fashion, could be the cause of Graves' disease [see review by Solomon and Kleeman (2)]. The field of thyroid autoimmunity was thus initiated and during the past 25 years has received particular impetus. The study of autoimmune thyroid disease has not only been valuable in itself but has also provided insight into the pathogenesis of autoimmune disease in general. This chapter is concerned primarily with two clinically disparate disorders of the human thyroid, i.e., Graves' disease and Hashimoto's thyroiditis (and its variants). Whereas the clinical expression of these two disorders may be markedly different, there are many genetic and pathogenetic elements which are similar, if not common, to them both, and indeed some workers (3–5) (although not this author) consider that these two conditions are merely opposite ends of a spectrum of the same condition. There are elements that are different between these disorders (6) and indeed even between the variants of thyroiditis (7), and these differences are discussed below.

Graves' disease (8–10) is currently defined as a form of hyperthyroidism with a diffuse hyperplastic goiter associated frequently with extrathyroidal manifestations, e.g., exophthalmos and occasionally pretibial myxedema. It is now accepted that the excess production of thyroid hormones in this disorder is due to the stimulation of the thyrotropin (thyroid-stimulating hormone; TSH) receptor on the thyroid cell membrane by an immunoglobulin termed thyroid-stimulating antibody (TSAb). Hence an appropriate new designation is "autoimmune hyperthyroidism" (6).

The second autoimmune thyroid disorder, autoimmune thyroiditis, was first described by Hashimoto (11) in 1912; he reported four patients with goiter in whom the histology of the thyroid gland was characterized by diffuse lymphocytic infiltration, atrophy of the parenchymal cells, fibrosis, and eosinophilic change in some of the parenchymal cells. Several variants of this picture have now been described, as noted in Table 1.

In the chronic fibrous thyroiditis variant, fibrosis predominates, and lymphocytic infiltration is less marked (12). In the lymphocytic thyroiditis group of childhood and adolescence, fibrosis, Askanazy cells, and even germinal centers are less obvious than in the adult (12). Moreover, the titers of thyroid autoantibodies are generally lower in this category than in the adult forms and are often negative (13). Postpartum thyroiditis is often a transient form of autoimmune thyroiditis, although it may culminate in a chronic form (14,15). In "idiopathic myxedema" the gland is characterized by atrophy, rather than hypertrophy. The

TABLE 1. *Autoimmune thyroid diseases*

(a) Graves' disease (synonyms: Parry's disease, Basedow's disease, exophthalmic goiter, autoimmune thyrotoxicosis)
(b) Chronic autoimmune thyroiditis
Variants
Hashimoto's (lymphocytic) thyroiditis
Lymphocytic thyroiditis of childhood and adolescence
Postpartum thyroiditis
Chronic fibrous variant
Idiopathic myxedema
Atrophic, asymptomatic thyroiditis

atrophic, asymptomatic form is clinically occult and often discovered at autopsy (16). There seem to be subtle genetic and pathogenetic differences between these variants (7) which are discussed below. Conversely, there is a large body of evidence favoring the view that all of the variants share at least a similar pathogenesis, and it is therefore time, in the view of the writer, to utilize the term "chronic autoimmune thyroiditis" as the generic term for this group.

For many years autoimmune thyroiditis was considered to be uncommon, and the diagnosis was often first made at thyroidectomy. Increased awareness, coupled with improved diagnostic procedures has certainly been an important factor in improving recognition of this disorder. There is also evidence that the disease may have increased in frequency, an increase that has been ascribed to increased iodine intake over the past few decades (17). It is now estimated that approximately 3 to 4% of the population has chronic autoimmune thyroiditis (4). Thyroid function in autoimmune thyroiditis may be normal, slightly reduced, or severely deficient (4). About 3% of the population has some functional deficiency of the thyroid secondary to autoimmune thyroiditis (18), whereas up to 16% of elderly females has at least some degree of lymphocytic infiltration in the thyroid gland, although this cannot be recognized clinically (19). Hawkins et al. (20,21) have reported a longitudinal study among the population of a Western Australian community. They found that 72% of subjects with persistent thyroid microsomal antibody had subclinical hypothyroidism. In their studies, thyroid microsomal antibody was found in 6.7% of the population. They thus calculated that 4.5% of the population can be expected to have clinical or subclinical hypothyroidism.

The first clear evidence demonstrating immunological abnormalities in Hashimoto's thyroiditis and in Graves' (Basedow's) disease was reported in 1956. At that time Roitt et al. (22) discovered antibodies to thyroglobulin in the serum of patients with Hashimoto's thyroiditis. Almost simultaneously, Rose and Witebsky (23) induced experimental autoimmune thyroiditis for the first time by injecting thyroid self-antigen mixed with Freund's adjuvant into rabbits. Concurrently, Adams and Purves (24), using a guinea pig bioassay, detected an abnormal thyroid stimulator in the sera of some patients with Graves' disease. Because this substance had a much longer duration of activity than TSH, it was later called "long-acting thyroid stimulator" (LATS) (25). In 1964 Kriss et al. (26) demonstrated that LATS was in fact an immunoglobulin. Thus both Hashimoto's thyroiditis and Graves' disease were associated with autoimmune processes.

IMMUNE SYSTEM

It is not possible in this brief review to discuss the immune system in depth (6). It is evident, however, that the large repertoire of lymphocytes is necessary to defend the organism against the equally large number of antigens with which it may come into contact. Thus throughout an organism's life, its lymphocytes undergo spontaneous mutation in order to produce a large number of new clones of lymphocytes, each of which would be potentially capable of interacting with (and being stimulated by) a specific antigen (27). This presentation of a unique immunogen to its complementary lymphocyte clone initiates a specific immune response. In developing the repertoire of lymphocyte clones so as to permit capability of interacting with every possible antigen, every so often self-reactive "forbidden" clones of lymphocytes arise which must be suppressed. Although all lymphocytes derive originally from bone marrow, there are ultimately two major forms of lymphocytes: ~60% of lymphocytes are processed by the thymus and thus become thymus-dependent (T) lymphocytes, whereas the remainder are not processed by the thymus and may actually mature in the microenvironment of the bone marrow itself; these are termed "bursa equivalent" (B) lymphocytes, analogous to the lymphocytes from the bursa of Fabricius in birds. The T lymphocytes are not capable of producing humoral antibodies but are involved in cell-mediated immune processes. There are at least two major subsets of T lymphocytes, i.e., helper T lymphocytes, which cooperate with groups of B lymphocytes, allowing the latter to produce immunoglobulin G (IgG), and suppressor T lymphocytes, which are regulatory lymphocytes preventing inappropriate immune responses. Individual clones of suppressor T lymphocytes are capable of suppressing individual clones of helper T lymphocytes, thereby preventing autoantibody production; they may also suppress individual clones of B lymphocytes (6). In addition, the third subset of T lymphocytes may be directly cytotoxic (DCC) (28,29). There is evidence that self-reactive B lymphocytes are present in organisms in fetal and postnatal life, but these are not stimulated to produce IgG unless self-reactive helper T lymphocytes arise to stimulate them to do so (6). In the normal situation, however, when "forbidden" clones of self-reactive helper T lymphocytes arise (by normal random mutation), they are immediately suppressed by specific clones of suppressor T lymphocytes (specific suppressor T lymphocytes versus specific helper T lymphocytes), resulting in tolerance and preventing autoimmune disease (6,29).

This system has been found to be increasingly complex, with messages continually passed among at least three types of lymphocytes: inducer cells, regulatory cells, and effector cells (30). Selective activation of regulatory T lymphocytes is required to avoid immunological reactions against self-antigens throughout adult life. A role for anti-idiotypic antibodies (i.e., antibodies against specific autoantibodies) has also been proposed (31–34).

Thus each organ-specific autoimmune disease may be thought to result from a single defect in immunoregulation, probably a specific defect in suppressor T lymphocytes (Fig. 1). This then permits the survival of the appropriate organ-specific self-reactive "forbidden" clone of helper T lymphocytes which has arisen by normal random mutation. The latter then interacts with its complementary antigen and is stimulated to perform "helper" functions, establishing a localized cell-mediated immune response and cooperating with appropriate self-directed, already present B lymphocytes, which in consequence produce the specific humoral antibodies. There would be no need for antigenic alteration in this system, merely the availability of the antigen (e.g., on the cell membrane of the thyroid cell) (6).

ASSOCIATION WITH OTHER AUTOIMMUNE DISEASES

There is now evidence that for each organ-specific autoimmune disorder there is one specific defect in immunoregulation (35). However, if a person inherited two or more specific defects in immunoregulation (due to their close genetic proximity), it would permit

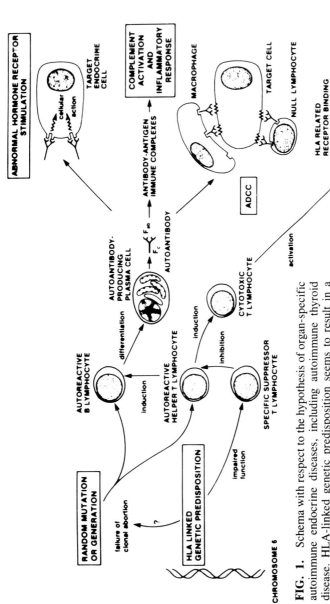

FIG. 1. Schema with respect to the hypothesis of organ-specific autoimmune endocrine diseases, including autoimmune thyroid disease. HLA-linked genetic predisposition seems to result in a specific defect in a clone of suppressor T lymphocytes (specific for each organ-specific autoimmune disease). Thus clonal abortion of autoreactive helper T lymphocytes does not properly occur when the latter arise by normal random mutation. If these auto-reactive helper T lymphocytes are not suppressed, they interact with appropriate and specific (already present) B lymphocytes that, in consequence, produce the appropriate antibodies. The effector mechanisms by which cellular action or target-cell damage occurs may vary. Such effects include stimulation of cellular action (as in the case of Graves' disease), the formation of antibody–antigen immune complexes, antibody-dependent cellular cytotoxicity (ADCC), and direct T-lymphocyte-induced cytotoxicity. (From ref. 279.)

TABLE 2. *Immune stigmata associated with Graves' disease and Hashimoto's thyroiditis*

Stigma	Graves' disease	Hashimoto's disease
Lymphocytic infiltration in thyroid	Frequently present	Almost invariable
Immunoglobulins in thyroid stoma	Yes	Yes
Type of infiltrating lymphocytes in thyroid	B and T lymphocytes, some unidentified lymphocytes	B and T lymphocytes, some unidentified lymphocytes
Immune complexes in circulation	Common	Common
Thymic enlargement	Common	Common
Lymphadenopathy and splenomegaly	Infrequent	—
Relative lymphocytosis	Common	—
Hypergammaglobulinemia	Occasional	Common
Benefit from corticosteroid therapy	Yes	Yes
Thyroid-stimulating immunoglobulin	Almost all	Infrequent
Exophthalmos	Common	Occasional
Evidence of cell-mediated immunity	Yes	Yes
Evidence for a specific defect in suppressor T lymphocytes	Yes	Yes
Other autoimmune diseases in patients	Pernicious anemia, vitiligo, diabetes mellitus, myasthenia gravis, Addison's disease, idiopathic thrombocytopenic purpura	Pernicious anemia, diabetes mellitus, Sjögren's syndrome, myasthenia gravis, Addison's disease, chronic active hepatitis
Thyroid antibodies in relatives	50%	50%
Thyroid and other autoimmune diseases in relatives	Common	Common
HLA genes (Caucasians)	HLA-B8-Dw3	Atrophic form: HLA-B8 and HLA-DRw3 Goitrous form: HLA-DR5
Animal models	—	Yes

the appearance of two or more autoimmune diseases and would explain the close association between the various organ-specific autoimmune diseases listed in Table 2. These conditions include insulin-dependent diabetes mellitus, pernicious anemia, myasthenia gravis, Addison's disease, autoimmune hypoparathyroidism, oophoritis or orchitis, vitiligo, Sjögren's syndrome, and lymphoid hypophysitis (6). These disorders occur in patients with autoimmune thyroid diseases much more often than chance alone would dictate. This is true for the overt forms of these conditions as well as the occult (serological evidence only) forms. There is also an increased incidence of these conditions in the families of patients with autoimmune thyroid disease. Many of these maladies are associated with an increased incidence of HLA-DR3 (6) (see section on genetics, below). Moreover, in the view of this author (6), exophthalmos probably represents an organ-specific autoimmune disorder which frequently overlaps with, but is nevertheless separate from, the thyroid abnormality of Graves' disease. This point is taken up elsewhere in this volume and thus is not discussed further in this chapter.

HUMORAL IMMUNITY IN HUMAN AUTOIMMUNE THYROID DISEASE

As mentioned previously, Roitt et al. (22) first detected antibodies to thyroglobulin in the serum of some patients with Hashimoto's thyroiditis in 1956. They initially used the agar precipitin test, which proved to be an excellent index of the chronic fibrous variant of Hashimoto's thyroiditis, where 96% of cases had positive precipitins as opposed to 4% in the euthyroid lymphocytic variant (35). At the present time, in addition to the thyroglobulin initially discovered, four other main antigen–antibody systems have been identified, including different constituents of the thyroid gland. They include not only thyroglobulin but also a microsomal antigen, a second antigen of the colloid, a cell-surface antigen, an antigen related to the TSH receptor, and antibodies reacting to the thyroid hormones thyroxine and triiodothyronine (36). In addition, thyroid growth-promoting (37) and growth-inhibiting antibodies (38) have been described, but the antigen for these antibodies is not yet known. The antigens involved, as well as the means for detecting the antibodies to these various antigens, are noted in Table 3.

A variety of antibodies to the various apparently normal constituents of the thyroid gland noted in Table 3 may be produced by patients with autoimmune thyroid disease. The number of epitopes on autologous molecules is far smaller than for foreign antigens, but it nevertheless seems that antibodies with different properties may all play a role in determining the pathogenetic mechanism involved in the clinical variants of autoimmune thyroiditis and Graves' disease (39). Thyroid autoantibodies have been found in all classes and subclasses of immunoglobulins (40). The complement-fixing antimicrosomal antibody has been shown to be cytotoxic (41). However, it is unclear if any of the other thyroid autoantibodies has deleterious effects on thyroid cells, at least when acting alone. Thyroglobulin antibody is generally noncomplement-fixing and is a precipitating antibody. IgE (reaginic) thyroid autoantibody is also detectable. Some antibodies may be involved in the normal disposal of degraded antigens in the physiological turnover of thyroid cells (42). Others may be involved in immune complexes and may produce tissue damage in this manner (43), or antibodies may cooperate with killer lymphocytes in producing an injury to thyroid tissue [antibody-dependent cellular cytoxicity (ADCC) (44)]; thus killer cells may have an adjunctive role in producing cellular damage (45) (Fig. 2). There is also evidence for direct damage by effector T lymphocytes [direct cellular cytotoxicity (DCC)] (29). At least two groups of workers have demonstrated the presence of lymphocytotoxic antibodies in many people with Graves' and Hashimoto's diseases (46,47). Whether these have any correlation with antibodies that are cytotoxic to thyroid cells remains to be established (46,47).

Each of the thyroid autoantibodies has been shown to be polyclonal (48–50). Although this was also thought to be true for TSAb, more recent evidence adduced by Zakarija and McKenzie (51–53) suggests that TSAb is oligoclonal at best and may even be monoclonal. Thyroid autoantibodies tend to decline during the last trimester of pregnancy, only to rebound to high levels 2 to 6 months postpartum, thus accounting for transient postpartum thyroiditis (14,15); this is discussed in detail elsewhere (6).

THYROGLOBULIN ANTIBODIES

It was once believed that thyroglobulin represented a "sequestered" antigen within the thyroid follicles which was not recognizable to the organism as "self," and that destruction of the follicles with escape of the thyroglobulin might lead into autoimmune thyroiditis (54). However, it is now known that thyroglobulin begins to leak into the circulation *in utero* in all persons and in fact is a normal circulating constituent even before birth (55). Thus the "secluded antigen" theory can be dismissed (56). Moreover, thyroglobulin-binding B lymphocytes can be shown to be present before birth (57).

Thyroglobulin antibodies are classically found in high titers in Hashimoto's and Graves' diseases; they are occasionally found in lower titers in other thyroid disorders (subacute

TABLE 3. *Antigen-antibody systems involved in humoral responses of thyroid autoimmune disease*[a]

Antigen	Antibody	Antibody detection
Thyroglobulin	Thyroglobulin	Precipitin technique
		Tanned red blood cell hemagglutination
		Immunofluorescence on fixed thyroid sections
		Competitive binding radioassay
		Coprecipitation with radioiodinated thyroglobulin
		Micro-enzyme-linked immunoassay (ELISA)
		Plaque-forming assay
Microsomal antigen	Microsomal	Complement fixation
		Immunofluorescence on unfixed thyroid sections
		Cytotoxicity test on cultured thyroid cells
		Competitive binding radioassay
		Tanned red blood cell hemagglutination
		Micro-ELISA
Second colloid component	CA_2	Immunofluorescence on fixed thyroid sections
Cell surface antigen(s)	Membrane	Immunofluorescence on viable thyroid cells
		Mixed hemadsorption
		Binding assays
Thyroxine and triiodothyronine	Thyroid hormone	Antigen-binding capacity
Antigen unclear	Growth-stimulating and growth-inhibiting	Effects on DNA content per thyroid cell nucleus or glucose-6-phosphate dehydrogenase (G6PD) activity per cell
TSH receptor-related	TSH receptor	*Stimulatory assays*
		LATS bioassay
		Colloid droplet formation in human thyroid slices
		Stimulation of human thyroid adenylate cyclase *in vitro*
		Cytochemical assay
		Current terms employed for stimulatory assays include:
		human thyroid stimulator, human thyroid stimulating immunoglobulin (TSI), thyroid-stimulating antibody (TSAb)
		Binding assays
		LATS protector assay
		Inhibition of ^{125}I-thyrotropin binding to human thyroid membranes
		Thyrotropin displacement activity (TDA), TSH-binding inhibitor immunoglobulin (TBII)
		Fat cell membrane radioligand assays
		Fat cell ELISA

[a]From ref. (201).

thyroiditis, nontoxic goiter, thyroid malignancy), in asymptomatic relatives of patients with autoimmune thyroid disease, in some nonthyroidal autoimmune conditions, and in some otherwise apparently normal persons (39,40). These antibodies may be of any class, although precipitins belong mostly to the IgG class. Thyroglobulin antibodies are noncomplement-fixing and for the most part are species-specific; however, they do show some cross-reactivity with monkey thyroglobulin (39). Currently the tanned red cell agglutination test is most often used for detecting these antibodies (39), although radioassays have also been utilized (58–60). Another technique being employed is the specific plaque-forming cell assay (61). A very sensitive technique for antithyroglobulin using a microenzyme-like immunoabsorbent assay (ELISA) has also been devised and is exceedingly sensitive (62). Pinchera et al. (36)

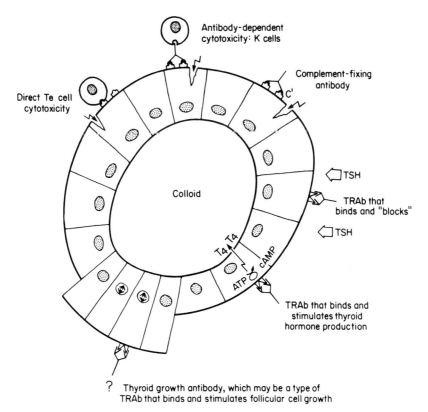

FIG. 2. Possible immune effector mechanisms in autoimmune thyroid disease. Cytotoxic mechanisms include direct cytotoxicity by sensitized effector *(Te)* cells, antibody-dependent cytotoxicity by killer *(K)* cells armed with antithyroid antibody, and cell lysis by complement-fixing thyroid antibody. The various types of thyrotropin-receptor antibody *(TRAb)* have different mechanisms of action. One type binds to the thyrotropin *(TSH)* receptor and blocks TSH from binding to the receptor. Another type—classic thyroid-stimulating antibody (TSAb)—binds to and stimulates the TSH receptor, which results in production of increased thyroid hormone by thyroid follicular cells. Thyroid growth antibody, which may be a type of TRAb, may bind to the TSH receptor and cause growth of thyroid follicular cells but not production of thyroid hormone. A variant of this antibody binds and blocks growth. (From ref. 29.)

have shown that antibodies to thyroglobulin may bind to various antigenic sites on the thyroglobulin molecule. Nevertheless, there is no evidence of an antigenic difference between the thyroglobulin found in autoimmune thyroid disease and that of normal persons (63,64).

By the common technique of tanned red cell hemagglutination, significant titers of antithyroglobulin are found in about 70% of patients with Hashimoto's thyroiditis or newly diagnosed idiopathic myxedema, about one-third of those with Graves' disease, and in a smaller percentage of those with thyroid carcinoma and other thyroid disorders (36). However, a large number of sera giving negative results by the hemagglutination technique were found to be positive by radioassay (36). The investigators could not explain the discrepancy by virtue of a greater sensitivity of the latter technique (36). Discrepancies between the two methods were mostly found in sera from patients with metastatic thyroid carcinoma, Graves' disease, or toxic adenoma. They suggested that these conditions may be associated with the presence in the serum of a substance which causes a positive radioassay response without producing hemagglutination. They further demonstrated that this substance could not be removed by immunoadsorption with thyroglobulin coupled to Sepharose. They proposed that the interfering substance could be thyroglobulin itself and indeed produced further data to indicate that increased serum thyroglobulin levels can produce false-positive results in the measurement of antithyroglobulin antibodies by radioassays. This problem was also encountered by Bayer and Kriss (65,66), who identified false-positive antithyroglobulin values by measuring the formation of thyroglobulin–antithyroglobulin complexes in the supernatants of the antithyroglobulin assay.

ANTIMICROSOMAL ANTIBODIES

The thyroid microsomal antigen has been localized by immunofluorescence in the apical cytoplasm of follicular cells (36). Roitt et al. (67) provided evidence that this antigen is an inherent part of the smooth endoplasmic reticulum and is apparently composed of the lipoprotein of the membrane of exocytotic vesicles supporting newly synthesized thyroglobulin from the Golgi apparatus to the colloid.

The precise antigen or antigens has/have been a matter of considerable investigation. Roitt and his colleagues (67) were unable to detect active antigen in solubilized preparations from human thyroid microsomes. However, Pinchera et al. (36) succeeded in solubilizing the appropriate antigen using various detergents, high-ionic-strength solution, and proteolytic enzymes as solubilizing agents. Despite continuing attempts to purify the solubilized microsomal antigen, the precise antigen has yet to be totally characterized. However, it is evident that an important component is cell membrane antigen(s) (36,68). In these investigations, a good correlation was found between the presence of antibodies reactive with the surface of human thyroid cells in tissue culture and the presence of antibodies reactive with thyroid microsomes. It suggests, in the case of thyroid cells, in contrast to pancreatic islet cells, either that microsomal antigens are also present in the thyroid cell surface membrane or that microsomal and cell surface antigens, although separate and distinct, are frequently associated with each other, with a strong tendency for autoantibodies to be formed against both antigens if they are formed at all.

Thus these antibodies have a close relationship to the antibodies to cell surface antigens, which have been found in a large proportion of patients with Hashimoto's thyroiditis, idiopathic myxedema, or Graves' disease utilizing either immunofluorescence (69) or a mixed hemadsorption technique using monocultures (70). Jonsson and Fagraeus (70) also demonstrated a close relationship between the presence of elevated microsomal antibody titers and elevated antibody to the cell surface antigens, as noted above (36,68). Nevertheless, in all of these studies, the relationship is not absolute and several discrepancies have been observed. Thus, it seems most likely that although there may be common antigens involved in both systems there are also some different antigens involved in these reactions. In any event, the cell surface antigen demonstrable in this manner seems to be separate and distinct from the antigen to which the TSAb or thyroid-stimulating immunoglobulin (TSI) is the antibody. For TSI and TSAb there is now good evidence that the antigen is the TSH receptor on the thyroid cell membrane (6).

Antibodies to the microsomal antigen have been shown to be complement-fixing (39) and have the ability to induce cytotoxic changes in monolayers of cultured thyroid cells (41). Correlation exists between the titers of this antibody and the histological lesions of Hashimoto's thyroiditis. The titers of thyroglobulin antibody do not correlate as well (39). Microsomal antibodies are also commonly associated with abnormalities of thyroid function

(20,21). Tanner et al. (71) have also shown evidence that when thyroid antibodies, particularly thyroid microsomal antibodies, are found unexpectedly a significant proportion of patients have biochemical evidence of hypothyroidism and may benefit from appropriate therapy. In a statistical sense, asymptomatic persons with thyroid microsomal antibodies stand an $\sim 10\%$ chance of ultimately having overt autoimmune thyroid disease (6). To that extent, the presence of such antibodies are predictive of overt disease.

Antimicrosomal antibodies may be detected by immunofluorescence, complement fixation, hemagglutination (6), or radioassay (58). Hemagglutination has become the favorite procedure for this antibody, but the micro-ELISA technique may become readily available in the near future (72). In any event, microsomal antibodies are detected in almost all patients with Hashimoto's thyroiditis, most of those with idiopathic myxedema or Graves' disease, and some asymptomatic relatives of patients with these disorders; they are found much less frequently in other thyroid disorders. There are marked discrepancies between the presence of antimicrosomal and antithyroglobulin antibody. Most commonly, antimicrosomal antibodies are detected, often in the absence of antithyroglobulin antibodies. Moreover, high levels of antithyroglobulin antibody may produce false-positive results in measurements of antimicrosomal antibodies by hemagglutination (36), but this interference may be easily overcome by adding an excess of thyroglobulin to the system. Fortunately, as mentioned above, because antimicrosomal antibodies are present much more commonly than antithyroglobulin antibodies, this problem is of minimal importance. Conversely, antithyroglobulin antibodies are rarely present in the absence of antimicrosomal antibodies. A preponderance of antimicrosomal antibodies was found by Pinchera et al. (36) to be even more pronounced in patients with Graves' disease.

The antigens present on human thyroid plasma membranes have been studied by Monzani et al. (73). These investigators showed that human thyroid plasma membrane possesses a limited number of antigenic determinants. Some are related to thyroglobulin, others to antigens which react to autoantibodies from patients with autoimmune thyroid disorders, and still others to antigens which produce thyroid antibodies experimentally in animals. It may also be pointed out that these antibodies do tend to fall in many, but not all, patients following antithyroid drug therapy for Graves' disease or after severe myxedema has occurred spontaneously in patients with Hashimoto's thyroiditis.

ANTIBODY TO A COLLOID COMPONENT
OTHER THAN THYROGLOBULIN

Sera from some patients with either Graves' or Hashimoto's disease show a uniform immunofluorescence in the colloid of fixed sections of thyroid tissue, even after adsorption with thyroglobulin (39). The antigen to which these antibodies are directed seems to be a noniodide-containing protein. This antibody is also found in some cases of thyroid malignancy and in subacute thyroiditis. Its significance is undetermined.

ANTIBODIES TO THYROID HORMONES

Antibodies are occasionally directed toward the thyroid hormones [thyroxine (T_4) and triiodothyronine (T_3)]. These are generally found in patients with Hashimoto's disease but also in those with Graves' disease and are generally found only when there is a high titer of antithyroglobulin. The titers of antibodies to T_4 and T_3 become important when measuring circulating levels of these thyroid hormones (74–76). Depending on the extraction and separation procedures, spuriously high or low T_4 or T_3 concentrations may result if the antibodies are present in sufficiently high titers. With polyethylene glycol radioimmunoassays the values are spuriously low, whereas when the hormones are extracted from serum with a Sephadex G-25 column the serum hormone concentrations are increased to their true high values (76). This may be particularly confusing when hypothyroid patients are treated with thyroid hormones, resulting in less than expected improvement, extremely high values of serum thyroxine, but continuing high levels of TSH (75). These antibodies do not affect thyroid function if the thyroid is capable of responding to TSH normally. Because these antibodies to the thyroid hormones have been shown to cross-react with thyroglobulin (77), it is possible that thyroglobulin acts as an adjuvant or a hapten in order to generate antibodies to the iodothyronines.

TSH RECEPTOR-RELATED ANTIGEN AND CELL SURFACE ANTIGENS: RELATIONSHIP TO THYROID-STIMULATING ANTIBODY

As mentioned above, antibodies to cell surface antigen have been identified by immunofluorescence on viable suspensions of human thyroid cells and by a mixed hemadsorption technique using monolayer cultures (69,70). However, this cell surface antigen seems to be unrelated to the antigen for thyroid-stimulating antibody (78).

It now seems increasingly evident that the thyrotropin (TSH) receptor in the plasma membrane of follicular cells is the antigen responsible for the production of thyroid-stimulating antibodies (TSAb, TSI, TSIg) which are present in the sera of patients with Graves' disease (79,80). These antibodies are detected by two basically different principles. First, the antibodies may be detected by methods based on their ability to stimulate thyroid function; this may be carried out by counting thyroidal intracellular colloid droplets (81), by measuring adenylate cyclase activity (80,82), or by a cytochemical assay (83–85). The stimulating activity has been given several names, including "human thyroid stimulator" (81), "human thyroid adenyl cyclase stimulator" (HTACS), "thyroid-stimulating antibody" (TSAb), or "thyroid-stimulating immunoglobulin" (TSI or TSIg) (80). The older term "long-acting thyroid stimulator" (LATS) now refers to a particular bioassay in the mouse (86).

These antibodies (and/or very closely related antibodies) may also be detected by their ability to bind to thyroid cell membranes. One such method is the LATS-protector (LATS-P) assay, and the other major radioligand assay measures the prevention of binding of TSH to the receptor site on the thyroid cell membrane by the IgG sample. The LATS-P assay is positive when binding to the thyroid prevents (protects) subsequent binding of LATS (87). The radioligand assay technique measuring the inhibition of binding of labeled TSH to its thyroid cell membrane binding site was first termed "thyroid-stimulating immunoglobulin" by Mukhtar et al. (88), but this term was not appropriate; some antibodies which bind to the thyroid cell membrane and prevent TSH binding thereto do *not* stimulate and some may even *inhibit* the action of TSH (see below). Hence this term has given way to other, more descriptive terms. Likewise the term "thyrotropin-displacement activity assay" (TDA) (89) is not quite accurate because in fact the assay measures the *prevention* of TSH binding by the receptor site, rather than its displacement. Hence the term which is now increasingly accepted for this assay system is "thyrotropin-binding-inhibitor immunoglobulin" (TBII) (6). In the remainder of this discussion, the term TBII is applied to this assay, no matter what term is employed by the particular authors. For the assays which actually measure cell stimulation, the term TSAb is utilized throughout the remainder of this discussion, again without relation to the term applied by the authors being cited. It is hoped that his maneuver reduces some of the terminological confusion which has surrounded this field. Moreover, because there is increasing evidence that the antibodies described in this section are directed to the TSH receptor, the generic term "thyrotropin receptor antibodies" (TRAb) is utilized as the all-encompassing term for this group of antibodies, whether they bind to the TSH receptor without any further action, they bind and then stimulate, or they bind and inhibit the action of TSH (29). Finally, it should be emphasized that assays which measure binding to the TSH receptor have been devised using certain *nonthyroidal tissues* which have TSH receptors, e.g., guinea pig fat cells (see below).

As suggested above, evidence is accruing that the binding of this antibody is indeed to the TSH receptor, although this has been a matter of controversy. Certainly it is clear that the antibody produces stimulation by interacting with the TSH receptor and thus stimulating adenyl cyclase and increasing cyclic AMP within the thyroid cell (90). Thus participation of the TSH receptor was always beyond doubt. However, these observations and the clear demonstration of the inhibition of TSH binding by the antibody did not settle the issue as to the actual site of binding of the immunoglobulin. Madsen and Bech (91) studied adenyl cyclase activity in human thyroid cell homogenates after stimulation with TSH or thyroid-stimulating antibodies. They found that TSAb prepared from different patients with Graves' disease showed different adenylate cyclase activation patterns, and a lag phase was frequently observed. TSH and TSAb seemed to cause mutually inhibitory activation of thyroid adenylate cyclase. The maximum adenylate cyclase activity was higher with TSH than with TSAb, although the authors thought that this might be due to contamination of TSAb preparations with an adenylate cyclase inhibitor. They also incubated thyroid homogenates with cortisol, which then produced a dose-dependent decrease in the adenylate cyclase response to TSAb, whereas the response to TSH was either increased or unchanged. These authors thought therefore that TSH and TSAb might activate thyroid adenylate cyclase through different pathways in the plasma membrane.

Fenzi et al. (92), however, attempted to characterize the various thyroid plasma membrane antigens and to study their interactions with thyroid autoantibodies and their relationship to the TSH receptor. They found that these membrane antigens could be freed of the TSH receptor by preabsorption with TSH-containing polymer. The preabsorbed thyroid plasma membrane material, however, still retained its binding to Graves' IgG as well as to Hashimoto's IgG, indicating that antigens different from the TSH receptor and present in thyroid plasma membrane interact with Graves' IgG. These membrane antigens, incidentally, included thyroglobulin and other lower-molecular-weight components. The important point from this study is that the Graves' IgG samples did bind to the thyroid plasma membrane even when it was devoid of the TSH receptor.

However, it should be remembered that Mori and Kriss (58) were unable to separate "antimicrosomal" antibody from LATS. One interpretation thus might be that although anti-cell-membrane antibodies may occur without thyroid-stimulating antibody, the reverse may not be true; that is, thyroid-stimulating antibody may always coexist with other antibodies directed against the thyroid cell membrane (see discussion of antimicrosomal antibodies above). Whether such antibodies represent two antibodies which cannot currently be separated or represent a single type of molecule acting on more than one antigenic site remains to be clarified. Because nonstimulating anti-cell-membrane antibody may occur alone, it is the author's speculation that two inseparable antibodies are involved when TSAb is present, accounting for the findings of Fenzi et al. (92) and Mori and Kriss (58).

There is now considerable direct evidence that the antibody does interact directly with the TSH receptor. Smith and Hall (93,94) have demonstrated that Graves' immunoglobulin seems to interact with the TSH receptors in thyroid membranes in a manner similar to its action with TSH receptors dispersed in detergent micelles. Moreover, they found that the binding of TSH and the immunoglobulins to the detergent-dispersed receptors seems to be mutually exclusive. Consequently, they concluded that the inhibition of TSH binding to thyroid membranes by Graves' immunoglobulins seems to be due to direct binding of the immunoglobulins to the TSH receptor. They conceded, however, that the immunoglobulins and TSH may interact with different sites on the same receptor molecule. Smith et al. (95) also demonstrated that TBII inhibits the binding of labeled TSH to thyroid membranes in a dose-dependent manner, and that this effect is localized in the Fab part of the TBII molecule. Analysis of the binding data suggested that TBII and TSH bound to the same receptor site. These authors were able to show that the effects of TBII and unlabeled TSH on the labeled hormone–membrane interaction were only additive and that no modification of the TSH binding process was induced by TBII. Moreover, kinetic studies indicated that the binding of TBII to the plasma membrane was not rate-limiting in the process of stimulating cyclic AMP production. De Bruin (96) showed that conditions for the measurement of optimal TSH binding are the same as those for the TBII assay. Smith and Buckland (97) summarized the evidence that the antibody binds directly to the TSH receptor, although they concede that a molecule as large as the receptor might be expected to have multiple antigenic binding sites. Furthermore, the binding of TSH and TSH receptor antibodies to the TSH receptor seems to be mutually exclusive in that there is no evidence for the formation of a complex consisting of all three components. It appears therefore that the antibody-binding sites are closely linked to the hormone-binding site (98). De Bruin (96) and Smith and Buckland (97) pointed out that there is more than one binding site in the TSH receptor, and thus there may be more than one class of immunoglobulins interacting with the TSH receptor. Moreover, further evidence leads one to believe that TSAb is truly an antibody to the TSH receptor: Wherever TSH receptors appear in tissues other than the thyroid (e.g., fat cells), TSAb binds to those receptors (99). This is also true for testicular cells (100). Farid et al. (101) and Islam et al. (102) showed that a heterologous anti-antithyrotropin (anti-idiotype) would bind to the thyroid membrane in a dose-dependent manner and was competitive with native TSH, stimulating cyclic AMP. They thus proposed that TSAb in human Graves' disease might be an anti-idiotype itself. This was also suggested by Beall and Kruger (103).

However, as mentioned above, whenever there is thyroid-stimulating antibody in patients with Graves' disease, it cannot be separated from anti-cell-membrane antibody (58), which strongly suggests that TSAb is an antibody directed to a cell membrane component and not an anti-idiotype. Moreover, Valente et al. (104,105) and Kohn et al. (106) demonstrated that monoclonal antibodies developed against soluble receptor preparations and using Graves' lymphocytes can simulate all of the actions of the natural TSAb. They also showed that those antibodies which stimulate the thyroid activity in cultured cell systems of most bioassays all interact with gangliosides on the TSH receptor. They provided evidence suggesting that TSH and TSAb might interact with slightly different sites on the TSH receptor (104–106).

It thus may be tentatively concluded that thyroid-stimulating antibodies constitute a family of antibodies directed against the human TSH receptor itself. It may be further concluded that it is not an anti-idiotype but is primarily directed against the TSH receptor component of the thyroid cell membrane.

There is certainly variable sensitivity and even specificity among the various assays. LATS, as measured by the mouse bioassay, is detectable only in ~50% of sera from patients with active untreated Graves' disease (107), and titers of LATS bear no relationship to the degree of thyrotoxicosis (90). It was for this reason that the role of LATS in the pathogenesis of Graves' disease was in some doubt for several years (108). Indeed, following the advent of human thyroid preparations in the various assay systems, there was a suggestion that LATS was only a mouse thyroid stimulator and that other, separate Graves' immunoglobulins stimulated the human thyroid alone (109). However, it soon became clear that the same molecule was indeed a stimulator of the human thyroid gland, and that the variation in response of the mouse thyroid to Graves' IgG was a problem of either variable mammalian cross-reactivity (110) or sensitivity (111,112). Strakosch et al. (113) have likewise shown that TSH-binding-inhibiting antibody represents an antibody against a single antigen at or near the TSH receptor and that the degree of reactivity with its antigen in other species depends mainly on the amount of antibody present in the serum.

There also has been a considerable variation from laboratory to laboratory in the results obtained for detection of the antibody. Even when the same techniques or modifications of the same procedure were employed, widely differing results were obtained. For example, Mukhtar et al. (88) found that with the radioligand assay for TBII virtually 100% of the patients with active untreated Graves' disease were positive. However, O'Donnell et al. (89) were able to find only 76% of patients positive in this assay, and Schleusener et al. (114) found such antibodies in only 54% of such patients with active untreated Graves' disease. Kuzuya et al. (115) found this antibody in 53% of a similar group of patients in Japan. Davies et al. (116) detected TBII in 73% of patients with active untreated Graves' disease, Docter et al. (117) in 63%, Teng and Yeung (118) in 84%, and Bliddal et al. (119–121) in 85%. Recent modifications have led to a yield of 86 to 94% positive results (122,123). On the other hand, the use of stimulatory assays for TSAb, e.g., measurement of the generation of cyclic AMP in thyroid slices or thyroid cells in culture, has brought a generally higher yield of positive results in active untreated Graves' disease. These have varied from 81% in the study of Sugenoya et al. (124), 82% in the study of Bech and Madsen (125), 95% in the reports by McKenzie and co-workers (79,80), and virtually 100% in the studies of Stockle et al. (126) and Hinds et al. (127).

In the hands of Smyth et al. (85), the cytochemical section bioassay for TSAb also yielded 100% positive results from patients with Graves' disease, but unfortunately several patients with toxic nodular goiters or even nontoxic goiter also had positive assays. Hence this technique seems to be very sensitive but to lack specificity.

When radioligand (TBII) and stimulating (TSAb) assays are carried out on the same specimens in the same laboratories, widely divergent results between the two assay systems are observed. In the study of Sugenoya et al. (124), even in active untreated Graves' disease there was no correlation between the radioligand assay (TBII) and a stimulatory assay measuring the generation of cyclic AMP in thyroid slices (TSAb) (Figs. 3 and 4). As in the study of Smith and Hall (128), correlation was obtained only in that subset of patients who were positive in both assay systems. Similar discrepancies were noted by Kuzuya et al. (115) and Pinchera et al. (129). Moreover, Shishiba et al. (130) also noted the discrepancy between TBII and TSAb using the murine TSH receptor and the McKenzie LATS bioassay, respectively.

Vitti et al. (131) showed no correlation between the stimulating activity and the ability of a Graves' immunoglobulin preparation to inhibit thyrotropin binding. On the other hand, Bliddal et al. (120) and Bech (132) were able to demonstrate a correlation between results from the assay systems in Graves' disease both before and during long-term anti-thyroid treatment, although even in this study discrepancies between the two assay systems were noted in some patients. This same group showed that after radioactive iodine many patients with Graves' disease showed a dissociation between results from the two assay systems (132,133).

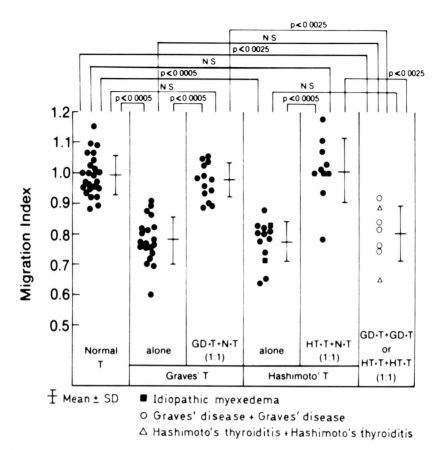

FIG. 3. The direct MIF test using T lymphocytes alone. This graph depicts the effect of adding normal T lymphocytes to Graves' or Hashimoto's T lymphocytes in a ratio of 1:1. Note that the production of MIF is abolished by the addition of the normal T lymphocytes, thus indicating that these normal cells seem able to suppress the Graves' or Hashimoto's T lymphocytes, thus preventing them from producing MIF in response to the thyroid antigen. (From ref. 213.)

In studies of subacute thyroiditis, Sugenoya et al. (124) and Wall et al. (134) likewise showed no correlation between the results of the two types of assay because it seemed that TBII demonstrated in subacute thyroiditis represents antibody which binds to but does not stimulate the TSH receptor. A curious discrepancy between laboratories has been noted when patients with Hashimoto's thyroiditis are studied. Bliddal et al. (121) reported that the TBII was detectable in 22% of patients with Hashimoto's thyroiditis, whereas TSAb was found in 51% of patients with this disorder. Although they concluded that TBII and TSAb are produced independently in Hashimoto's thyroiditis, their findings are contradictory to those described by Sugenoya et al. (124) and Pinchera et al. (135), who found the TBII to be positive in some patients with Hashimoto's thyroiditis, whereas the TSAb results were generally negative.

The reason for these various discrepancies is not entirely clear. It would be more comprehensible if at least consistent results in the various assays were obtained from laboratory to laboratory, but even that is not the case. It is thus possible that technical problems in both assay systems may be one factor in bringing about discrepancies. This is particularly

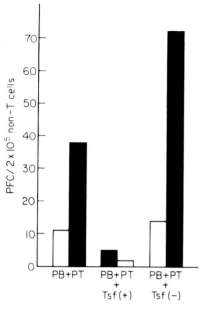

FIG. 4. Suppression of thyroglobulin (Tg) specific plaque forming cells *(PFC)* by culture supernatant from Tg-stimulated cells. *P* = patient. *B* = non-T cells. *T* = T cells. *Tsf(+)* = supernatant of Tg-stimulated cells. *Tsf(−)* = supernatant of Tg-unstimulated cells. *Closed bar* = Tg-stimulated assay. *Open bar* = Tg-unstimulated assay. (From ref. 189.)

of importance when it is recollected that normal IgG variably binds to the cell membrane and prevents TSH binding, and this inhibition of TSH binding by normal IgG occasionally can be marked (79,80). It is also possible that there may be some TSAb molecules which bind to the thyroid cell membrane, interact with the TSH receptor, and thus stimulate the thyroid cells without at the same time inhibiting the binding of TSH any more than do normal IgG samples (29). This suggestion might give credence to the notion that the binding of TSAb is not necessarily directed to the TSH receptor itself. However, as mentioned above, increasing evidence has accrued to indicate that binding is directly to the TSH receptor. Moreover, because Endo et al. (136) and Konishi et al. (137) described antibodies positive in the TBII assay which block TSH activity, leading to atrophy of the thyroid gland and actual hypothyroidism, it is clear that TBII cannot equate to TSAb. Hence results from the radioligand assay cannot be termed thyroid-*stimulating* immunoglobulin or antibody. Discrepancies where TBII is positive and TSAb is negative can be explained in this fashion. In addition, Carayon et al. (138) demonstrated heterogeneity in Graves' immunoglobulins with regard to binding constants and to the stimulating/blocking effects on adenylate cyclase.

    This explanation may well account for some of the observations in disorders other than Graves' disease which have called into question the specificity of the TBII. Positive results in the radioligand assay have been obtained in a small proportion of patients with Hashimoto's thyroiditis, in significant numbers of patients with subacute thyroiditis, and in a small proportion of patients with thyroid carcinoma (88,93,121,124,134,135). The TBII was also found to be positive by Brown et al. (139) in nontoxic goiters and nontoxic multinodular goiters, but others have not found positive results in those particular categories (89,96,140). Thus the disease specificity of the TBII is in some doubt; it is in less doubt for the TSAb assay, which is generally positive only in Graves' disease. Only the results of Bliddal et al. (121) and Smyth et al. (85) are discrepant in the latter respect.

    The organ specificity of TSAb for the thyroid cell membrane has been a subject of some study and is described briefly above. It is known that TSH binds to and has effects on other organs, e.g., monocytes, testes, fat cells, and the adrenal (100). It has also been shown that there is an effect of TSAb on testis and fat cells (99,100,141,142). The latter studies lend support to the argument that TSAb is an antibody to the TSAb receptor, and thus wherever TSAb receptors are found one might expect TSAb–TSH receptor interaction. Moreover, the use of fat cell membranes has led to the development of a much more sensitive and specific radioligand assay than was possible using the TBII technique (143), as well as a sensitive enzyme immunoassay (ELISA) technique (144).

It is increasingly evident that there is a direct TSAb–TSH receptor interaction and that the antibody is directed to some part of the TSH receptor itself as well as perhaps to contiguous parts of the cell membrane. Kohn et al. (106) provided evidence, using monoclonal antibodies developed against soluble thyroid TSH receptor preparations (and using Graves' lymphocytes), that the antibodies which stimulate thyroid activity in cultured cell systems or mouse bioassays interact with gangliosides. Other monoclonal antibodies have no intrinsic stimulatory action in assays of thyroid function but were able to inhibit TSH activity in the assays tested. These data established the pluritopic nature of the immunoglobulins in Graves' disease and related individual components or determinants of the thyrotropic receptor structure with specific autoimmune immunoglobulins (104,105).

A central role for this antibody in causing the stimulation of the thyroid cells and thus the hyperthyroidism of Graves' disease seems inescapable (Fig. 2). First, TSAb can now be demonstrated in virtually all cases of active untreated Graves' disease (79,80,126,127). Moreover, the effects on the thyroid which are shared by TSAb and TSH included the uptake, discharge, and release of radioactive iodine *in vivo* and *in vitro*, colloid droplet formation in follicular cells, glucose oxidation and incorporation of ^{32}P into phospholipids, adenyl cyclase activity, and cyclic AMP accumulation (90). Although there has been no unanimity with respect to a good correlation between the various assay systems and the severity of hyperthyroidism (132), some groups have shown a fair correlation with respect to early thyroidal uptake of ^{131}I or ^{99m}Tc (88,136). More importantly, if the assay for thyroid-stimulating antibody remains positive after patients have been controlled with propylthiouracil for a long interval, cessation of the therapy will almost invariably bring about a recurrence (80,89,112,118,145,146). Moreover, neonatal Graves' disease, which is almost always a transient disorder lasting less than 3 months, has been shown to have a very good correlation with the presence of high titers of thyroid-stimulating immunoglobulin (or LATS protector) in the mothers and (by passive transfer) in the newborns (79,80,90,147,148). It is thus contended that TSAb reflects the immune disorder which is the basis of Graves' disease and the cause of the hyperthyroidism of this disorder. At times it seems that very closely related antibodies can act as "blocking" antibodies, thereby causing hypothyroidism (136,137), and there is also some evidence that this blocking antibody could have caused the delayed onset of neonatal hyperthyroidism in two children (146).

The uniqueness of TSAb, an antibody which interacts with a receptor and stimulates it (i.e., acting as an agonist) has been a matter of concern among skeptics. Other antireceptor antibodies, e.g., the antibody against the acetylcholine receptor in myasthenia gravis (149) or against the insulin receptor in certain forms of diabetes mellitus (150,151), are generally blocking (antagonistic) antibodies. However, occasionally the anti-insulin receptor antibody can act as an agonist (resulting in hypoglycemia), thereby diminishing the uniqueness of TSAb (150).

The thyroid-stimulating antibodies are generally not found in relatives of patients with Graves' disease who are asymptomatic (80,152,153). The presence of thyroid antibodies of all kinds in relation to exophthalmos is discussed separately elsewhere in this volume.

IMMUNE COMPLEXES, RHEUMATOID FACTORS, OTHER ANTIBODIES

Circulating immune complexes have been detected in the sera from patients with Hashimoto's thyroiditis and Graves' disease (154–158). Immune complexes within the thyroid gland itself and their possible cytolytic effect have already been discussed above (43). Mariotti et al. (156) have shown data suggesting that both thyroglobulin–antithyroglobulin complexes and complexes unrelated to thyroglobulin are present in sera of patients with thyroid autoimmune disorders and thyroid carcinoma. Using the Raji cell method, Mariotti et al. (156) showed that immune complexes unrelated to thyroglobulin were frequently present. Although thyroglobulin–antithyroglobulin complexes are also frequently detectable, there is no evidence that they fix complement. This may explain why immune complex disease is not characteristic of autoimmune thyroid disease, although immune complex glomerulonephritis associated with autoimmune thyroiditis has been rarely reported (159–161). Van der Heide et al. (162) studied immune complexes in relation to TSI in patients with Graves' disease before and after antithyroid drug therapy. They found that immune complexes were present in all untreated patients who had a normal or subnormal TBII index, whereas they were absent in all patients with an abnormal TBII index. There thus seemed to be an inverse correlation with TBII and immune complexes in Graves' disease. If the immune complex included TBII, thus rendering it incapable of interacting with the TSH receptor, this conceivably could be an explanation for at least one type of remission. It is of interest that Endo et al. (163) reported an inverse correlation between the presence of immune complexes in autoimmune thyroid diseases and the numbers of peripheral killer (K) cells, perhaps due to saturation of K cell Fc receptors by binding immune complexes. Circulating immune complexes in relation to exophthalmos are discussed elsewhere in this volume.

Drexhage et al. (37) detected the presence of a thyroid growth-promoting antibody in some patients with goitrous Hashimoto's thyroiditis, possibly accounting for the thyroid hypertrophy in this condition. Moreover, they were also able to demonstrate antibodies which *inhibited* the trophic effect of TSH in most cases of atrophic primary myxedema. This antibody apparently did not prevent the binding of TSH to its receptor, only its trophic effect (38). However, the histology of atrophic myxedema does *not* resemble that of an unstimulated thyroid but, rather, appears to represent a destructive process; this does *not* seem to result from an antibody which inhibits growth. Thus in any event, there seem to be antibodies in these disorders which *may* account for atrophy or hypertrophy, although in view of the histological observations it remains to be shown if this is correct and if these antibodies are distinct from previously demonstrated antibodies.

Antibodies to *Yersinia enterocolitica* have been found in increased frequency in Graves' disease (∼59%), compared with ∼20% in control groups (164). Indeed, Bech et al. (164,165) also found a positive correlation between migration inhibition in response to thyroid and *Yersinia* antigens in a group of patients with Graves' disease, whereas no correlation could be demonstrated in the control population. Moreover, direct immunofluorescence techniques revealed a high frequency of thyroid cell-membrane-directed antibodies in sera with *Yersinia* agglutinating antibodies. This led Bech et al. (165) to conclude that there was no actual *Yersinia* infection in patients with thyroid disease, but that there was a cross-reaction between antigenic components of the thyroid and *Yersinia* (164,165). Indeed Weiss et al. (166) demonstrated cross-reactivity between *Yersinia* membrane and mammalian TSH receptor, and later showed it between *Escherichia coli* and mammalian TSH receptor (167). Moreover, Shenkman and Bottone (168) demonstrated that antibodies to *Yersinia* were found in populations of patients with Graves' disease in North America, despite the fact that *Yersinia* infections are much less common in North America than in Europe. This also seemed to favor the view that *Yersinia* was playing no role whatever in these patients, but that there was some cross-reactivity between thyroid and *Yersinia* antigens. Thus the detection of antibodies to *Yersinia* may be an artifact and of no relevance to the pathogenesis of Graves' disease.

Other antibodies should also be mentioned. Rheumatoid factor has been detected in Graves' disease (169,170), and lymphocytotoxic antibodies have been demonstrated in both Graves' and Hashimoto's diseases (46,47). Tao and Kriss (171) demonstrated, in patients with Graves' disease and other autoimmune diseases, antibodies which bind to membranes containing TSH receptors, although these did not correlate consistently with either the presence of TBII or the clinical estimate of thyrotoxicity in Graves' disease. Antibodies to other organs are also found in some patients with Graves' and Hashimoto's diseases (as well as their relatives), e.g., autoantibodies to gastric antigens, islet cell antigens, adrenal antigens, and others (172).

CELLULAR ASPECTS OF GRAVES' AND HASHIMOTO'S DISEASES

Thyroid Lymphocytes

Graves' disease and Hashimoto's thyroiditis have several cellular aspects in common. In both conditions the gland is infiltrated with lymphocytes, frequently organized as germinal centers (3,173), and the two conditions may coexist in the same thyroid gland (174,175). As mentioned above, the clinical expression in the presence of TSAb (i.e., hyperthyroidism, euthyroidism, or hypothyroidism) depends on the availability of the thyroid follicular cells which then can respond to TSAb (6). If there are simply too few cells to respond, the patient is of course hypothyroid (176). In 1978 Totterman et al. (177,178) first reported the distribution of T, B, and thyroglobulin-binding lymphocytes infiltrating the thyroid gland of Graves' disease, Hashimoto's thyroiditis, and De Quervain's subacute thyroiditis. He showed that in both Graves' and Hashimoto's diseases ~40% of the lymphocytes were T lymphocytes with an equal proportion of B lymphocytes. (In De Quervain's thyroiditis, incidentally, the majority of thyroid infiltrating cells were T lymphocytes with only a few B lymphocytes.) The frequency of thyroglobulin-binding lymphocytes was also studied by Totterman (177) and was found to be high in the thyroid infiltrates of patients with both Graves' and Hashimoto's diseases. Subsequently, Totterman et al. (179) showed (by means of a leukocyte migration inhibition test) that the infiltrating T lymphocytes from patients with Graves' disease were sensitized against thyroid antigen in cells obtained at fine needle aspiration biopsy. Surprisingly, they could not demonstrate that the infiltrating lymphocytes from the thyroid gland of Hashimoto's thyroiditis were positive in this test procedure, although they pointed out that this lack of reactivity could be caused by an excess of antigen.

Totterman et al. (179) also argued that the considerably increased frequency of thyroglobulin-binding lymphocytes within the thyroid gland of both disorders argues against the possibility that the thyroid-infiltrating lymphocytes are merely "passive bystanders" secondarily trapped in the thyroid after some unknown traumatic mechanism. Moreover, the striking accumulation of thyroglobulin-binding B lymphocytes plus the finding of mature plasma cells in the gland of Hashimoto's thyroiditis suggested intrathyroidal synthesis of autoantibody. These findings were subsequently amply confirmed (180–185). In several of these studies there seemed to be a decrease in the number of suppressor T lymphocytes isolated from the thyroid tissue obtained at surgery relative to the number of helper T lymphocytes. However, as Wall and his colleagues (184) pointed out, this was found not only in Graves' disease but in the thyroid glands from multinodular nontoxic goiters, not considered to be autoimmune in nature. Thus it is important that appropriate controls in terms of thyroid tissue from various *nonimmune* disorders be compared to the findings of lymphocyte subsets from the thyroid gland in autoimmune thyroid disease. Nevertheless, McLachlan et al. (181) and Weetman et al. (183) were able to demonstrate that thyroid autoantibody production is much more readily demonstrable when lymphocytes from the thyroid gland of autoimmune thyroid disease are cultured *in vitro*, when compared to similar studies with peripheral blood lymphocytes from the same patients. This is discussed further below. However, it seems inescapable that a major source of thyroid autoantibody production in autoimmune thyroid disease is from lymphocytes within the thyroid gland itself.

Peripheral Blood Lymphocytes

Totterman (177) showed that patients with either Graves' or Hashimoto's disease have about twice as many thyroglobulin-binding lymphocytes in the peripheral blood as do healthy subjects; most of these were B lymphocytes, although a few T lymphocytes which would bind to thyroglobulin were also found in the blood and infiltrates of patients with these disorders. This finding has been confirmed by several other workers (186–188). Although there was a definite increase in thyroglobulin-binding lymphocytes in such patients in these studies, there was no correlation between these cells and the presence or titer of the various thyroid autoantibodies, particularly antibodies against thyroglobulin. Moreover, similar cells, albeit in small numbers, are also found in normal healthy control persons.

Several studies have attempted to determine the numbers, type, activity, and function of peripheral blood lymphocytes circulating in patients with Graves' or Hashimoto's disease. Studies of subsets of T lymphocytes have shown variable results, partly dependent on the technique employed to measure them and partly (possibly) on the state of the metabolic disturbance. Mori et al. (189) showed a significant reduction in peripheral immunoglobulin G (IgG) Fc receptor-bearing T lymphocytes (Tγ) in patients with hyperthyroid Graves' disease, but this situation returned to normal when the patients became euthyroid. The function of these cells was thought to include suppressor activity, natural cytotoxicity, and antibody-dependent cell-mediated cellular cytotoxicity. The numbers of Tγ were likewise normal in Hashimoto's thyroiditis. The authors speculated that the finding of reduced Tγ in hyperthyroidism was secondary to the hyperthyroidism itself, but that it might act as a self-perpetuating factor in the expression of the disease.

Sridama et al. (190) demonstrated a decreased percentage of OKT8-positive cells (considered to be suppressor T lymphocytes) in both Graves' disease and Hashimoto's thyroiditis, similar to the observation of Thielemans et al. (191), who found a slightly decreased proportion of OKT8-positive cells in a small number of patients with Hashimoto's thyroiditis. In contrast, however, Canonica et al. (192,193) found no imbalance of OKT4 (mainly helper) and OKT8 T lymphocytes; they have, however, shown (using a new monoclonal antibody termed 5/9) an increased proportion of helper T lymphocytes in Hashimoto's disease. Canonica's results are similar to those described by Wall et al. (184). An increased proportion of OKIa-positive cells have been found in patients with untreated Graves' disease; these cells include B lymphocytes, monocytes, null cells, and activated T lymphocytes; again, these changes may be secondary to the hyperthyroidism per se. Iwatani et al. (194) showed a significant decrease in the peak position on Leu 2a lymphocytes (considered to be suppressor-cytotoxic lymphocytes) in patients with thyrotoxic Graves' disease, although once again this situation returned to normal when patients were treated and was also normal in patients with Hashimoto's thyroiditis who happened to be euthyroid.

Because of the discrepancies between these reports, it is very difficult to collate and interpret the findings clearly. As is discussed below, there is evidence for an antigen-specific disorder in a single clone or a few clones of suppressor T lymphocytes which would not be expected to be detected by studies of generalized suppressor T lymphocyte function or by enumerating the total number of such cells. That is, such a small defect would not likely be reflected in any reduction in the absolute number of suppressor T lymphocytes. Thus to attempt to resolve the conflicting reports noted above, it may well be that generalized suppressor T lymphocyte numbers can be decreased as a result of a severe metabolic disturbance, as would occur in hyperthyroidism or other active metabolic diseases, but do not represent the immune abnormality responsible for autoimmune thyroid disease in the first place.

Similarly, the response of lymphocytes to mitogens and to thyroid antigen has also been a subject of great interest in these autoimmune disorders.

Aoki and De Groot (195) studied the blastogenic response of lymphocytes to human thyroglobulin in autoimmune thyroid disease and reviewed contradictory reports of the results of this procedure. These authors found that lymphocytes from patients with autoimmune thyroid disease responded by more blastogenesis than did lymphocytes from patients with other thyroid disorders or healthy controls. Similar findings with various thyroid antigenic preparations have been noted by Makinen et al. (196), Wenzel et al. (197), and Balazs et al. (198). Although it seemed difficult previously to show increased thyroid autoantibody production by peripheral blood lymphocytes in response to thyroglobulin, this has now been clearly demonstrated by Noma et al. (199) and Benveniste et al. (200). However, it must be conceded that lymphocytes from the thyroid of patients with autoimmune thyroid disease respond much more readily to the antigenic stimulus of thyroglobulin than do peripheral blood lymphocytes (181).

Several workers have studied the response of peripheral blood lymphocytes to mitogens in autoimmune thyroid disease. Because these are concerned with the regulation of thyroid autoantibody production, they are discussed below under the heading "Suppressor T Lymphocyte Function." The studies cited above certainly indicate that there is sensitization of lymphocytes in response to thyroid antigen but do not make it clear what subsets (helper T lymphocytes, B lymphocytes, or both) are in fact sensitized. However, studies of the migration inhibition factor (MIF) test using isolated preparations of T lymphocytes alone have shown clearly that patients with Graves' disease or Hashimoto's thyroiditis manifest MIF production in response to human thyroid antigen (201). T lymphocytes from normal persons do not respond in this manner when exposed to the same thyroid antigen, nor do T lymphocytes from nontoxic goiter or thyroid carcinoma. Moreover, the T lymphocytes from patients with Graves' disease or Hashimoto's thyroiditis do not produce MIF when in contact with human liver antigen or purified protein derivative (PPD) (201). From these observations, therefore, it seems clear that there are indeed T lymphocytes in these disorders which are sensitized specifically to the thyroid antigen (201). Furthermore, Okita et al. (202) reported that lymphocytes from patients with Graves' or Hashimoto's disease release MIF lymphokine into the medium, which then can be added to normal human T lymphocytes and cause the latter to undergo inhibition of migration. This study thus confirms that the lymphokine MIF is indeed being produced by sensitized T lymphocytes in response to thyroid antigen in autoimmune thyroid disease, confirming once again that T lymphocytes are specifically sensitized to thyroid antigen in these disorders.

Because we can now conclude that there are indeed sensitized T lymphocytes in both Graves' and Hashimoto's diseases, the question arises as to the nature of the function of these sensitized cells. It may be proposed that these cells are almost certainly sensitized helper T lymphocytes which are then capable of interacting with appropriate and already-present, thyroid-directed autoreactive B lymphocytes. It was pointed out above that auto-reactive thyroid-directed B lymphocytes are present in normal persons; indeed it can be assumed that many other types of self-reactive B lymphocytes are also always present. What is thus required to stimulate groups of these B lymphocytes to produce autoantibodies is the emergence of specific helper T lymphocytes, which are then capable of mounting an autoimmune process.

Evidence for a Defect in Suppressor T Lymphocytes

The current author proposed several years ago that both Graves' and Hashimoto's diseases probably represent disorders in immunoregulation (56,108,203). However, those proposals were based on circumstantial rather than direct evidence. It seemed probable, however, that both disorders could be due to specific genetic defects in clones of suppressor T lymphocytes. There is no evidence for generalized hypersensitivity in Graves' disease; this would militate against the possibility that there is a causative *generalized* defect in suppressor T lymphocytes (204). It may thus have been predicted that if there is a single defect in the immune system which is responsible for either Graves' or Hashimoto's disease, procedures which test the whole system should be normal and those which test for a specific defect should be abnormal. Accordingly, we might expect that each of the organ-specific autoimmune diseases is caused by a single defect in immunoregulation. One would still have to account for the association of more than one autoimmune thyroid disease in the same person because, as mentioned above, the coincidence of two or more such autoimmune diseases in association with autoimmune thyroid disease occurs much more commonly than chance alone would dictate (although only a minority of patients have such combined diseases). Because these combined diseases, when present in one patient, occur at different times in relation to one another, it seems likely that even in patients with multiple associated organ-specific autoimmune diseases there has been inheritance of several closely related defects in immunoregulation; that is, several specific but separate defects in suppressor T lymphocyte function may be present. However, even in such patients there is evidence that there is not *generalized hypersensitivity*.

It was mentioned above (see "Peripheral Blood Lymphocytes") in relation to enumeration of subsets of T lymphocytes that some studies show a reduction in the number of suppressor T lymphocytes in active untreated Graves' disease; this tends to return to normal when the patients are treated (189,190,194). On the other hand, in most studies normal proportions of T lymphocyte subsets have been found in euthyroid Hashimoto's thyroiditis (189,194). It was pointed out above that there are many discrepancies in these various studies, although the above represents the overall consensus. Similarly, in studies of generalized suppressor T lymphocyte *function*, many discrepancies appear in the literature (198,205–212). Most of these studies have to do with the action of mitogens, e.g., pokeweed or concanavalin A, to stimulate appropriate subsets of T lymphocytes. Once again, the overall consensus of such studies seem to suggest that in active untreated Graves' disease there is a mild generalized deficiency in suppressor T lymphocyte function which is restored to normal when patients with Graves' disease are rendered euthyroid over long periods of time. Results have generally been normal in patients with euthyroid Hashimoto's disease (198,205–212).

It is entirely likely that this mild generalized deficiency in suppressor T lymphocyte function, as demonstrated by several workers, represents the consequences of hyperthyroidism, i.e., the metabolic disturbance of thyroid disease, and does not represent a *de novo* primary immunological disturbance. There is some supporting evidence to indicate that hyperthyroidism per se either directly or indirectly (through the stimulation of adrenocortical function) can have an adverse effect on suppressor T lymphocytes and thus may explain these findings (6). Indeed, this effect may serve as a self-perpetuating factor in the disease (see "Nature of Remissions in Graves' Disease," below).

These comments are certainly not offered to obviate the possible role for an antigen-specific suppressor T lymphocyte dysfunction in the pathogenesis of Graves' and Hashimoto's diseases. What has been required are techniques which can detect an isolated antigen specific defect in immunoregulation, i.e., an isolated defect in suppressor T lymphocytes. Thus Okita et al. (213) reported a new approach to the study of suppressor T lymphocytes. They modified the MIF procedure using preparations of T lymphocytes alone. As mentioned above, they have shown that T lymphocytes from patients with Graves' or Hashimoto's disease produce MIF in response to thyroid antigen. If, however, one adds normal T lymphocytes to the Graves' or Hashimoto's T lymphocytes in ratios as low as 1:9, the ability of the latter sensitized T lymphocytes to produce MIF in response to the thyroid antigen is abolished (Fig. 3). However, if Graves' T lymphocytes are added to Graves' T lymphocytes from a second patient in similar ratios, the ability of the lymphocytes to produce MIF is retained, thus ruling out the mixed lymphocyte reaction as the cause of the original abolition of the MIF effect. Conversely, if the normal T lymphocytes are initially incubated with mitomycin C and subsequently added to the Graves' lymphocytes, the normal T lymphocytes lose their ability to influence the Graves' lymphocytes, which then produce MIF as before when in contact with their appropriate antigen (213).

Our group has shown that irradiation of normal T lymphocytes with 1,000 rads (sufficient to inhibit suppressor T lymphocyte function without damaging the viability of the lymphocytes or affecting helper T lymphocyte function) abolishes the normal suppressor T lymphocyte activity when these cells are added to Graves' or Hashimoto's T lymphocytes; thus once again, the sensitized T lymphocytes produce MIF as before when in contact with the appropriate antigen (214). It also seems that H2 receptor integrity is necessary for the suppressor T lymphocytes to function, as the H2 receptor blocker cimetidine completely abolishes the ability of the normal suppressor T lymphocytes to function in this system (215). These data have been confirmed by Vento et al. (280).

We have endeavored to determine if there are single specific defects in immunosuppression for each of the organ-specific diseases by mixing T lymphocytes from one organ-specific autoimmune disease (insulin-dependent diabetes mellitus) with the T lymphocytes from patients with Graves' disease; we then observed the response in the MIF test to thyroid antigen on the one hand and to islet cell antigen on the other. The lymphocytes from the diabetic patients produced an MIF response to islet cell antigen, but this was abrogated when Graves' disease T lymphocytes (positive against thyroid antigen but negative against islet cell antigen in the MIF system) were added. Thus the Graves' disease T lymphocytes acted as "normal" T lymphocytes in the system in which the diabetic T lymphocytes were incubated with islet cell antigen. This indicates that the defect of suppressor T lymphocytes is not the same in Graves' disease as in diabetes mellitus (35).

Certainly this disease-specific and organ-specific defect in suppressor T lymphocytes is not influenced by thyroid function. How et al. (216) showed that this defect may last for decades after treatment of Graves' disease. Moreover, as mentioned above, the defect is also detected in patients with Hashimoto's thyroiditis, either treated or untreated and either hypothyroid or euthyroid (213). Thus although there may be some evidence that there are abnormalities of *generalized* suppressor T lymphocyte function in relation to the *metabolic disturbance* associated with autoimmune thyroid disease, the *antigen-specific* disorder certainly has no relationship whatever to thyroid function and is thus much more likely to be pathogenic in its significance.

Noma et al. (199) used the production of antithyroglobulin antibody by peripheral blood lymphocytes *in vitro*, detected by the plaque-forming cell assay system, in studies similar in principle to those of Okita et al. (213). First, they were able to show that helper T lymphocytes were required for autoantibody formation. The generation of thyroglobulin-specific plaque-forming cells from lymphocytes of patients with Hashimoto's thyroiditis was markedly suppressed by the addition of normal T lymphocytes or of T lymphocytes from other patients whose lymphocytes had not produced plaque-forming cells in the first place. On the other hand, T lymphocytes from patients with lymphocytes which had produced plaque-forming cells initially were not able to show such suppressor effects. These data indicated once again that the regulatory T lymphocyte function that prevents thyroglobulin autoantibody formation is impaired in Hashimoto's thyroiditis. Of interest was their further finding of the same level of suppression upon the addition of culture supernatants from thyroglobulin-antigen-stimulated normal lymphocytes [suppressor factor (SF)] (Fig. 4). No such suppression was observed, however, in the presence of supernatants of thyroglobulin-stimulated T lymphocytes of Hashimoto's patients whose lymphocytes had previously produced plaque-forming cells (199). These results, if confirmed, will lend considerable support to the concept that there is indeed an antigen-specific defect in suppressor T lymphocyte function in autoimmune thyroid disease in humans.

Balazs et al. (198) also studied antigen-specific (as well as nonspecific) suppressor T lymphocyte function in a set of identical twins discordant for Graves' disease (i.e., one had active Graves' disease, one was healthy). The first step was to culture lymphocytes with concanavalin A or thyroid membrane antigen for 24 hr. The workers then added these lymphocytes to second groups of lymphocytes (lymphocyte indicator cells) which had been stimulated by concanavalin A for 72 hr, or thyroid membrane antigen for 96 hr; they measured the uptake of tritiated thymidine as an index of nonspecific or specific suppressor T lymphocyte function, respectively. In the twin with active Graves' disease there was a specific suppressor T lymphocyte defect accompanied by a much less severe nonspecific suppressor T lymphocyte defect; no such abnormalities could be detected in the healthy twin under these conditions.

These various studies can be interpreted only as indicating that in Graves' and Hashimoto's diseases there is a loss of specific suppressor T lymphocyte activity. This seems to imply that suppressor factor produced by normal suppressor T lymphocytes in response to specific antigens must itself be antigen-specific. If each suppressor factor is indeed antigen-specific, this may have major therapeutic implications in the decades to come.

Other Cellular Elements

A role for other cellular elements is also clearly evident. "Killer" (K) cells may be defined as antibody-dependent cytotoxic lymphoid cells which possess the surface membrane receptors for the Fc region of IgG. Evidence suggests that these cells have a role in thyroid cell destruction, which may be the means by which antibody-mediated cellular destruction occurs (44,45,163). Natural killer (NK) cells, which show cytotoxicity against target cells without prior sensitization, have been the topic of intensive investigation because of their possible role in immune surveillance against malignancy, resistance against microbial infection, and regulation of lymphohematopoiesis and the immune response. In human peripheral blood, they are considered to be the lymphocytes that are nonadherent and nonphagocytic and which bear Fc receptors for IgG and mostly low-affinity receptors for sheep erythrocytes (217). Their role in autoimmune thyroid disease has yet to be clearly defined. The role of macrophages, although nonspecific, is clearly essential as an intermediary in the immune response, but is not further discussed herein (218).

ROLE OF THE ANTIGEN

It is thus increasingly evident that there is indeed a primary defect in immunoregulation which serves as the predisposition for Graves' and Hashimoto's diseases; this seems to be due to a specific defect in a clone or clones of suppressor T lymphocytes. The proposal that anti-idiotype antibodies (32–34) may play a role in immunoregulation is within the realm of possibility, but there is little evidence for such a defect in this putative form of immunoregulation as yet demonstrated in these disorders. Thus accepting that there is a specific disorder in suppressor T lymphocytes, it does not seem necessary to invoke antigenic stimulation as a necessary initiator of these conditions but, rather, merely the presence and availability of the appropriate antigen (in its usual normal location and state).

Nevertheless, Werner and Fierer (219) suggested that there might be an occult antigenic change within the thyroid (possibly virus-induced) to which the immunological phenomena are secondary. Indeed, Joassoo et al. (220) observed an increased frequency of antibodies to influenza B in a group of thyrotoxic patients compared to that in normal persons. There have also been cases of Graves' disease following viral and bacterial infections (221–223). Moreover, virus-like particles have been demonstrated in the thyroid of autoimmune thyroiditis in chickens (224), a finding which permits the postulate that the immune disturbance in human chronic thyroiditis may be initiated by a virus with secondary occult thyroidal antigenic change. Furthermore, similar virus-like particles have been observed in thyroid tissue in the human disease (225). However, they can also be demonstrated in normal thyroid as well as in other tissues (225). It seems therefore that these particles are almost ubiquitous.

Weiss et al. (166), having noted that there are often agglutinating antibodies to *Yersinia enterocolitica* in Graves' disease (see "Immune Complexes, Rheumatoid Factor, Other Antibodies," above), described the presence of a specific saturable binding site for the mammalian peptide hormone thyrotropin in the same bacillus. They suggested that the initiating event in susceptible individuals might be infection with an organism such as *Y. enterocolitica* that bears antigens which cross-react with those of the human thyroid gland. However, antibodies to *Yersinia* have been found in populations of patients with Graves' disease in North America (168) in equal proportions to those in Europe (164,165) despite the fact that the *Yersinia* infections are much less common in North America than in Europe. It may well be therefore that *Yersinia* is playing no role whatever in these patients, but that there is cross-reactivity between the human thyroid TSH receptor and *Yersinia* antigens. It seems more likely that the detection of antibodies to *Yersinia* is almost certainly an artifact and of no relevance to the pathogenesis of Graves' disease. Similarly, Weiss et al. (167) demonstrated TSH binding sites in *E. coli*, with the same ramifications as those mentioned above for *Yersinia*.

In 1979 Werner (226) returned to his earlier argument during the course of describing a case of Graves' disease following acute (subacute) thyroiditis, i.e., that an occult antigenic change in the thyroid may be the initiating factor for autoimmune thyroid disease. Indeed Sheets (227) and Perloff (228) had also reported similar findings, and Volpé et al. (229) reported the rare incidence of Hashimoto's thyroiditis following subacute thyroiditis. It is true that in subacute thyroiditis secondary immunological phenomena may be observed, e.g., thyroid autoantibodies, the appearance of TBII, and the appearance of sensitized T lymphocytes (230). Thyroid autoantibodies occur in less than half the patients, appearing some weeks after onset, rarely reaching high titers, and then subsiding spontaneously (229). TBII has been demonstrated during the course of subacute thyroiditis by several workers (230). However, in those instances in which it was detected, there was no correlation with the presence of hyperthyroidism, nor was there evidence that the TBII represented a true thyroid stimulator; that is, it was negative in the TSAb assay (230). Similarly, evidence of cell-mediated immunity has been shown to be transitory and secondary in this disorder (230,231). Moreover, Totterman et al. (177,178) showed that antigen-reactive T lymphocytes are present in large numbers within the thyroid gland in subacute thyroiditis. Nevertheless, it is exceedingly unlikely that this inflammatory reaction or its immune response is responsible for the Graves' disease that only rarely occurs following the thyroiditis. It should be pointed out that only a few cases of autoimmune thyroid disease have followed subacute thyroiditis; over 99% of the patients go on to full recovery. Thus clearly autoimmune thyroid disease is precipitated only in those patients who are already predisposed to it, and thus the finding of the frequently positive HLA-Bw35, as is seen in subacute thyroiditis (230), bears no relationship whatever to the Graves' disease that occurs in Caucasians (see "Genetics of Autoimmune Thyroid Disease").

Because on the one hand almost all patients with subacute thyroiditis go on to recovery and not on to autoimmune thyroid disease, whereas virtually all cases of Graves' and Hashimoto's diseases arise *de novo*, it is much more likely that in those few cases where the disorders have followed subacute thyroiditis or another viral infection these inflammatory disorders have acted as a nonspecific "stress" to precipitate the hyperthyroidism, as is discussed below (see "Precipitation of the Disease").

There is no evidence that the thyroid antigenic alteration induced by the viral infection plays any special role in precipitating the autoimmune process. Thus any infection, acute trauma, emotional disturbance, or even the administration of thyroid hormone itself may be sufficient to precipitate hyperthyroidism in a predisposed person by virtue of effects on the immunoregulatory system, rather than on the target organ (6) (see below).

Normal thyroid cell membrane antigenic preparations have been shown to stimulate lymphocyte cultures from patients with Graves' disease to produce thyroid-stimulating antibody (232). Moreover, thyroid-stimulating antibody, whether produced *in vivo* or *in vitro*, interacts with perfectly normal thyroid tissue in the various assay systems. In addition, von Westarp et al. (63) were unable to demonstrate any antigenic differences between Hashimoto's and normal antigens. Knight and Adams (233) similarly were unable to show any variation in the autoantigen for the thyroid-stimulating autoantibodies in a variety of thyroid tissues. These authors concluded that there was no antigenic alteration necessary to initiate Graves' disease.

In addition, Carayon et al. (234) showed that the thyrotropin receptor adenylate cyclase system is unchanged in the thyroid glands of Graves' disease compared to normal thyroid glands. They stated therefore that an antigenic abnormality has not been demonstrated in the Graves' thyroid gland and thus could not act as the initiator of this disorder. Newer techniques are now being employed to purify and characterize the receptor (106,235,236), but a completely "pure" receptor preparation has yet to be prepared. Such an ultimate preparation may permit more precise investigations into the role of the TSH receptor in the initiation and pathophysiology of Graves' disease. The use of fat cell membranes as a source of TSH receptor may facilitate this process (237).

Actually there are several reasons for considering that it is not necessary to invoke an occult antigenic change as the initiator for Graves' or Hashimoto's disease. First, this presupposes a genetically based hyperimmune response not only to the thyroid antigens but also to gastric antigen, islet cell antigen, and a few other organ-specific antigens (to account for the overlap of other organ-specific autoimmune diseases)—and yet not to all of the host of other possible autoantigens, as generalized hypersensitivity is not a feature of Graves' or Hashimoto's disease (204). Second, because the immune response to what has been postulated as an occult thyroidal antigenic change is excessive, this would necessitate a defect in immunoregulation, as discussed above. Indeed such a defect has now been demonstrated (see "Evidence for a Defect in Suppressor T Lymphocytes," above). With such a disorder in immunoregulation, there is no need for any alteration of the antigen, merely the availability of the antigen. Third, as we noted above, there is no evidence of any thyroidal antigenic change demonstrable. Finally, where there is severe thyroidal antigenic change, as in severe subacute thyroiditis, only very rarely is there progression to either Graves' or Hashimoto's disease. For these reasons, there is no need to invoke thyroidal antigenic change as a *sine qua non* in initiating either disorder.

GENETICS OF AUTOIMMUNE THYROID DISEASE

It is interesting to attempt to understand why some people and not others have this apparent defect in the response of a specific clone of suppressor T lymphocytes to thyroid antigen which consequently renders them susceptible to autoimmune thyroid disease. In mice, genes that map in the region which corresponds to the HLA-D locus in human beings are responsible for controlling the response of helper or suppressor T lymphocytes to a given antigen (6). In Caucasians, Graves' hyperthyroidism is associated with HLA-DR3, goitrous Hashimoto's thyroiditis with HLA-DR5, and atrophic thyroiditis apparently with HLA-DR3 (238). In Oriental races, the HLA markers are different than in those seen in Caucasians, as it seems that different genes have different functions in different human races. Previous findings that link Graves' disease with HLA-B8 in Caucasians probably reflected a linkage disequilibrium between HLA-DR3 and B8. These associations are not absolute. Many patients with Graves' disease do not have the HLA-DR3 genotype, and most persons with HLA-DR3 (approximately 20% of the Caucasian population) do not have Graves' disease. Thus it seems that the gene associated with susceptibility for Graves' disease is not HLA-DR3 but may be very near it, also in linkage disequilibrium. It seems likely that patients with certain genotypes are predisposed to have a defect in the response of suppressor T lymphocytes to thyroid antigen. How the genotype causes an abnormality in a specific clone of suppressor T lymphocytes is unknown, as is the molecular nature of the abnormality. Further details of the familial and sex incidence (F/M 4:1), the genetic aspects, and the relationship of nongenetic factors are documented elsewhere (6,239).

PRECIPITATION OF THE DISEASE

If it may be assumed that there is a genetically determined antigen-specific defect in suppressor T lymphocytes in autoimmune thyroid disease, the next problem is understanding what factors result in initiation of the disorder. Most studies of this particular aspect have investigated Graves' disease, as its onset is much more dramatic than those of the other autoimmune thyroid disorders and both remissions and relapses are common. It has been demonstrated that both Graves' disease and Hashimoto's thyroiditis appear at random in genetically predisposed populations (56,108). More than one mechanism could initiate either disorder. One such mechanism could be the random appearance of the appropriate autoreactive helper T lymphocyte for which control is inadequate (6,239).

This event in itself would be sufficient to initiate the disease. In other instances, suppressor T lymphocyte function may be only partially affected, and with optimal conditions their function may be sufficient to completely suppress the disease (6,239). An age-related decline in the function of suppressor T lymphocytes in a person who already has such a partial abnormality in a clone of suppressor T lymphocytes may also be sufficient to allow the disease to be precipitated. One of the first reports of Graves' disease, by Parry (8) in the early nineteenth century, pointed out an association between the onset of the disorder and stress. Although early reports were anecdotal, substantial indirect evidence now links stress and the onset of the disease (6,239). Bereavement depresses the lymphocyte response to mitogens in human beings, and stress diminishes the lymphocyte response in animals (29). It is possible that stress brings about its effects on suppressor T lymphocytes via an increase in cortisol that occurs as a result of the stress, although this point remains to be proved (6). In any event, various types of stress have been reported to precipitate Graves' disease, including bereavement, infections, car accidents, and dieting (6,240). Thus in this context, stress could be emotional or biological (e.g., a viral infection). Stress may thus cause decompensation of an already genetically compromised population of suppressor T lymphocytes, thus allowing helper T lymphocytes to cooperate with B lymphocytes, with the ultimate result of producing autoantibodies, as well as allowing cytotoxic effects by effector lymphocytes.

In Graves' disease the production of thyroid-stimulating antibody induces elevated levels of thyroid hormones. Evidence was presented above that thyrotoxicosis also may depress the function of suppressor T lymphocytes; indeed thyroid hormone therapy itself has been thought to precipitate hyperthyroidism in predisposed persons (241). The tendency in Graves' disease for defective *generalized* suppressor T lymphocyte function to become normal after treatment, as documented above, indicates that the hyperthyroid state itself affects the immune system. This effect, although not related to the pathogenesis of the disease, may be important in the *self-perpetuation* of hyperthyroidism.

NATURE OF REMISSIONS IN GRAVES' DISEASE

Even in early accounts of Graves' (Basedow's) disease, it was recognized that the disorder was one of remissions and exacerbations (242,243). Indeed, remissions also occur in Hashimoto's thyroiditis not uncommonly (244,249). However, the nature of such remissions has been heretofore unclear, and only recently has it been possible to at least formulate a hypothesis regarding the mechanisms involved.

It is clear that in Graves' disease there may be several forms of clinical remissions (250). One may be due to radioactive iodine ablation or surgical removal of sufficient tissue to prevent recurrence by virtue of an insufficient thyroid remnant. However, even without such destructive therapy, continuing spontaneous thyroid damage may bring about remission, presumably because of a continuing immunological process (246,251–254). Other possibilities in the context of continuing immunological processes included the possibility of an alteration of a thyroid-stimulating antibody to another, nonstimulating form of TBII, even with TSH blocking propensities as described by Endo et al. (136) and Konishi et al. (137).

This sequence of events has not yet been proved to actually occur, but at least it is within the realm of possibility. Another possibility, suggested by Van der Heide et al. (162) and Feldt-Rasmussen et al. (255), is that immune complexes may arise which interfere with the ability of the antibody to produce its effects.

Another form of remission is one of which all immunological stigmata of the disease disappear, including thyroid antibodies (36), TBII (88,89,145,146,256,257), and evidence of sensitization of T lymphocytes (201,202,213,216). It seems possible that this form of remission can occur only in those patients with a partial defect in immunoregulation, a defect susceptible to further depression by "stress" (see section immediately above) and which is therefore reversible when that circumstance is overcome. Restoration of a euthyroid state by whatever means (antithyroid drugs, radioactive iodine, or surgery) should serve to improve suppressor T lymphocyte function, as the possible deleterious effects of excessive thyroid hormones themselves directly on the immune system, as well as indirect effects of thyroid hormones on the adrenocortical system (and thus on the immune system), would be reversed under these circumstances (6). In addition, social factors, rest, passage of time, the clearing of infection, and the use of sedation and other nonspecific measures (e.g., beta-adrenergic blockers) would each serve to reduce "stress," thereby allowing the partially defective immunoregulatory system to be restored to its previous functional capacity. Thus the thyroid-directed "forbidden" clone of helper T lymphocytes would again be suppressed, and the disease would consequently go into *immunological* remission. Such mechanisms could also account for the spontaneous remissions which were observed long before any specific therapy became available (242,243). Of course, such patients would be prone to recurrence if similar "stressful" events were experienced later. Clearly, "stress" is important only as it is perceived by the organism and in relation to the physiological (hormonal, immunological, etc.) response to it. What is thus required to prove this theory is some sensitive means of measuring suppressor T lymphocyte function in response to such events (258) in appropriate genetically predisposed persons.

Those persons with a presumed *complete* defect would not be expected to go into *immunological* remission, no matter how long his/her antithyroid drug was continued or what form of therapy was employed. Only those remissions associated with continuing immunological activity directed to the thyroid and/or thyroid destruction would occur in this group. This would be in accord with the continuing evidence of humoral and cell-mediated immunity in some patients following antithyroid or other forms of therapy (216).

There is some genetic evidence consistent with this concept. Irvine et al. (259) first showed that those patients with Graves' disease who lacked HLA-B8 are more likely to go into remission, whereas those positive for HLA-B8 are likely to relapse. Similarly, Bech et al. (260) showed that the presence of HLA-Dw3 is found in significantly higher numbers in those who relapse, and conversely its incidence is much lower in those who remit.

This finding has been confirmed by MacGregor et al. (145) (Fig. 5). Thus there seems to be a genetic basis for the ability to remit (or relapse) which is also consistent with the hypothesis for remission advanced above. Those with the presumed complete defect in immunoregulation are more closely related to HLA-B8 and Dw3 (DR3) when compared to those who have only a partial defect and hence the possibility to undergo immunological remission.

INTERRELATIONSHIPS BETWEEN GRAVES' AND HASHIMOTO'S DISEASES

As pointed out above, there is much in common between Graves' disease and Hashimoto's thyroiditis to the extent that some observers have considered that these two conditions

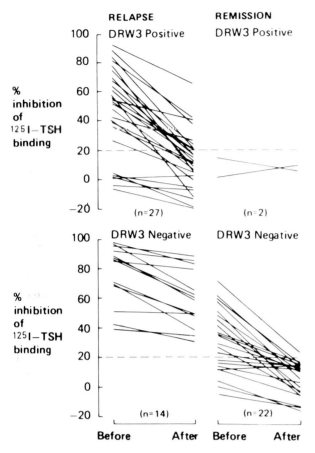

FIG. 5. TBII activity immediately prior to and shortly after cessation of antithyroid drug therapy, respectively, in Graves' disease. The graph shows the relationship to remission and the presence or absence of HLA-DRw3. Note that positive results are <80, negative results >80. (From McGregor et al., ref. 145.)

represent opposite ends of the same spectrum of a single entity (3,5). Indeed depending on one's perspective of what variants a "single entity" may reasonably include, this notion may be acceptable. The evidence for at least genetic, pathogenetic, and immunological overlap between the two disorders is overwhelming and is discussed in the following paragraphs. Yet there are elements in each condition which are clearly different, and the author's perception at present is that Graves' disease and Hashimoto's thyroiditis are two different entities, no matter how closely related they are to one another (6).

Evidence for common features include the observation that both conditions may aggregate in the same families (39,261) or even coexist within the same thyroid gland (89,174). In some identical twin sets, one twin may have Graves' disease and the other Hashimoto's thyroiditis (262,263). Lymphocytic infiltration of the thyroid is observed in both conditions (3,264,265). Various immunoglobulins may be observed in the thyroid stroma of each malady (43,266). Thymic enlargement is common to both (267), and "conventional thyroid autoantibodies" (i.e., thyroid autoantibodies other than TSAb) are commonly found in both conditions (58). Studies of asymptomatic relatives of patients with each disorder yield similar functional and immunological abnormalities. As mentioned above, Graves' disease may spontaneously culminate in Hashimoto's thyroiditis (and hypothyroidism); conversely, Hashimoto's thyroiditis with or without hypothyroidism may ultimately change into Graves' disease associated with hyperthyroidism. The studies of Torfs et al. (261) and Tamai et al. (264) also show that common immunogenetic factors are involved in the pathogenesis of both Graves' and Hashimoto's diseases. Additionally, tests of sensitized T lymphocytes (in response to thyroid antigens) and tests which demonstrate a specific defect in suppressor T lymphocyte function are likewise common to both (35,213–215).

However, the differences that can be discerned between these two autoimmune diseases may be of fundamental importance. Of course, at the extremes the clinical presentation may be quite disparate, with hyperthyroidism as the expression of Graves' disease, and hypothyroidism reflecting Hashimoto's thyroiditis (i.e., stimulation of the thyroid gland versus destruction of the thyroid gland, respectively). In terms of HLA association, Moens and Farid (268) showed that the atrophic form of autoimmune thyroiditis is associated with HLA-B8 and HLA-DR3, similar to the HLA findings in Graves' disease (238). In the goitrous form of thyroiditis, however, there seems to be an association with HLA-DR5 (238,269). [Schleusener et al. (270) reported that a subtype of hyperthyroidism is also associated with HLA-DR5—see above.] Moreover, exophthalmos, which is commonly associated with Graves' disease, is observed only occasionally in patients with Hashimoto's thyroiditis (271–277). TBII, found in most patients with active untreated Graves' disease, is detectable by most groups in only a small proportion of those with Hashimoto's thyroiditis (see "TSH Receptor-Related Antigen...," above). Indeed if a stimulatory rather than a radioligand assay is performed, many of the Hashimoto's patients with a positive TBII have a negative TSAb (6). The incidence of various associated organ-specific autoimmune diseases seems to differ significantly between the two diseases; for example, Sjögren's syndrome is associated much more commonly with Hashimoto's thyroiditis than with Graves' disease (278). These discrepancies suggest that there may be subtle genetic and pathogenetic differences between these two disorders and, if this is so, further suggest that lymphocyte populations (and thus precise antigens) are slightly different.

However, with currently available thyroidal antigenic preparations, it is not possible to separate the two putative antigen systems. Even with preparations labeled "solubilized TSH receptor" from human thyroid tissue, it is clear that this is merely a preparation rich in cell membranes (and thus rich in TSH receptor protein) composed of many membrane antigens (as well as some nonmembrane antigens) (213–215). Hence it should come as no surprise that tests of cell-mediated immunity employing such preparations provide similar results for the two diseases. However, when fat cell membrane preparations are employed, Shinozawa and Ingbar (143) showed a clear separation between Graves' and Hashimoto's diseases in terms of antibody binding. Eguchi and Ingbar (237) further showed that lymphocytes from Graves' disease (but not from Hashimoto's thyroiditis) have a mitogenic response (measured by incorporation of ^{125}I-deoxyuridine) when exposed to guinea pig fat cell membrane (presumably the TSH receptor). Doniach (7) suggested that there are even subtle genetic and pathogenetic differences between the atrophic form of autoimmune thyroiditis and the goitrous form. She pointed out that in the atrophic form not only is the HLA complement somewhat different than in the goitrous form but that there are different antibodies present as well; thyroid growth-inhibiting antibodies have been detected in the atrophic form, whereas thyroid growth-promoting antibodies have been observed in the goitrous form.

It is the author's current view, therefore, that Graves' disease and Hashimoto's thyroiditis are separate disorders, however close they are to one another genetically and pathogenetically and however much they may overlap. Speculatively, both conditions may involve antigens closely related on the thyroid cell membrane. Whether these thyroid antigens will yield technically to procedures to separate them remains to be seen. However, Eguchi and Ingbar (237), using guinea pig fat cell membranes (which have TSH receptors but which do not seem to have other thyroid-like membrane antigens), suggest that the TSH receptor is the appropriate antigen for Graves' disease whereas presumably other thyroid antigens are appropriate for Hashimoto's thyroiditis. The genes which cause each disorder, if indeed separate, must be very closely related to one another, with inheritance of both genes being common enough to cause frequent overlap. The concurrence of the two conditions in identical twins (i.e., one twin with Graves' disease, the other with Hashimoto's thyroiditis) may be explained by the inheritance of both genes in each; the subsequent random appearance of slightly different thyroid-directed "forbidden clones" of helper T lymphocytes for which immunoregulation is genetically inadequate might dictate which of the two entities is finally expressed (despite the identical available genetic predisposition to both diseases in each twin). Similarly, there seem to be very subtle genetic and pathogenetic differences between even some of the variants of autoimmune thyroiditis, e.g., atrophic myxedema on the one hand and goitrous Hashimoto's thyroiditis on the other. It will be some time, however before the precise genetic background of these disorders and their possible differences are completely elucidated.

SUMMARY

The author views Graves' hyperthyroidism and Hashimoto's thyroiditis as very closely related but nevertheless *separate* organ-specific autoimmune diseases. A new term for Graves' disease is "autoimmune thyrotoxicosis," and a more fitting term for Hashimoto's thyroiditis and its variants is "autoimmune thyroiditis." Incidentally, the author also views exophthalmos as a very closely related but separate organ-specific autoimmune disease which is *not* directly due to thyroid disease. Autoimmune thyroid diseases, as well as other closely related organ-specific autoimmune disorders, may each be attributable to separate, albeit closely related, inherited isolated defects in immunoregulation. Evidence presented above indicates that there is an antigen-specific defect in a population of suppressor T lymphocytes (which would ordinarily suppress a clone of thyroid-directed autoreactive helper T lymphocytes) in the patients predisposed to have either Graves' or Hashimoto's disease. The defect which is present in the specific clones of suppressor T lymphocytes may well be present from birth onward, although there has been no proof of this point. If one had such a defect, however, this would permit a normally randomly mutating "forbidden" clone of thyroid-directed helper T lymphocytes arising at random to survive and to interact with its complementary antigen on the thyroid cell membrane, and then to set up a localized cell-mediated immune response. This would not require any alteration of the antigen, only the mere availability of the specific antigen. The clone of self-reactive lymphocytes so arising and escaping immunoregulation would presumably then expand upon interaction with this antigen and consequently direct and cooperate with groups of (already present) thyroid-directed appropriate B lymphocytes, which in turn would produce specific immunoglobulin that seems necessary for the full expression of these conditions.

There seems to be slight genetic differences between Graves' and Hashimoto's disease and perhaps even among the variants of autoimmune thyroiditis. The gene responsible for Graves' disease may lie in close linkage disequilibrium with HLA-DR3 on chromosome 6 in Caucasians. Evidence suggests that there is an association with HLA-DR5 in goitrous Hashimoto's thyroiditis. However, in families in which Hashimoto's thyroiditis coexists with Graves' disease, the haplotype is the same for both (HLA-DR3). Although it is true that results of cell-mediated immunity and abnormalities of suppressor T lymphocytes presented in this chapter have been common to both Graves' and Hashimoto's diseases, this may well be because it has been impossible to separate the putative antigens on the thyroid cell membrane in the two disorders. There are enough differences in the two conditions to at least suggest that they do not represent the opposite ends of a spectrum of a single entity but, rather, represent differing entities. It would take purification of specific antigens to prove this suggestion.

The role of anti-idiotypic antibodies in these conditions is still somewhat speculative as there are few data yet reported. Adjunctive roles for immune complexes, nonspecific cells (macrophages, "killer" cells), and chemical mediators are undoubtedly important. The role of thyroid-stimulating antibody in the induction of the hyperthyroidism of Graves' disease is of crucial interest and importance; new evidence now relates its activity to specific binding sites on the TSH receptor. This antibody acts as an agonist, a very unusual characteristic for antireceptor antibodies, which usually act as antagonists. Some antibodies which have the ability to prevent the binding of TSH to its receptor have been shown to be antagonistic to the effects of TSH and thus produce some confusion in assessing the results of the radioligand assay for Graves' immunoglobulins.

The role of stress in the induction of hyperthyroidism may be by means of its effect in further reducing immunosuppression in those persons with only a partial isolated defect. It is entirely possible in such persons that there is a clone of suppressor T lymphocytes which is *partially* defective but which is ordinarily capable of suppressing the "forbidden" clone of thyroid-directed autoreactive helper T lymphocytes under optimal conditions. However, if the conditions are not optimal for those suppressor T lymphocytes, their occult defect would become overt. Such a situation may occur with a slight increase in cortisol (resulting from stress), or other chemical mediators could be implicated. Once the disease has been initiated, it might remain self-perpetuating by virtue of the effect of the disease itself on the immune system, i.e., through an indirect effect of hyperthyroidism on the adrenal cortex or a direct effect of thyroid hormones on suppressor T lymphocytes. On the other hand, remissions may be brought about by restoring immunoregulation to its previous state, normalizing the hyperthyroidism, and/or relieving the "stress." Those persons having an isolated *complete* defect in immunoregulation would not be expected to achieve remissions except by destruction of thyroid parenchyma. It is of interest that those patients who retain a positive test for thyroid-stimulating antibody can be expected to relapse after discontinuance of antithyroid drug therapy, whereas the relapse rate is much lower when thyroid-stimulating antibody has disappeared. Moreover, there is evidence that there is an increase in HLA-Dw3 (or HLA-DR3) in those patients who relapse compared to those who remain in remission. This would be consistent with the view that there is a genetic basis for the ability to relapse or remit.

Finally, it is considered likely that there is one defect (therefore one gene) responsible for Graves' disease and one defect responsible for each of the other organ-specific autoimmune diseases. Because it seems evident that each of these genes lies close to the others, it is altogether possible that a person could inherit one, two, or more such genes and therefore have a predisposition to more than one of the closely related autoimmune conditions.

REFERENCES

1. Ehrlich, P. (1900): On Autoimmunity with special reference to cell life. *Proc. R. Soc. Med.*, 66B:424–448.
2. Solomon, D. H., and Kleeman, K. E. (1977): Concepts of pathogenesis of Graves' disease. *Adv. Intern. Med.*, 22:273–299.
3. Bastenie, P. A., and Ermans, A. M. (1972): Thyroiditis and thyroid function: clinical, morphological and physiopathological studies. In: *International Series of Monographs on Pure and Applied Biology, Modern Trends in Physiological Sciences*, Vol. 36. Pergamon, Oxford.
4. Fisher, D., and Beall, G. N. (1976): Hashimoto's thyroiditis. *Pharmacol. Ther.*, 83:170–176.

5. Davies, T. F., and De Bernardo, E. (1983): Thyroid autoantibodies and disease: An overview. In: *Autoimmune Endocrine Disease*, edited by T. F. Davies, pp. 127–137. Wiley, New York.
6. Volpé, R. (1981): Autoimmunity in the endocrine system. In: *Monographs in Endocrinology*, No. 20. Springer Verlag, New York.
7. Doniach, D. (1981): Hashimoto's thyroiditis and primary myxoedema viewed as separate entities. *Eur. J. Clin. Invest.*, 11:245–247.
8. Parry, C. H. (1825): *Collections from the Unpublished Medical Writings of the Late Caleb Hillier Parry*, Vol. 2, pp. 111–128. Underwood, London.
9. Graves, R. J. (1835): Clinical lectures. *Lond. Med. Surg.*, 7:516–517.
10. Von Basedow, C. A. (1840): Exophthalmos durch Hypertrophie des Zellgewebes in der Augenhöle Woch-enschr. *Gesamte. Hellkd.*, 13:198–228.
11. Hashimoto, H. (1912): Zur Kenntris der lymphomatosen veranderung der Schilddruse (Struma lymphomatosa). *Arch. Klin. Chir.*, 97:219–248.
12. Hazard, J. B. (1955): Thyroiditis: a review. *Am. J. Clin. Pathol.*, 25:289–298, 399–426.
13. Loeb, P. B., Drash, A. L., and Kenny, F. M. (1973): Prevalence of low titre and "negative" antithyroglobulin antibodies in biopsy-proved juvenile Hashimoto's thyroiditis. *J. Pediatr.*, 82:17–21.
14. Amino, N., Mori, H., Iwatani, Y., Tanizawa, O., Kawashima, M., Tsuge, I., Ibaragi, K., Kumahara, Y., and Miyai, K. (1982): High prevalence of transient postpartum thyrotoxicosis and hypothyroidism. *N. Engl. J. Med.*, 306:849–852.
15. Fein, H. G., Goldman, J. M., and Weintraub, B. D. (1980): Postpartum lymphocytic thyroiditis in American women: a spectrum of thyroid dysfunction. *Am. J. Obstet. Gynecol.*, 138:504–510.
16. Bastenie, P. A., Nove, P., Bonnyns, M., Van Gaekst, K., and Chailly, M. (1967): Clinical and pathological significance of asymptomatic atrophic thyroiditis; a condition of latent hypothyroidism. *Lancet*, 1:915–919.
17. Beierwaltes, W. H. (1969): Iodine and lymphocytic thyroiditis. *Bull All-India Inst. Med. Sci.*, 3:145–152.
18. Tunbridge, W. M. G. (1979): The epidemiology of hypothyroidism. *Clin. Endocrinol. Metab.*, 8:21–27.
19. Yoshida, H., Amino, N., Yagawa, K., Uemura, K., Satoh, M., Miyai, K., and Kumahara, Y. (1978): Association of serum antithyroid antibodies with lymphocytic infiltration of the thyroid gland: study of 70 autopsied cases. *J. Clin. Endocrinol. Metab.*, 46:859–862.
20. Hawkins, B. R., O'Connor, K. J., Dawkins, R. L., Dawkins, B., and Rodger, B. (1979): Autoantibodies in an Australian population. I. Prevalence and persistence. *J. Clin. Lab. Immunol.*, 2:211–215.
21. Hawkins, B. R., Cheah, P. S., Burger, H. G., Patel, Y., MacKay, I. R., and Welborn, T. A. (1980): Diagnostic significance of thyroid microsomal antibodies in a randomly selected population. *Lancet*, 8203:1057–1059.
22. Roitt, I. M., Doniach, D., Campbell, R. N., and Hudson, R. V. (1956): Autoantibodies in Hashimoto's disease (lymphadenoid goitre). *Lancet*, 2:820–821.
23. Rose, N. R., and Witebsky, E. (1956): Studies on organ specificity. V. Changes in the thyroid gland of rabbits following active immunization with rabbit thyroid extracts. *J. Immunol.*, 76:417–427.
24. Adams, D. D., and Purves, H. D. (1956): Abnormal response in the assay of thyrotrophin. *Univ. Otago Med. School Proc.*, 34:11–12.
25. McKenzie, J. M. (1960): Further evidence for a thyroid activator in hyperthyroidism. *J. Clin. Endocrinol. Metab.*, 20:380–388.
26. Kriss, J. P., Pleshakov, V., and Chien, J. R. (1964): Isolation and identification of the long acting thyroid stimulator and its relationship to hyperthyroidism and circumscribed pretibial myxedema. *J. Clin. Endocrinol. Metab.*, 24:1005–1028.
27. Burnet, F. M. (1959): *The Clonal Selection Theory of Acquired Immunity*. Vanderbilt University Press, Nashville, Tenn.
28. Rose, N. R., Kong, Y. M., Okayasu, I., Geraldo, A. A., Beisel, K., and Sundick, R. S. (1981): T cell regulation in autoimmune thyroiditis. *Immunol. Rev.*, 55:219–314.
29. Strakosch, C. R., Wenzel, B. E., Row, V. V., and Volpé, R. (1982): Immunology of autoimmune thyroid diseases. *N. Engl. J. Med.*, 307:1499–1507.
30. Gershon, R. K. (1979): "Clonal selection and after" and after. *N. Engl. J. Med.*, 300:1105–1107.
31. Wigzell, H., Binz, H., Frischknecht, H., Peterson, P., and Sege, K. (1978): Possible roles of auto-anti-idiotypic immunity in autoimmune disease. In: *Genetic Control of Autoimmune Disease*, edited by R. N. Rose, P. E., Bigazzi, and N. L. Warner, pp. 327–342. Elsevier/North Holland, New York.
32. Urbain, J., and Wuilmart, C. (1982): Some thoughts on idiotypic networks and immunoregulation. *Immunol. Today*, 3:88–92, 125–128.
33. Zanetti, M., Barton, R. W., and Bigazzi, P. E. (1983): Anti-idiotypic immunity and autoimmunity. II. Idiotypic determinants of autoantibodies and lymphocytes in spontaneous and experimental induced autoimmune thyroiditis. *Cell. Immunol.*, 75:292–299.
34. McCoy, J. P., Michaelson, J. H., and Bigazzi, P. E. (1983): Anti-idiotype immunity and autoimmunity. III. Investigations in human autoimmune thyroiditis. *Life Sci.*, 32:109–118.
35. Topliss, D. J., How, J., Lewis, M., Row, V. V., and Volpé, R. (1983): Evidence for cell-mediated immunity and specific suppressor T lymphocyte dysfunction in Graves' disease and diabetes mellitus. *J. Clin. Endocrinol. Metab.*, 57:700–705.
36. Pinchera, A., Fenzi, G. F., Bartalena, L., Chiovato, L., Marcocci, C., and Pacini, F. (1979): Thyroid

antigens involved in autoimmune thyroid disorders. In: *Autoimmunity in Thyroid Diseases*, edited by E. Klein and F. A. Horster, pp. 49–67. Schattauer, Stuttgart.

37. Drexhage, H. A., Bottazzo, G. F., Bitemsky, L., Chayen, J., and Doniach, D. (1980): Evidence for thyroid growth stimulating immunoglobulins in some goitrous thyroid diseases. *Lancet*, 2:281–292.

38. Drexhage, H. A., Bottazzo, G. F., Bitemsky, L., Chayen, J., and Doniach, D. (1981): Thyroid growth blocking antibodies in primary myxoedema. *Nature*, 289:594–596.

39. Doniach, D. (1975): Humoral and genetic aspects of thyroid autoimmunity. *Clin. Endocrinol. Metab.*, 4:267–285.

40. Hay, F. C., and Torrigiani, G. (1973): The distribution of antithyroglobulin antibodies in the immunoglobulin G subclasses. *Clin. Exp. Immunol.*, 15:517–521.

41. Pulvertaft, R. J. V., Doniach, D., and Roitt, I. M. (1959): Cytotoxic effect of Hashimoto's serum on human thyroid cells in tissue culture. *Lancet*, 2:214–216.

42. Grabar, P. (1974): "Self" and "not self" in immunology. *Lancet*, 1:1320–1322.

43. Kalderon, A. E., and Bogaars, H. A. (1977): Immune complex deposits in Graves' disease and Hashimoto's thyroiditis. *Am. J. Med.*, 63:729–734.

44. Calder, E. A., Urbaniak, S. J., Penhale, W. J., and Irvine, W. J. (1974): Characterization of human lymphoid cell-mediated antibody-dependent cytotoxicity (LDAC). *Clin. Exp. Immunol.*, 18:597–598.

45. Calder, E. A., Irvine, W. J., Davidson, N. M., and Wu, F. (1976): T, B and K cells in autoimmune thyroid disease. *Clin. Exp. Immunol.*, 25:17–22.

46. Pruzanski, W., Capes, H., Row, V. V., and Volpé, R. (1984): Lymphocytotoxic and phagocytotoxic activity in Graves' disease and Hashimoto's thyroiditis. *J. Endocrinol. Invest.*, 7:7–14.

47. Eguchi, K., Kanazawa, H., Ishikawa, N., Fukuda, T., Mine, M., Izumi, M., and Nagataki, S. (1982): Lymphocytotoxic antibodies in autoimmune thyroid disease. In: *Proc. 64th Meeting, Endocrine Society, June 16–18, San Francisco*, p. 112. abstract 132.

48. Kriss, J. P. (1968): Inactivation of long acting thyroid stimulator (LATS) by anti-kappa and anti-lambda antisera. *J. Clin. Endocrinol. Metab.*, 28:1440–1444.

49. Fahey, J. L., and Goodman, H. (1964): Antibody activity in six classes of human immunoglobulin. *Science*, 143:588–590.

50. Adlkofer, F., Schleusener, H., Uher, L., and Amanos, A. (1973): Heterogeneity of long acting thyroid stimulating (LATS) activity, thyroglobulin antibodies and thyroid microsomal antibodies. *Acta Endocrinol. (Copenh.)*, 73:483–488.

51. Zakarija, M. (1980): The thyroid stimulating antibody (TSAb) of Graves' disease: evidence for restricted heterogeneity. *Horm. Res.*, 13:1–15.

52. Zakarija, M., and McKenzie, J. M. (1980): Immunochemical characterization of thyroid stimulating antibody (TSAb). In: *Thyroid Research VIII*, edited by J. R. Stockigt and S. Nagataki, pp. 669–672. Australian Academy of Science, Canberra.

53. Zakarija, M., and McKenzie, J. M. (1983): Thyroid stimulating antibody in Graves' disease. *Life Sci.*, 32:31–44.

54. Owen, C. A. (1958): A review of autoimmunization in Hashimoto's disease. *J. Clin. Endocrinol. Metab.*, 18:1015–1023.

55. Roitt, I. M., and Torrigiani, G. (1967): Identification and estimation of undegraded thyroglobulin in human serum. *Endocrinology*, 81:421–429.

56. Volpé, R., Farid, N. R., von Westarp, C., and Row, V. V. (1974): The pathogenesis of Graves' disease and Hashimoto's thyroiditis. *Clin. Endocrinol. (Oxf.)*, 3:239–261.

57. Roberts, I. M., Whittingham, S., and MacKay, I. R. (1973): Tolerance to an autoantigen-thyroglobulin-antigen-binding lymphocytes in thymus and blood in health and autoimmune disease. *Lancet*, 2:936–940.

58. Mori, T., and Kriss, J. P. (1971): Measurements by competitive binding radioassays of serum antimicrosomal and antithyroglobulin antibodies in Graves' disease and other thyroid disorders. *J. Clin. Endocrinol. Metab.*, 33:688–698.

59. Peake, R. L., Willis, D. B., Asimakis, G. K., Jr., and Deiss, W. P., Jr. (1974): Radioimmunologic assay for antithyroglobulin antibodies. *J. Lab. Clin. Med.*, 84:907–919.

60. Salabe, G. B., Salabe, H., Dominici, R., Daroli, C., and Andreoli, M. (1974): Radioimmunoassay for human antithyroglobulin antibodies. II. Determination of antigen-binding capacity. *J. Clin. Endocrinol. Metab.*, 39:1125–1132.

61. Weiss, I., and Davies, T. F. (1982): A specific plaque forming assay for human thyroglobulin antibody secreting immunocytes. *J. Clin. Endocrinol. Metab.*, 54:282–285.

62. McLachlan, S. M., Clark, S., Stimson, W. H., Clark, F., and Rees Smith, B. (1982): Studies of thyroglobulin antibody synthesis using a micro-ELISA assay. *Immunol. Lett.*, 4:27–33.

63. Von Westarp, C., Knox, A. J. S., Row, V. V., and Volpé, R. (1977): Comparison of thyroid antigens by the experimental production of precipitating antibodies to human thyroid fractions and the identification of an antibody which competes with long acting thyroid stimulator for thyroid binding. *Acta Endocrinol. (Copenh.)*, 84:759–769.

64. Izumi, M., Morita, S., Yamashita, Y., Horayu, H., Taura, M., Sato, K., Okamoto, S., Morimoto, I., and

Nagataki, S. (1982): Comparison of serum thyroglobulin of various diseases. In: *Proc. 58th Meeting, American Thyroid Assoc., Quebec City, September 22–25*, T21.

65. Bayer, M. F., and Kriss, J. P. (1979): Immunoradiometric assay for serum thyroglobulin semiquantitative measurement of thyroglobulin in antithyroglobulin-positive sera. *J. Clin. Endocrinol. Metab.*, 49:557–564.

66. Bayer, M. F., and Kriss, J. P. (1979): A solid phase sandwich type radioimmunoassay for antithyroglobulin: elimination of false positive results and semi-quantitative measurement of antithyroglobulin in the presence of elevated thyroglobulin. *J. Clin. Endocrinol. Metab.*, 49:565–570.

67. Roitt, I. M., Ling, N. R., Doniach, D., and Couchman, K. G. (1964): The cytoplasmic autoantigen of the human thyroid. I. Immunological and biochemical characteristics. *Immunology*, 7:375–393.

68. Butler, S., and Irvine, W. J. (1981): The correlation between the results of tests for thyroid autoantibodies to cell surface and microsomal antigens and to thyroglobulin. *J. Clin. Lab. Immunol.*, 6.237–239.

69. Fagraeus, A., and Jonsson, J. (1970): Distribution of organ antigens over the surface of thyroid cells as examined by the immunofluorescence test. *Immunology*, 18:413–416.

70. Jonsson, J., and Fagraeus, A. (1969): On the mechanism of the ring zone effect obtained with the mixed haemadsorption technique: studies with human antithyroid sera reacting with thyroid monolayer culture. *Immunology*, 17:387–411.

71. Tanner, A. R., Scott Morgan, L., Mardell, R., and Lloyd, R. S. (1982): The incidence of occult thyroid disease associated with thyroid antibodies identified on routine autoantibody screening. *Acta Endocrinol. (Copenh.)*, 100:31–35.

72. Schardt, C. W., McLachlan, S. M., Matheson, J., and Rees-Smith, B. (1982): An enzyme-linked immunoassay for thyroid microsomal antibodies. *J. Immunol. Methods*, 55:155–168.

73. Monzani, F., Fenzi, G. F., Lippi, F., Bartalena, L., Matchia, E., Pinchera, A., and Baschieri, L. (1982): Studies on human plasma membrane antigens. *Ann. Endocrinol. (Paris)*, 43:55A (abstract 90).

74. Staeheli, V., Vallotton, M. B., and Burger, A. (1975): Detection of human anti-thyroxine and anti-triiodo-thyronine antibodies in different thyroid conditions. *J. Clin. Endocrinol. Metab.*, 41:669–675.

75. Ginsberg, J., Segal, D., Erlich, R. M., and Walfish, P. G. (1978): Inappropriate triiodothyronine (T_3) and thyroxine (T_4) radioimmunoassay levels secondary to circulating thyroid hormone autoantibodies. *Clin. Endocrinol. (Oxf.)*, 8:133–139.

76. Inada, M., Nishikawa, M., Naito, K., Oishi, M., Kurata, S., and Imura, H. (1980): Triiodothyronine binding immunoglobulin in a patient with Graves' disease and its effect on metabolism and radioimmunoassay of triiodothyronine. *Am. J. Med.*, 68:787–792.

77. Pearce, C. J., Byfield, P. G. H., Edmonds, C. J., Lalloz, M. R. A., and Himsworth, R. L. (1981): Autoantibodies to thyroglobulin crossreacting with iodothyronines. *Clin. Endocrinol. (Oxf.)*, 15:1–10.

78. Fagraeus, A., Jonsson, J., and El Kahir, D. J. (1970): What is the antibody specificity of LATS? *J. Clin. Endocrinol. Metab.*, 31:445–447.

79. McKenzie, J. M., and Zakarija, M. (1977): LATS in Graves' disease. *Recent Prog. Horm. Res.*, 33:29–57.

80. McKenzie, J. M., Zakarija, M., and Sato, A. (1978): Humoral immunity in Graves' disease. *Clin. Endocrinol. Metab.*, 7:31–45.

81. Onaya, T., Kotani, M., Yamada, T., and Ochi, Y. (1973): New in vitro tests to detect the thyroid stimulator in sera from hyperthyroid patients by measuring colloid droplet formation and cyclic AMP in human thyroid slices. *J. Clin. Endocrinol. Metab.*, 36:859–866.

82. Orgiazzi, J. D. C., Chopra, I. J., and Solomon, D. H. (1976): Human thyroid adenyl cyclase by antisera to thyroid plasma membrane preparations. *Endocrinology*, 98:880–885.

83. Bitensky, L., Alaghband-Zadeh, J., and Chayen, J. (1974): Studies in thyroid stimulating hormone and long acting thyroid stimulator. *Clin. Endocrinol. (Oxf.)*, 3:363–374.

84. Chayen, J. (1980): The cytochemical bioassay of polypeptide hormones. In: *Monographs in Endocrinology*. Springer Verlag, New York.

85. Smyth, P. P. A., Neylan, D., and O'Donovan, D. K. (1982): The prevalence of thyroid stimulating antibodies in goitrous disease assessed by cytochemical section bioassay. *J. Clin. Endocrinol. Metab.*, 54:357–361.

86. McKenzie, J. M. (1968): Humoral factors in the pathogenesis of Graves' disease. *Physiol. Rev.*, 48:252–310.

87. Adams, D. D., and Kennedy, T. H. (1971): Evidence to suggest that LATS protector stimulates the human thyroid gland. *J. Clin. Endocrinol. Metab.*, 33:47–51.

88. Mukhtar, E. D., Smith, B. R., Pyle, G. A., Hall, R., and Vice, R. (1975): Relationship of thyroid stimulating immunoglobulin to thyroid function and effects of surgery, radioiodine and antithyroid drugs. *Lancet*, 1:713–715.

89. O'Donnell, J., Trokoudes, K., Silverberg, J., Row, V. V., and Volpé, R. (1978): Thyrotropin displacement activity (TDA) of serum immunoglobulin from patients with Graves' disease. *J. Clin. Endocrinol. Metab.*, 46:770–777.

90. Kendall-Taylor, P. (1975): LATS and human specific thyroid stimulator: their relation to Graves' disease. *Clin. Endocrinol. Metab.*, 4:319–339.

91. Madsen, S. N., and Bech, K. (1979): TSH and thyroid stimulating antibodies (TSAb) activate thyroid adenylate cyclase through different pathways. *Acta Med. Scand. [Suppl.]*, 624:35–42.

92. Fenzi, G. F., Pinchera, A., Bartalena, I., Monzani, F., Macchia, E., Mammoli, C., and Baschieri, L. (1980):

Thyroid plasma membrane antigens and TSH receptor. In: *Thyroid Research VIII*, edited by J. R. Stockigt and S. Nagataki, pp. 703–706. Australian Academy of Science, Canberra.

93. Smith, B. R. (1976): Immunology of the thyrotrophin receptor. *Immunol. Commun.*, 5:345–360.

94. Smith, B. R., and Hall, R. (1980): The interaction of Graves' immunoglobulin with the TSH receptor. In: *Thyroid Research VIII*, edited by J. Stockigt and S. Nagataki, pp. 715–716. Australian Academy of Science, Canberra.

95. Smith, B. R., Pyle, G. A., Peterson, V. B., and Hall, R. (1977): Interaction of thyroid stimulating antibodies with the human thyrotropin receptor. *J. Endocrinol.*, 75:401–407.

96. De Bruin, T. W. A. (1982): Thyrotropin receptors and antithyrotropin receptor antibodies in Graves' disease. Thesis, University of Leiden, Holland (ISBN 90-9000326-6).

97. Smith, B. R., and Buckland, P. R. (1982): Structure-function of the thyrotropin receptor. In: *Receptors, Antibodies and Disease*, edited by D. Evered, pp. 114–132. Ciba Foundation Symposium 90, Pitman, London.

98. Rickards, C., Buckland, P., Rees-Smith, B., and Hall, R. (1981): The interaction of Graves' IgG with the thyrotropin receptor. *FEBS Lett.*, 127:17–21.

99. Endo, K., Amir, S. M., and Ingbar, S. H. (1981): Development and evaluation of a method for the partial purification of immunoglobulins specific for Graves' disease. *J. Clin. Endocrinol. Metab.*, 52:1113–1123.

100. Trokoudes, K. M., Sugenoya, A., Hazani, E., Row, V. V., and Volpé, R. (1979): Thyroid stimulating hormone binding to extrathyroidal human tissues: TSH and thyroid stimulating immunoglobulin effects on adenosine 3', 5'-monophosphate in testicular and adrenal tissue. *J. Clin. Endocrinol. Metab.*, 48:919–923.

101. Farid, N. R., Briones-Urbina, R., and Nazrul-Islam, M. (1982): Biologic activity of anti-thyrotropin anti-idiotype antibody. *J. Cell. Biochem.*, 19:305–313.

102. Islam, M. N., Pepper, B. M., Briones-Urbina, R., and Farid, N. R. (1983): Biological activity of anti-thyrotropin anti-idiotypic antibody. *Eur. J. Immunol.*, 13:57–63.

103. Beall, G. N., and Kruger, S. R. (1983): Binding of ^{125}I-human TSH by gamma globulin of sera containing thyroid stimulating immunoglobulin. *Life Sci.*, 32:77–83.

104. Valente, W. A., Vitti, P., Yavin, E., Rotella, C. M., Grollman, E., Toccafondi, R. S., and Kohn, L. D. (1982): Monoclonal antibodies to the thyrotropin receptor. *Proc. Natl. Acad. Sci. USA*, 79:6680–6684.

105. Valente, W. A., Yavin, Z., Yavin, E., Grollman, E. F., Schneider, M., Rotella, C. M., Zonefrati, R., Toccafondi, R. S., and Kohn, L. D. (1982): Monoclonal antibodies to the thyrotropin receptor: the identification of blocking and stimulating antibodies. *J. Endocrinol. Invest.*, 5:293–301.

106. Kohn, L. D., Valente, W. A., Laccetti, P., Cohen, J. L., Aloj, S. M., and Grollman, E. F. (1983): Multicomponent structure of the thyrotropin receptor. *Life Sci.*, 32:15–30.

107. Major, P. M., and Munro, D. S. (1962): Observations on the stimulation of thyroid function in mice by the injection of serum from normal subjects and from patients with thyroid disorders. *Clin. Sci.*, 23:463–475.

108. Volpé, R., Edmonds, M. W., Lamki, L., Clarke, P. V., and Row, V. V. (1972): The pathogenesis of Graves' disease: a disorder of delayed hypersensitivity? *Mayo Clin. Proc.*, 47:824–834.

109. Adams, D. D., Dirmikis, S., Doniach, D., El Kabir, D. J., Hall, R., Ibbertson, H. K., Irvine, W. J., Kendall-Taylor, P., Manley, S. W., Mehdi, S. Q., Munro, D. S., Purves, H. D., Smith, B. P., and Stewart, R. D. H. (1975): Nomenclature of thyroid stimulating antibodies. *Lancet*, 1:1201.

110. Zakarija, M., and McKenzie, J. M. (1978): Adsorption of thyroid stimulating antibody (TSAb) of Graves' disease by homologous and heterologous thyroid tissue. *J. Clin. Endocrinol. Metab.*, 47:906–908.

111. Zakarija, M., and McKenzie, J. M. (1978): Zoological specificity of human thyroid stimulating antibody. *J. Clin. Endocrinol. Metab.*, 47:249–254.

112. McKenzie, J. M., and Zakarija, M. (1979): Factors and concepts in autoimmune stimulation of the thyroid. In: *Autoimmunity in Thyroid Disease*, edited by E. Klein and F. A. Horster, pp. 107–115. Schattauer, Stuttgart.

113. Strakosch, C. R., Joyner, D., Manley, S. W. W., and Wall, J. R. (1982): The species specificity of TSH receptor binding antibodies as measured by the radioreceptor assay. *Clin. Endocrinol. (Oxf.)*, 17:173–179.

114. Schleusener, H., Kotulla, P., Kruck, I., Kruck, G., Geissler, D., and Adlkofer, F. (1976): Comparison and revaluation of radioligand receptor assay and the mouse bioassay for the protection of human thyroid stimulating immunoglobulins. In: *Thyroid Research*, edited by J. Robbins and L. E. Braverman, pp. 414–416. Excerpta Medica, Amsterdam.

115. Kuzuya, N., Chiu, S. C., Ikeda, H., Uchimura, H., Ito, K., and Nagataki, S. (1979): Correlation between thyroid stimulators and 3,5,3-triiodothyronine suppressibility in patients during treatment for hyperthyroidism with thionamide drugs: comparison of assays by thyroid stimulating and thyrotropin displacement activities. *J. Clin. Metab.*, 48:706–711.

116. Davies, T. F., Yeo, P. P. B., Evered, D. C., Clark, F., Smith, B. R., and Hall, R. (1977): Value of thyroid stimulating antibody determinations in predicting short term thyrotoxic relapse in Graves' disease. *Lancet*, 1:1181–1182.

117. Docter, R., Bos, G., Visser, T. J., and Henneman, G. (1980): Thyrotrophin binding inhibiting immunoglobulins in Graves' disease before, during and after therapy, and its relation to long acting thyroid stimulator. *Clin. Endocrinol. (Oxf.)*, 12:143–153.

118. Teng, C. S., and Yeung, R. T. T. (1980): Changes in thyroid stimulating antibody activity in Graves' disease

treated with antithyroid drugs and its relationship to relapse: a prospective study. *J. Clin. Endocrinol. Metab.*, 50:144–147.

119. Bliddal, H., Kirkegaard, C., Siersback-Neilsen, K., and Friis, T. (1981): Prognostic value of thyrotropin binding inhibiting immunoglobulin (TBII) in long term antithyroid drug therapy, ^{131}I therapy given with methimazole and in euthyroid ophthalmopathy. *Acta Endocrinol. (Copenh.)*, 98:364–369.

120. Bliddal, H., Bech, K., Petersen, P. H., Siersback-Neilsen, K., and Friis, T. (1982): Evidence for a correlation between thyrotropin receptor binding inhibition and thyroid adenylate cyclase activation by immunoglobulins in Graves' disease before and after long term antithyroid drug treatment. *Acta Endocrinol. (Copenh.)*, 101:35–40.

121. Bliddal, H., Bech, K., Feldt-Rasmussen, U., Thomson, M., Ryder, L. P., Molholm-Hansen, J., Siersback-Neilsen, K., and Friis, T. (1982): Thyroid stimulating immunoglobulins in Hashimoto's thyroiditis measured by radioreceptor assay and adenylate cyclase stimulation and their relationship to HLA-D alleles. *J. Clin. Endocrinol. Metab.*, 55:995–1001.

122. Kleinman, R. E., Braverman, L. E., Vagenakis, A. G., Butcher, R. W., and Clark, R. B. (1980): A new method for measurement of human thyroid stimulating immunoglobulins. *J. Lab. Clin. Med.*, 95:581–585.

123. Borges, M., Ingbar, J. C., Endo, K., Amir, S., Uchimura, H., Nagataki, S., and Ingbar, S. H. (1982): A new method for the thyrotropin binding inhibitory activity in the immunoglobulin and whole serum of patients with Graves' disease. *J. Clin. Endocrinol. Metab.*, 54:552–558.

124 Sugenoya, A., Kidd, A., Trokoudes, K., Row, V. V., and Volpé, R. (1979): Correlation between thyrotropin displacing activity (TDA) and human thyroid stimulating activity (TSA) by immunoglobulins from patients with Graves' disease and other thyroid disorders. *J. Clin. Endocrinol. Metab.*, 48:398–402.

125. Bech, K., and Madsen, S. N. (1979): Thyroid adenylate cyclase stimulating immunoglobulin in thyroid diseases. *Clin. Endocrinol. (Oxf.)*, 11:47–58.

126. Stockle, G., Wahl, R., and Seif, F. J. (1981): Micromethod of human thyrocyte cultures for detection of thyroid stimulating antibodies and thyrotropin. *Acta Endocrinol. (Copenh.)*, 97:369–375.

127. Hinds, W. E., Takai, N., Rapoport, B., Filetti, S., and Clark, O. H. (1981): Thyroid stimulating immunoglobulin assay using cultured human thyroid cells. *J. Clin. Endocrinol. Metab.*, 53:1263–1266.

128. Smith, B. R., and Hall, R. (1974): Thyroid stimulating immunoglobulins in Graves' disease. *Lancet*, 2:427–431.

129. Pinchera, A., Fenzi, G. F., Bartalena, L., Chiovato, L., Marcocci, C., Toccafondi, R., Rotella, A. C. M., and Zonefrati, R. (1980): Thyroid cell surface and thyroid stimulating antibody in patients with thyroid autoimmune disease. In: *Thyroid Research VIII*, edited by J. R. Stockigt and S. Nagataki, pp. 707–710. Australian Academy of Science, Canberra.

130. Shishiba, Y., Ozawa, Y., Ohtsuki, N., and Shimizu, T. (1982): Discrepancy between thyroid stimulating and thyrotropic inhibitory activities of Graves' IgG's, assessed in the mouse. *J. Clin. Endocrinol. Metab.*, 54:858–862.

131. Vitti, P., Valente, W. A., Ambesi-Impiobato, F. S., Fenzi, G. F., Pinchera, A., and Kohn, L. D. (1982): Graves' IgG stimulation of continuously cultured rat thyroid cells. *J. Endocrinol. Invest.*, 5:179–182.

132. Bech, K. (1983): Immunological aspects of Graves' disease and importance of thyroid stimulating immunoglobulins. *Acta Endocrinol. (Copenh.) [Suppl. 254]*, 103:1–38.

133. Bech, K., Bliddal, H., Siersback-Nielsen, K., and Friis, T. (1982): Production of non-stimulating immunoglobulin that inhibits the TSH binding in Graves' disease. *Clin. Endocrinol. (Oxf.)*, 13:417–424.

134. Wall, J. R., Strakosch, C. R., Bandy, P., and Bayly, R. (1982): Nature of thyrotropin displacement activity in subacute thyroiditis. *J. Clin. Endocrinol. Metab.*, 54:349–353.

135. Pinchera, A., Fenzi, G. F., Macchia E., Bartalena, A., Mariotti, S., and Monzano, F. (1982): Thyroid stimulating immunoglobulins. *Horm. Res.*, 16:317–328.

136. Endo, K., Kasagi, T., Konishi, J., Ikekubo, K., Okuno, T., Takeda, Y., Mori, T., and Torizuka, K. (1978): Detection and properties of TSH binding inhibitor immunoglobulins in patients with Graves' disease and Hashimoto's thyroiditis. *J. Clin. Endocrinol. Metab.*, 52:1113–1123.

137. Konishi, J., Kasagi, K., Endo, K., Mori, T., Torizuka, K., Yamada, Y., Nohara, Y., Matsura, N., and Kajiama, H. (1980): TSH binding inhibitor immunoglobulins in Hashimoto's disease and neonatal transient hypothyroidism. In: *Thyroid Research VIII*, edited by J. R. Stockigt and S. Nagataki, pp. 555–558. Australian Academy of Science, Canberra.

138. Carayon, P., Adler, G., Roulier, R., and Lissitzky, S. (1983): Heterogeneity of the Graves' immunoglobulins directed towards the thyrotropin receptor-adenylate cyclase system. *J. Clin. Endocrinol. Metab.*, 56:1202–1208.

139. Brown, R. S., Jackson, I. M. B., Pohl, S. L., and Reichlin, S. (1978): Do thyroid stimulating immunoglobulins cause non-toxic and toxic multinodular goitres? *Lancet*, 1:904–906.

140. Bolk, J. H., Elte, J. W. F., Bussemaker, J. K., Haak, A., and Vander Heide, D. (1979): Thyroid stimulating immunoglobulins do not cause non-autonomous, autonomous, or toxic multinodular goitre. *Lancet*, 2:61–63.

141. Hart, I. R., and McKenzie, J. M. (1971): Comparison of the effects of thyrotrophin and long acting thyroid stimulator on guinea pig adipose tissue. *Endocrinology*, 88:26–30.

142. Kishihara, M., Nakao, Y., Baba, Y., Matsukura, S., Kuma, K., and Fujita, T. (1979): Interaction between

thyroid stimulating immunoglobulins and thyrotropin receptors in fat cell membranes. *J. Clin. Endocrinol. Metab.*, 49:706–711.

143. Shinozawa, T., and Ingbar, S. (1984): A new serum based assay for fat cell-binding immunoglobulins: application to the detection of the TSH receptor antibodies of Graves' disease. *J. Clin. Endocrinol. Metab. (in press)*.

144. Baker, J. R., Lukes, Y. G., Smallbridge, R. C., Berger, M., and Burman, K. D. (1984): Partial characterization and clinical correlation of specific TSH receptor binding human immunoglobulins as evaluated by direct enzyme immunoassay. *J. Clin. Invest. (in press)*.

145. McGregor, A. M., Dewar, P. J., Petersen, M. M., Miller, M., Rees-Smith, B., and Hall, R. (1980): Prediction of relapse in hyperthyroid Graves' disease. *Lancet*, 2:1101–1103.

146. Zakarija, M., and McKenzie, J. M. (1983): Thyroid stimulating antibody in Graves' disease. *Life Sci.*, 32:31–44.

147. Dirmikis, S. M., and Munro, D. S. (1975): Placental transmission of thyroid stimulating immunoglobulin. *Br. Med. J.*, 2:665–666.

148. Dirmikis, S. M., Kendal-Taylor, P., and Munro, D. S. (1976): The nature and significance of LATS protector. In: *Thyroid Research*, edited by J. Robbins and L. E. Braverman, pp. 403–406. Excerpta Medica, Amsterdam.

149. Seybold, M. E., and Lindstrom, J. M. (1982): Immunopathology of acetylcholine receptors in myaesthenia gravis. *Springer Semin. Immunopathol.*, 5:389–412.

150. Flier, J. S., Kahn, C. R., and Roth, J. (1979): Receptors, antireceptor antibodies and mechanisms of insulin resistance. *N. Engl. J. Med.*, 300:413–419.

151. Harrison, L. (1982): Autoantibodies to hormone receptors. *Springer Semin. Immunopathol.*, 5:447–462.

152. Banovac, K., Zakarija, M., McKenzie, J. M., Witte, A., and Sekso, M. (1981): Absence of thyroid stimulating antibody and long acting thyroid stimulator in relatives of Graves' disease patients. *J. Clin. Endocrinol. Metab.*, 53:651–653.

153. Wall, J. R., Strakosch, C. R., Wellby, M. L., Gooden, J., Joyner, D., and Bayly, R. (1982): Thyroid stimulating hormone receptor antibodies and antibodies stimulating adenyl cyclase in relatives from two families with a high prevalence of Graves' hyperthyroidism. *J Clin. Immunol.*, 2:15–19.

154. Calder, G. A., Penhale, W. J., Barnes, E. W., and Irvine, W. J. (1974): Evidence for circulating immune complexes in thyroid diseases. *Br. Med. J.*, 2:30–31.

155. Cano, P. O., Chertman, M. M., Jerry, L. M., and McKenzie, J. M. (1976): Circulating immune complexes in Graves' disease. *Endocrinol. Res. Commun.*, 3:307–317.

156. Mariotti, S., De Groot, L. J., Scarborough, D., and Mehof, M. E. (1979): Study of circulating immune complexes in thyroid diseases: comparison of the Raji cell radioimmunoassay and specific thyroglobulin-antithyroglobulin radioassay. *J. Clin. Endocrinol. Metab.*, 49:679–686.

157. Ohtaki, S., Endo, Y., Horniuchi, K., Yoshitake, S., and Ishikawa, E. (1981): Circulating thyroglobulin-antithyroglobulin immune complexes in thyroid disease using enzyme linked immunoassays. *J. Clin. Endocrinol. Metab.*, 52:239–246.

158. Thomas, J. L., Montagne, P., Heimfert, C., Cuilliere, M. L., Le Clere, J., Harteman, P., and Duheile, J. (1982): Complexes immuns circulants et dysthyroidies autoimmunes. *Horm. Res.*, 16:345–352.

159. Horvath, F., Teague, P., Gaffney, E. F., Maro, D. R., and Fuller, T. G. (1979): Thyroid antigen associated immune complex glomerulonephritis in Graves' disease. *Am. J. Med.*, 67:891–904.

160. Jordan, S. C., Buckingham, B., Sakai, R., and Olson, D. (1981): Studies of immune complex glomerulonephritis mediated by human thyroglobulin. *N. Engl. J. Med.*, 304:1212–1215.

161. Churchill, D., and Farid, N. R. (1981): Proteinuria in Hashimoto's thyroiditis. *N. Engl. J. Med.*, 305:1286.

162. Van der Heide, D., Daha, M. R., Bolk, J. H., Bussemaker, J. K., De Bruin, T. W. A., Goslings, B. M., and Van Es, L. A. (1980): Circulating immune complexes and thyroid stimulating immunoglobulins before, during and after antithyroid drug therapy in patients with Graves' disease. *Lancet*, 1:1376–1379.

163. Endo, Y., Arstake, Y., Yamamoto, I., Nakagawa, H., Kurbayashi, T., and Ohtaki, S. (1983): Peripheral K cells in Graves' disease and Hashimoto's thyroiditis in relation to circulating immune complexes. *Clin. Endocrinol.*, 18:187–194.

164. Bech, K., Nerup, J., and Larsen, J. H. (1977): Yersinia enterocolitica infection and thyroid disease. *Acta Endocrinol. (Copenh.)*, 84:87–92.

165. Bech, K., Clemmensen, O., Larsen, J. H., and Bendixen, G. (1977): Thyroid disease and Yersinia. *Lancet*, 1:1060–1061.

166. Weiss, M., Ingbar, S. H. Winblad, S., and Kasper, D. L. (1983): Demonstration of a saturable binding site for thyrotropin in Yersinia enterocolitica. *Science*, 219:1331–1333.

167. Weiss, M., Kasper, D., and Ingbar, S. H. (1983): Antigenic cross-reactivity of thyroid membranes and certain gram-negative bacteria. In: *Proc. 65th Meeting, Endocr. Soc., San Antonio Texas, June 8–10*, p. 208, abstract 511.

168. Shenkman, L., and Bottone, E. J. (1976): Antibodies to Yersinia enterocolitica in thyroid disease. *Ann. Intern. Med.*, 85:735–739.

169. Silverberg, J., Row, V. V., and Volpé, R. (1978): Rheumatoid factors in Graves' disease. *Ann. Intern. Med.*, 88:216.

170. Scherbaum, W., Rosenau, K. O., and Seif, F. J. (1978): Rheumatoid factors and thyroid antibodies in Graves'-Basedow disease. *Acta Endocrinol. (Copenh.) [Suppl.215]*, 89:77–78.
171. Tao, T. W., and Kriss, J. P. (1982): Membrane binding antibodies in patients with Graves' disease and other autoimmune diseases. *J. Clin. Endocrinol. Metab.*, 55:935–939.
172. Irvine, W. J. (1975): Autoimmunity in endocrine disease. *Clin. Endocrinol. Metab.*, 4:227–499.
173. Livolsi, J. A., and Lo Grefo, P. (1981): *Thyroiditis*. CRC Press, Boca Raton, FL.
174. Fatourechi, V., McConahey, W. M., and Woolner, L. B. (1971): Hyperthyroidism associated with histological Hashimoto's thyroiditis. *Mayo Clin. Proc.*, 46:682–689.
175. Doniach, D. (1975): Humoral and genetic aspects of thyroid autoimmunity. *Clin. Endocrinol. Metab.*, 4:267–285.
176. Christy, J. H., and Morse, R. S. (1977): Hypothyroid Graves' disease. *Am. J. Med.*, 62:291–296.
177. Totterman, T. H. (1978): Distribution of T, B and thyroglobulin-binding lymphocytes infiltrating the thyroid gland in Graves' disease, Hashimoto's thyroiditis and De Quervain's thyroiditis. *Clin. Immunol. Immunopathol.*, 10:270–277.
178. Totterman, T. H., Gordin, A., Hayry, P., Andersson, L. C., and Makinen, T. (1978): Accumulation of thyroid antigen-reactive T lymphocytes in the gland of patients with subacute thyroiditis. *Clin. Exp. Immunol.*, 32:153–158.
179. Totterman, T. H., Andersson, L. C., and Hayry, P. (1979): Evidence for thyroid antigen-reactive T lymphocytes infiltrating the thyroid gland in Graves' disease. *Clin. Endocrinol. (Oxf.)*, 11:59–68.
180. Skoldstam, L., Anderberg, B., and Norrby, K. (1978): B and T lymphocytes in toxic diffuse goitre. *Clin. Exp. Immunol.*, 31:524–528.
181. McLachlan, S. M., Dickinson, A. M., Malcolm, A., Farndon, J. R., Young, E., Proctor, S. J., and Rees-Smith, B. (1983): Thyroid autoantibody synthesis by cultures of thyroid and peripheral blood lymphocytes. I. Lymphocyte markers and responses to pokeweed mitogen. *Clin. Exp. Immunol.*, 52:45–53.
182. Jansson, R., Totterman, T. H., Sallstrom, J., and Dahlberg, P. A. (1973): Thyroid infiltrating T lymphocyte subsets in Hashimoto's thyroiditis. *J. Clin. Endocrinol. Metab.*, 56:1164–1168.
183. Weetman, A. P., McGregor, A. M., Lazarus, J. H., and Hall, R. (1982): Thyroid antibodies are produced by thyroid-derived lymphocytes. *Clin. Exp. Immunol.*, 48:196–200.
184. Wall, J. R., Baur, R., Schleusener, H., and Bandy-Dafoe, P. (1983): Peripheral blood and intrathyroidal mononuclear cell populations in patients with autoimmune thyroid disorders enumerated by monoclonal antibodies. *J. Clin. Endocrinol. Metab.*, 56:164–169.
185. Canonica, G. W., Bagnasco, M., Cosulich, M. E., Torre, E., McLachlan, S. M., and Rees-Smith, B. (1983): Why thyroid is the major site for thyroid autoantibody synthesis in autoimmune thyroid disease. *Lancet*, 1:163.
186. Richter, E., Wick, G., Zambelis, N., Ludwig, H., and Schernthaner, G. (1978): Demonstration and characterization of thyroglobulin binding peripheral blood cells in Hashimoto's patients by fluoroimmunocytoadherence. *Clin. Immunol. Immunopathol.*, 11:178–189.
187. Ludwig, H., Schernthaner, G., Richter, E., Zambelis, N., and Wick, G. (1978): Thyroglobulin binding cells—a diagnostic marker for Hashimoto's thyroiditis. *Acta Endocrinol. (Copenh.) [Suppl. 215]*, 87:78–79.
188. Gordin, A., Maenpaa, J., Makinen, T., Totterman, T. H., and Tilikainen, A. (1979): Immunological and genetic markers in a family with Hashimoto's disease. *Clin. Endocrinol. (Oxf.)*, 11:425–435.
189. Mori, H., Amino, N., Iwatani, Y., Asari, S., Izuniguchi, Y.,Kumahara, Y., and Miyai, K. (1982): Decrease of immunoglobulin G-Fc receptor bearing T lymphocytes. *J. Clin. Endocrinol. Metab.*, 55:399–402.
190. Sridama, D., Pacini, F., and De Groot, L. J. (1982): Decreased suppressor T lymphocytes in autoimmune thyroid diseases detected by monoclonal antibodies. *J. Clin. Endocrinol. Metab.*, 54:316–322.
191. Thielemans, C., Van Haelst, L., De Waele, M., Jonckheer, M., and Van Camp, B. (1981): Autoimmune thyroiditis—a condition related to decreased T suppressor cells. *Clin. Endocrinol. (Oxf.)*, 15:259–265.
192. Canonica, G., Bagnasco, M., Moretta, L., Cocco, R., Ferrini, O., and Giordano, G. (1981): Human T lymphocyte subpopulations in Hashimoto's disease. *J. Clin. Endocrinol. Metab.*, 52:553–556.
193. Canonica, G. W., Bagnasco, M., Korte, G., Ferrini, S., Ferrini, O., and Giordano, G. (1982): Circulating T lymphocytes in Hashimoto's disease: imbalance of subsets and presence of activated cells. *Clin. Immunol. Immunopathol.*, 23:616–625.
194. Iwatani, Y., Amino, N., Mori, H., Asari, S., Izumiguch, Y., Kumahara, Y., and Mujai, K. (1983): T lymphocyte subsets in autoimmune thyroid disease and subacute thyroiditis detected by monoclonal antibodies. *J. Clin. Endocrinol. Metab.*, 56:251–254.
195. Aoki, N., and De Groot, L. J. (1979): Lymphocyte blastogenic response to human thyroglobulin in Graves' disease, Hashimoto's thyroiditis and metastatic thyroid carcinoma. *Clin. Exp. Immunol.*, 38:523–530.
196. Makinen, T., Wagar, G., Apter, L., Von Willebrand, E., and Pekonen, F. (1978): Evidence that the TSH receptor acts as a mitogenic antigen in Graves' disease. *Nature*, 275:314–315.
197. Wenzel, B., Kotulla, P., Wenzel, K. W., Fink, R., and Schleusener, H. (1981): Mitogenic response of peripheral blood lymphocytes from patients with Graves' disease incubated with solubilized thyroid cell membranes containing TSH receptor and with thyroglobulin. *Immunobiology*, 160:302–310.
198. Balazs, C. S., Stenszky, V., Kozma, L., and Farid, N. R. (1983): Specific suppressor T cell defect in Graves' disease. In: *Proc. 65th meeting, Endocr. Soc., San Antonio, Texas, June 8–10*, p. 207, abstract 507.

199. Noma, T., Yata, J., Shishiba, Y., and Inatsuki, B. (1982): In vitro detection of antithyroglobulin antibody forming cells from the lymphocytes of chronic thyroiditis patients and analysis of their regulation. *Clin. Exp. Immunol.*, 49:565–571.

200. Benveniste, P., Khalil, A., Wenzel, B., Row, V. V., and Volpé, R. (1984): Spontaneous *in vitro* production of thyroid antibodies from peripheral blood lymphocytes of Hashimoto's thyroiditis detected by micro ELISA techniques. In: *Clin. Exper. Immunol. (in press)*.

201. Okita, N., Kidd, A., Row, V. V., and Volpé, R. (1980): Sensitization of T lymphocytes in Graves' and Hashimoto's diseases. *J. Clin. Endocrinol. Metab.*, 51:316–320.

202. Okita, N., Kidd, A., Row, V. V., and Volpé, R. (1981): T lymphocyte sensitization in Graves' and Hashimoto's diseases confirmed by an indirect migration inhibition factor (MIF) test using normal-T lymphocytes as indirect cells. *J. Clin. Endocrinol. Metab.*, 52:523–527.

203. Volpé, R., Edmonds, M. W., Clarke, P. V., and Row, V. V. (1970): A viewpoint regarding the nature of the emergence of long acting thyroid stimulator of Graves' disease. *Acta Endocrinol. Panam.*, 1:155–170.

204. Robinson, R. G., Guttler, R. B., Rhea, T. H., and Nicoloff, J. T. (1974): Delayed hypersensitivity in Graves' disease. *J. Clin. Endocrinol. Metab.*, 38:322–324.

205. Aoki, N., Pinnamaneni, K. M., and De Groot, L. J. (1979): Studies of suppressor cell function in thyroid diseases. *J. Clin. Endocrinol. Metab.*, 48:803–810.

206. Balazs, C. S., Leovey, A., and Borden, L. (1979): Decrease of concanavalin-A activated and short-lived suppressor T cell function in thyrotoxicosis. *Biomedicine*, 30:143–147.

207. Goldrath, N., Shoham, J., Bank, H., and Eisenstein, Z. (1982): Anti-thyroid drugs and lymphocyte function. II. The in vivo effect on blastogenesis and suppressor cell activity in Graves' disease. *Clin. Exp. Immunol.*, 50:62–69.

208. Hallengren, B., and Forsgren, A. (1982): Suppressor T lymphocyte function in Graves' disease. *Acta Endocrinol. (Copenh.)*, 101:354–358.

209. Jones, B. M., Teng, C. S., and Yeung, R. (1982): Evaluation of B cells, T helper and suppressor cell function in patients with Graves' disease before and after treatment with antithyroid drugs. *Clin. Immunol. Immunopathol.*, 25:232–242.

210. McLean, D. B., Miller, K. B., Brown, R., and Reichlin, S. (1981): Normal immunoregulation of in vitro antibody secretion in autoimmune thyroid disease. *J. Clin. Endocrinol. Metab.*, 53:801–805.

211. Pacini, F., and De Groot, L. J. (1983): Studies of immunoglobulin synthesis in cultures of peripheral T and B lymphocytes: reduced T suppressor cell activity in Graves' disease. *Clin. Endocrinol. (Oxf.)*, 18:219–232.

212. Wall, J. R., and Ryan, E. A. (1980): Leukocyte migration inhibition factor production in response to bacterial and fungal antigens in patients with Graves' hyperthyroidism suppression by concanavalin A induced suppressor cells. In: *Autoimmune Aspects of Endocrine Disorders*, edited by A. Pinchera, pp. 235–240. Academic Press, New York.

213. Okita, N., Row, V. V., and Volpé, R. (1981): Suppressor T lymphocyte deficiency in Graves' disease and Hashimoto's thyroiditis. *J. Clin. Endocrinol. Metab.*, 52:528–533.

214. Topliss, D. J., Okita, N., Lewis, M., Row, V. V., and Volpé, R. (1981): Allosuppressor T lymphocytes abolish migration inhibition factor production in autoimmune thyroid disease: evidence from radiosensitivity studies. *Clin. Endocrinol. (Oxf.)*, 15:335–341.

215. Okita, N., How, J., Topliss, D., Lewis, M., Row, V. V., and Volpé, R. (1981): Suppressor T lymphocyte dysfunction in Graves' disease: role of the H-2 histamine receptor-bearing suppressor T lymphocytes. *J. Clin. Endocrinol. Metab.*, 53:1002–1007.

216. How, J., Topliss, D. J., Strakosch, C., Lewis, M., Row, V. V., and Volpé, R. (1983): T lymphocyte sensitization and suppressor T lymphocyte defect in patients long after treatment for Graves' disease. *Clin. Endocrinol. (Oxf.)*, 18:61–72.

217. Wall, J. R., Bear, B., Schleusener, H., and Bandy-Dafoe, P. (1983): Peripheral blood and intrathyroidal mononuclear cell populations in patients with autoimmune thyroid disorders enumerated by monoclonal antibodies. *J. Clin. Endocrinol. Metab.*, 56:164–169.

218. Moller, G. (1978): Role of macrophages in the immune response. *Immunol. Rev.*, 30:1–255.

219. Werner, S. C., and Fierer, J. A. (1972): Cell mediated immunity in Graves' disease? *N. Engl. J. Med.*, 287:1251.

220. Joassoo, A., Robertson, P., and Murray, I. P. C. (1975): Viral antibodies in thyrotoxicosis. *Lancet*, 2:125.

221. Alexander, W. D., Harden, R., and Shimmins, J. (1968): Emotion and non-specific infection as possible aetiological factors in Graves' disease: their relation to thyroid suppressibility. *Lancet*, 2:196–197.

222. Salisbury, S., and Embril, J. A. (1978): Graves' disease following congenital cytomegalovirus infection. *J. Pediatr.*, 92:954–955.

223. Ziring, P. R., Fedun, B. H., and Cooper, L. A. (1975): Thyrotoxicosis in congenital rubella. *J. Pediatr.*, 87:1002.

224. Wick, G., and Graf, J. (1972): Electron-microscopic studies in chickens of the obese strain with spontaneous hereditary autoimmune thyroiditis. *Lab. Invest.*, 27:400–411.

225. Kahn, L. D., and Dale, J. (1973): Virus like particles in Hashimoto's disease and a variety of other tissues. *Lab. Invest.*, 29:350–351.

226. Werner, S. C. (1979): Graves' disease following acute (subacute) thyroiditis. *Arch. Intern. Med.*, 139:1313–1315.
227. Sheets, R. F. (1955): The sequential occurrence of acute thyroiditis and thyrotoxicosis. *JAMA*, 157:139–140.
228. Perloff, W. H. (1956): Thyrotoxicosis following acute thyroiditis: a report of five cases. *J. Clin. Endocrinol. Metab.*, 16:542–546.
229. Volpé, R., Row, V. V., and Ezrin, C. (1967): Circulating viral and thyroid antibodies in subacute thyroiditis. *J. Clin. Endocrinol. Metab.*, 27:1275–1284.
230. Volpé, R. (1979): Subacute (De Quervain's) thyroiditis. *Clin. Endocrinol. Metab.*, 8:81–96.
231. Galluzzo Giordano, C., Andronico, F., Filardo, C., Andronico, G., and Bompiano, G. (1980): Leukocyte migration test in subacute thyroiditis: hypothetical role of cell-mediated immunity. *J. Clin. Endocrinol. Metab.*, 50:1038–1041.
232. Sugenoya, A., Trokoudes, K., Row, V. V., and Volpé, R. (1978): The production of thyroid stimulating immunoglobulin by lymphocytes from patients with Graves' disease cultured with human thyroid subcellular fractions. *J. Endocrinol. Invest.*, 1:245–251.
233. Knight, A., and Adams, D. D. (1983): Lack of allotypic variation in the autoantigen of the thyroid stimulating antibodies. *Clin. Exp. Immunol.*, 52:317–324.
234. Carayon, P., Grubon, T. M., and Lissitzky, S. (1978): Thyrotropin receptor adenylate cyclase system in plasma membranes from normal and diseased thyroid glands. *J. Endocrinol. Invest.*, 1:321–328.
235. Manley, S. W. W., Knight, A., and Adams, D. D. (1982): The thyrotrophin receptor. *Springer Semin. Immunopathol.*, 5:413–432.
236. Garcia, M. A. (1983): The thyrotropin receptor in Graves' disease. Ph.D. thesis, University of Alberta, Edmonton, Alberta, Canada.
237. Eguchi, K., and Ingbar, S. H. (1983): Disease-specific sensitization of Graves' disease lymphocytes in guinea pig fat cell membranes. *Clin. Res.*, 31:527A.
238. Farid, N. R., and Bear, J. C. (1981): The human major histocompatibility complex and endocrine disease. *Endocrinol. Rev.*, 2:50–86.
239. Volpé, R. (1985): Immunology of autoimmune thyroid disease. In: *Autoimmunity in Endocrine Disorders*, edited by R. Volpé. Marcel Dekker, New York.
240. Morillo, E., and Gardner, L. I. (1980): Activation of latent Graves' disease in children. *Clin. Pediatr.*, 19:160–163.
241. Cooper, D. S., Ridgway, E. C., and Maloof, F. (1978): Unusual types of hyperthyroidism. *Clin. Endocrinol. Metab.*, 7:199–220.
242. Murray, G. R. (1903): The clinical history and symptoms of exophthalmic goitre. *Med. Chir. Trans.*, 8:141–153.
243. Sattler, H. (1952): *Basedow's Disease*, Grune & Stratton, New York.
244. Rallison, M. L., Dohyns, B. M., Keating, F. R., Rall, J. E., and Tyler, F. H. (1975): Occurrence and natural history of chronic lymphocytic thyroiditis in children. *J. Pediatr.*, 86:675–682.
245. Yamamoto, T., and Sakamoto, H. (1978): Spontaneous remission from primary hypothyroidism. *Ann. Intern. Med.*, 88:808–809.
246. De Papendieck, L. R., Iorcansky, S., Rivarola, M. A., and Bergada, C. (1982): Variations in clinical hormonal and serological expressions of chronic lymphocytic thyroiditis in children and adolescents. *Clin. Endocrinol. (Oxf.)*, 16:19–28.
247. Gordin, A., and Lamberg, B. A. (1975): Natural course of symptomless autoimmune thyroiditis. *Lancet*, 2:1234–1238.
248. Maagoe, H., Reintoft, I., Christensen, H. E., Simonsen, J., and Magenson, E. F. (1977): Lymphocytic thyroiditis. II. The course of the disease in relation to morphologic, immunologic and clinical findings at the time of biopsy. *Acta Med. Scand.*, 202:469–473.
249. Frey, H. (1981): Intermittent course of chronic goitrous autoimmune thyroiditis. *Acta Endocrinol. (Copenh.)*, 98:210–214.
250. Buerklin, E. M., Schimmel, M., and Wiger, R. D. (1976): Pituitary-thyroid regulation in euthyroid patients with Graves' disease previously treated with antithyroid drugs. *J. Clin. Endocrinol. Metab.*, 43:419–427.
251. Wood, L. C., and Maloof, F. (1975): Thyroid failure after potassium iodide treatment of diffuse toxic goitre. *Trans. Assoc. Am. Physicians*, 88:235–247.
252. Wood, L. C., and Ingbar, S. H. (1979): Hypothyroidism as a late sequela in patients with Graves' disease treated with antithyroid agents. *J. Clin. Invest.*, 64:1429–1436.
253. Jaffiol, C., Baldet, L., Pages, A., Clot, J., and Wilkin, T. J. (1982): Hypothyroidie par thyroidite lymphocytaire: evolution d'une hyperthyroidie Basedowienne traitée medicalement. *Horm. Res.*, 16:345–352.
254. Lamberg, B. A., Salmi, J., Wagar, G., and Makinen, T. (1981): Spontaneous hypothyroidism after antithyroid treatment of hyperthyroid Graves' disease. *J. Endocrinol. Invest.*, 4:399–402.
255. Feldt-Rasmussen, U., Hyltoft Petersen, P., Date, J., and Madsen, C. M. (1980): Sequential changes in serum thyroglobulin and its autoantibodies following subtotal thyroidectomy of patients with preoperatively detectable antithyroglobulin. *Clin. Endocrinol. (Oxf.)*, 12:29–38.
256. Fenzi, G. F., Hashizume, K., Roudebush, C. B., and De Groot, L. J. (1979): Changes in thyroid stimulating immunoglobulin during antithyroid drug therapy. *J. Clin. Endocrinol. Metab.*, 48:572–576.

257. Teng, C. S., and Yeung, R. T. T. (1980): Changes in thyroid stimulating antibody activity in Graves' disease treated with antithyroid drugs and its relationship to relapse: a prospective study. *J. Clin. Endocrinol. Metab.*, 50:144–147.

258. Ader, R. (1981): *Psychoneuroimmunology*, pp. 1–688. Academic Press, New York, ISBN O-12-043780-S.

259. Irvine, W. J., Gray, R. S., Morris, P. J., and Ting, A. (1977): Correlation of HLA and thyroid antibodies with the clinical course of thyrotoxicosis treated with antithyroid drugs. *Lancet*, 2:898–900.

260. Bech, K., Lumholtz, B., Nerup, J., Thomsen, M., Platz, P., Ryder, L. P., Svejgaard, A., Siersback-Neilsen, K., Hansen, J. M., and Larsen, J. H. (1977): HLA antigens in Graves' disease. *Acta Endocrinol. (Copenh.)*, 86:510–516.

261. Torfs, C., King, M. C., Thompson, G., Grumet, F. C., and Okerlund, M. (1982): Evidence for an autosomal dominant inheritance in autoimmune thyroid disease. In: *Proc. 58th Meeting, Am. Thyroid Assoc., Sept. 22–25, Quebec City*, p. T-9.

262. Jayson, M. I. V., Doniach, D., Benhamou-Glynn, N., Roitt, I. M., and El Kabir, D. J. (1976): Thyrotoxicosis and Hashimoto's goitre in a pair of monozygotic twins with serum long active thyroid stimulator. *Lancet*, 2:15–18.

263. Chertow, B. S., Fidler, W. J., and Fariss, B. L. (1973): Graves' disease and Hashimoto's thyroiditis in monozygous twins. *Acta Endocrinol. (Copenh.)*, 72:18–74.

264. Tamai, H., Ohsako, N., Takeno, K., Tukino, O., Takahashi, H., Kuma, K., Kumagai, L. F., and Nagataki, S. (1980): Changes in thyroid function in euthyroid subjects with a family history of Graves' disease: a follow-up study of 69 patients. *J. Clin. Endocrinol.*, 51:1123–1127.

265. Beck, J. S., Young, R. T., Simpson, J. G., and Michie, W. (1973): Lymphoid tissue in the thyroid gland and thymus of patients with primary thyrotoxicosis. *Br. J. Surg.*, 60:769–771.

266. Werner, S. C., Wegelius, O., Fierer, J. A., and Hsu, C. (1972): Immunoglobulins (E,M,G) and complement in the connective tissues of the thyroid in Graves' disease. *N. Engl. J. Med.*, 287:421–425.

267. Michie, W., and Gunn, A. (1966): The thyroid, the thymus and autoimmunity. *Br. J. Clin. Pract.*, 20:9–13.

268. Moens, H., and Farid, N. R. (1978): Hashimoto's thyroiditis is associated with HLA-DRw3. *N. Engl. J. Med.*, 299:133–135.

269. Weissel, M., Hofer, R., Zasmeta, H., and Mayr, W. R. (1980): HLA-DR and Hashimoto's thyroiditis. *Tissue Antigens*, 16:256–257.

270. Schleusener, H., Schernthaner, G., Mayr, W. R., Kotulla, P., Bogner, U., Finke, R., Meinhold, H., Koppenhagen, K., and Wenzel, K. W. (1983): HLA-DR3 and HLA-DR5 associated thyrotoxicosis—two different types of toxic diffuse goitre. *J. Clin. Endocrinol. Metab.*, 56:781–785.

271. Mahaux, J. (1961): L'association exophthalmie ophthalmoplegique-thyroidite chronique avec reactions d'autoimmunite antithyroide. *Acta Clin. Belg.*, 16:292–296.

272. Mason, R. E., and Walsh, F. B. (1963): Exophthalmos in hyperthyroidism due to Hashimoto's thyroiditis. *Bull. Johns Hopkins Hosp.*, 112:323–327.

273. Eversman, J. J., Skillern, P. G., and Senhauser, D. A. (1966): Hashimoto's thyroiditis and Graves' disease with exophthalmos without hyperthyroidism. *Cleve. Clin. Q.*, 33:179–182.

274. Anderson, S. R., Seedorff, H. H., and Halberg, P. (1963): Thyroiditis with myxoedema and orbital pseudotumor. *Acta Ophthalmol. (Copenh.)*, 112:323–327.

275. Wyse, E. P., McConahey, W. M., Woolner, L. B., Scholz, D. A., and Kearns, T. P. (1968): Ophthalmopathy without hyperthyroidism in patients with histologic Hashimoto's thyroiditis. *J. Clin. Endocrinol. Metab.*, 28:1623–1629.

276. Cathelineau, G., and Fribourg-Desi, M. (1974): Ophthalmopathie de type basedowien et hypothyroidie primitive. *Nouv. Presse Med.*, 332:1995–1998.

277. Brownlie, B. E. W., Newton, O. A. G., and Singh, P. (1975): Ophthalmopathy associated with primary hypothyroidism. *Acta Endocrinol. (Copenh.)*, 97:691–699.

278. Martinez-Lavin, M., Vaughan, J. H., and Tan, E. M. (1979): Antibodies and the spectrum of Sjögren's syndrome. *Ann. Intern. Med.*, 91:185–190.

279. Topliss, D. J., Lewis, M., How, J., Row, V. V., and Volpé, R. (1981): Autoimmunity in endocrine disease. *Med. North Am.*, 10:1053–1064.

280. Vento, S., Hegarty, J. E., Bottazzo, G., Macchia, E., Williams, R., and Eddleston, W. F. (1984): Antigen-specific suppressor call function in autoimmune chronic active hepatitis. *Lancet*, 8388:1200–1204.

The Eye and Orbit in Thyroid Disease, edited by
C. A. Gorman et al. Raven Press, New York 1984.

Autoimmunity and Graves' Ophthalmopathy

J. R. Wall

The Montreal General Hospital Research Institute, Montreal, Quebec H3G 1A4, Canada

Although there is considerable evidence that Graves' ophthalmopathy is an autoimmune disorder, the identity and nature of the putative orbital autoantigens have been unknown until recently, and corresponding autoantibodies had not been detected in patients' serum. Moreover, the mechanism for the well-known relationship between ophthalmopathy and hyperthyroidism is unclear. Although Graves' ophthalmopathy usually occurs in association with Graves' hyperthyroidism (though they may be separate in time by many years), the eye disease definitely occurs in the absence of thyroid abnormalities in a small proportion of patients, and in most patients with hyperthyroidism and ophthalmopathy the eye disease tends not to be influenced by treatment of the hyperthyroidism.

Much of the earlier research into the pathogenesis of Graves' ophthalmopathy focused on its association with hyperthyroidism and a possible role of long-acting thyroid stimulator (LATS) (30,36,47,50,55–57,69,94), an immunoglobulin G (IgG) of lymphoid origin that seems to be an antibody directed against some component of the thyroid cell plasma membrane receptor for thyroid-stimulating hormone (TSH) (115). It now seems likely, however, that the eye disease is a separate autoimmune disorder and is not caused by LATS or other TSH receptor antibodies.

The eye changes of Graves' disease have been classified by a subcommittee of the American Thyroid Association (102,103) according to the severity of the changes and the extent of the orbital tissue involvement. There are two main subdivisions: (a) mild ophthalmopathy (lid lag and stare), thought to be due to increased sensitivity of the sympathetic nervous system to catecholamines and attributed to hyperthyroidism per se; and (b) severe ophthalmopathy, a distinct autoimmune disorder which is called Graves' ophthalmopathy in this chapter. When lid lag and stare persist after the patient has become euthyroid, they may indicate immunologically mediated ophthalmopathy.

The clinical features of Graves' ophthalmopathy are due mainly to the orbital inflammation associated with the putative immunologically mediated reactions. The main features—epiphora, conjunctival injection, chemosis, periorbital swelling, and double vision—reflect the sites of the inflammatory reactions. Optic nerve involvement is secondary to orbital congestion and vascular obstruction. Untreated, this may lead to blindness. Corneal ulceration or keratitis due to exposure may also occur. Because of the presumed autoimmune nature of the disease, unilateral ophthalmopathy is expected not to occur, although it is certainly possible that the disease can progress more rapidly in one eye than in the other.

About 80% of patients with progressive inflammation of the orbital tissues have associated hyperthyroidism, and 10% have Hashimoto's thyroiditis, or primary hypothyroidism; the other 10% have no demonstrable thyroid disease, and their ophthalmopathy is called euthyroid Graves' disease or ophthalmic Graves' disease. The true prevalence of ophthalmopathy in hyperthyroid patients is unknown and depends on the parameters examined when making the diagnosis. Discussion of the mechanism of the eye disease clearly depends on a knowledge of this, as its occurrence even rarely in the absence of thyroid disease or in patients with other autoimmune disorders would be highly relevant in respect to its possible pathogenesis. Presently, the diagnosis of Graves' ophthalmopathy is mainly clinical and is based on the demonstration of the characteristic bilateral eye signs in patients with, usually, associated thyroid disease. In difficult cases the diagnosis can be helped by computerized tomography or ultrasonography, which may demonstrate the increased muscle bulk characteristic of the disease (25,104,114), even though these tests may also show a general increase in the volume of the orbital contents which is not specific for ophthalmopathy. Gamblin et al. (29), using raised intraocular pressure (IOP) on upward gaze as the parameter for eye muscle involvement, showed that most patients with Graves' disease have eye muscle disease, and almost all patients with ophthalmopathy have eye muscle involvement. They also showed a high prevalence of eye muscle disease in patients with Hashimoto's thyroiditis (28). Although these findings certainly suggest a close relationship between ophthalmopathy and Graves' disease, they can also be interpreted as providing strong evidence that Graves' hyperthyroidism, Hashimoto's thyroiditis, and ophthalmopathy are three separate autoimmune disorders. Although these findings must be confirmed by others and evidence shown that raised IOP on upward gaze correlates with other parameters of eye muscle dysfunction, this test offers hope for a simple diagnostic clinical procedure. Clearly the controversy concerning the relationship between ophthalmopathy and thyroid disorders will not be resolved for some time, particularly as the parameters for ophthalmopathy are not well established. Thus one needs not only a very sensitive and specific clinical test for eye muscle disease but also biochemical tests to confirm the diagnosis (19). As is discussed here, blood tests for eye muscle antibodies may provide the latter. Indeed, studies correlating IOP on upward gaze with serum levels of antibodies against eye muscle antigens are in progress in the author's laboratory.

Ophthalmopathy in the absence of Graves' disease (opthalmic Graves' disease) was first described in 1945 by Rundle and Wilson (75). Subsequently, Hall and colleagues (30) extended the definition and described the clinical manifestations. They included thyroid enlargement as one of the manifestations. Ormston and associates (67) showed lack of TSH control of thyroid function in some patients with ophthalmic Graves' disease who did not have an overt thyroid disorder. Tamai and co-workers (87) confirmed this and described the natural history of ophthalmic Graves' disease in 27 patients who had been clinically euthyroid initially. Of these, nine became hyperthyroid and two overtly hypothyroid during a 3-year follow-up period. Other groups have shown thyroid abnormalities in patients with ophthalmic Graves' disease and apparently normal thyroid function, including an increased prevalence of thyroid antibodies (67,94) and lack of suppression by T_3 of thyroidal uptake of ^{131}I (67, 87,94,101), suggesting to Liddle and colleagues (49) a "limited thyroid reserve" with the inability to respond to thyroid-stimulating antibodies. Tamai et al. (87) demonstrated thyroid abnormalities in most such patients.

Most investigators have detected LATS and other thyroid-stimulating antibodies in ~40% of patients with euthyroid Graves' disease (12,49,66,85,88,101), although in one study with a radioreceptor assay the prevalence was found to be only 11% (96). Certainly some patients with isolated ophthalmopathy have normal thyroid function, normal thyroid control, and no detectable serum thyroid antibodies (12,67,85,88,96). Thus the evidence suggests that some patients with isolated ophthalmopathy may never have a thyroid disorder. Solomon and associates (85) subdivided euthyroid Graves' disease into three groups: group 1 patients with associated Hashimoto's thyroiditis or Graves' disease detected by thyrotropin-releasing hormone (TRH) response tests, LATS protector (LATS-P), and thyroid nonsuppressibility; group 2 patients with isolated Graves' ophthalmopathy and no associated thyroid disease or detectable thyroid antibodies; and group 3 patients, who show a dissociation between detectable LATS-P and thyroid nonsuppressibility. In summary, these studies suggest that ophthalmic Graves' disease is heterogeneous, either because patients in different phases of the disease were included or because the pathogenesis in the subgroups differed. Again, use of gaze IOP and antibody tests help confirm the existence of ophthalmopathy in the absence of any thyroid abnormality.

This chapter focuses on the underlying mechanisms of Graves' ophthalmopathy, examines theories about its pathogenesis, and discusses in detail new information concerning recently identified eye muscle autoantigens and their corresponding circulating autoantibodies. In so doing, the criteria for autoimmunity, established in 1962 by Milgrom and Witebsky (59), are used as a basis for the discussion.

PATHOLOGY

Histologic findings in the orbital tissues of patients with Graves' ophthalmopathy certainly suggest an immunologically mediated inflammatory reaction. Thus there is widespread infiltration of mast cells, lymphocytes, and plasma cells (48,72,84) as well as an increase in the amount of ground substance and interstitial tissue (2,62,63,100) and of fat and collagen in the connective tissue (73,74,89). Sisson and colleagues (81) showed that lymphocytes from patients with ophthalmopathy can stimulate the production of glycosaminoglycans by cultured fibroblasts obtained from normal human retro-orbital connective tissue, which suggests an interaction between the immune system and the orbital tissues. One of the major sites of the inflammation is the eye muscles, where there is marked lymphocytic infiltration and edema. Indeed, the muscles are enlarged to several times their original size (48,72,81,89). There is also lacrimal gland enlargement [although no increase in lymphocyte infiltration was noted in biopsy specimens of the lacrimal glands of three patients with Graves' ophthalmopathy in one study (97)], and the patients have increased tearing. Later in the course of the disease these glands may become fibrous and atrophic. After the initial inflammatory phase, orbital fibroblasts produce excess collagen and there is scarring. Double vision and permanent proptosis are probably due to scarring of the eye muscles, although this has not been proved by biopsy. A possible cause of the prominent collagen production and scarring may be secretion, *in situ*, of lymphokines that stimulate fibroblasts.

Thus although its association with autoimmune thyroid disorders and the typical histologic findings strongly suggest that Graves' ophthalmopathy is immunologically mediated, the mechanism(s) for the orbital tissue damage is unclear. There are four main possibilities.

First, the disorder may be initiated by reaction of circulating antithyroglobulin autoantibodies with thyroid-derived thyroglobulin (Tg) inserted in eye muscle membranes. The basis for this theory is that thyroglobulin has been demonstrated in normal human eye muscle membranes by immunofluorescence, Ouchterlony precipitation, and binding of [^{125}I]anti-Tg antibody (Ig) prepared from rabbits to normal human eye muscle. Konishi and co-workers (42) showed that retro-orbital muscle has an affinity for both thyroglobulin and thyroglobulin–antithyroglobulin immune complexes, and Mullin and colleagues (60) confirmed the binding of immune complexes to eye muscle membranes and claimed to have shown that thyroglobulin was a component of normal human eye muscle. Furthermore, Kriss and Medhi (46), using a system of artificial lipid vesicles containing eye muscle protein, showed that lymphocytes are involved in reactions against thyroglobulin inserted into the vesicle surface.

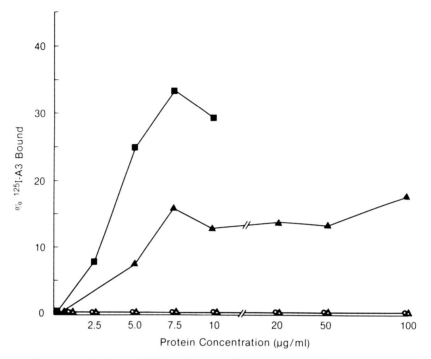

FIG. 1. Percentage binding of [^{125}I]antithyroglobulin monoclonal antibody (Ig) to normal human thyroid (▲), eye muscle (△), and liver (○) membranes (100,000×g pellet) and human thyroglobulin (■). Individual values represent means of three replicates. (From ref. 39.)

These workers postulated that thyroglobulin from the thyroid reaches the orbit by means of the lymphatics which connect the thyroid and orbital tissues (42,76), and when it is deposited in eye muscle membranes (42,44–46) it initiates an inflammatory reaction that involves lymphocytes and killer cells. The evidence against a role of thyroglobulin is considerable, however. Thus the eye disease occurs occasionally in the absence of any thyroid disorder, and there is no close relationship between ophthalmopathy and: (a) the presence or levels of serum thyroglobulin [except in a study by Cupini and colleagues (13)]; (b) titers of antithyroglobulin antibodies; or (c) levels of immune complexes (8). Moreover, because normal T lymphocytes were also able to lyse the vesicles in Kriss and Medhi's study (46), the reactions against thyroglobulin inserted into membranes cannot be specific. Indeed a study by Blau et al. (4) showed that killing of cultured human eye muscle cells by lymphocytes from patients with ophthalmopathy was thyroglobulin-independent.

In our studies, monoclonal antibodies (MCAb) against human thyroglobulin were used as probes to: (a) identify thyroglobulin in eye muscle membranes prepared from normal subjects; and (b) measure binding of human thyroglobulin and thyroglobulin–antithyroglobulin immune complexes to eye muscle membranes. Reactivity of antithyroglobulin MCAb with human thyroglobulin was determined as binding of [^{125}I]antithyroglobulin monoclonal antibody (Ig) and using an enzyme-linked immunosorbent assay (ELISA) and the indirect immunofluorescence technique (39). Seven membrane fractions, prepared by differential and sucrose gradient centrifugation, were used. Whereas significant binding of [^{125}I]antithyroglobulin MCAb was demonstrated for all thyroid membrane fractions tested, including a 100,000×g pellet (Fig. 1), this was not the case for eye muscle membranes.

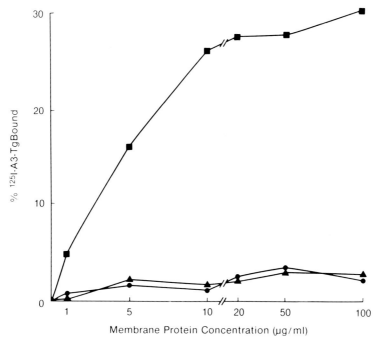

FIG. 2. Binding of [^{125}I]antithyroglobulin monoclonal antibody (Ig)-thyroglobulin immune complexes to human thyroid (■), eye muscle (▲), and liver (●) membranes (100,000 × g). Immune complexes were formed *in vitro* by incubating [^{125}I]monoclonal antibody (Ig) and thyroglobulin in the presence of 13% normal human serum and EDTA/HCl buffer pH 7.2 and in the absence of phosphate. Individual values represent means of three replicates. (From ref. 39.)

Similarly, reactivity of antithyroglobulin MCAb with eye muscle membranes was not demonstrated in ELISA or immunofluorescence tests. Whereas significant binding of thyroglobulin–antithyroglobulin immune complexes to thyroid membranes was demonstrated, this was not the case for eye muscle membranes where binding was not greater than background (Fig. 2). Significant binding of [^{125}I]thyroglobulin to eye muscle or thyroid membranes was not demonstrated for any membrane preparation. On the other hand, modest (but significant) binding to skeletal muscle was shown. Similar results were found using an ELISA. Binding of [^{125}I]antithyroglobulin(Ig)–thyroglobulin or [^{125}I]thyroglobulin to thyroid and eye muscle membranes was not affected by the presence of normal human serum or phosphate, the final pH, or the incubation temperature, conditions claimed by Konishi et al. (42) to be critical for both thyroglobulin and thyroglobulin–antithyroglobulin immune complex binding to thyroid and eye muscle membranes. We have carried out similar experiments using [^{125}I]polyclonal antithyroglobulin antibody (Ig). Significant binding of [^{125}I]polyclonal and antithyroglobulin (Ig) to all thyroid membrane preparations was demonstrated, although the percent binding was generally low. On the other hand, no specific binding to any eye muscle or skeletal muscle membrane fraction was demonstrated (39). In conclusion, because thyroglobulin is not present in normal human eye muscle and neither thyroglobulin nor immune complexes bind to eye muscle, a major role of thyroglobulin or thyroglobulin–antithyroglobulin immune complexes in the pathogenesis of Graves' ophthalmopathy seems to have been excluded by these findings.

Second, Graves' ophthalmopathy may be initiated by the interaction, in eye muscle membranes, of TSH or TSH subfragments (also referred to as "exophthalmogenic factors") with "an abnormal immunoglobulin" (presumed to be an antibody against an eye muscle antigen). Thus for many years it was thought that ophthalmopathy was either an unusual manifestation of Graves' disease or secondary to a pituitary factor secreted in excess by hyperthyroid patients. Several workers had provided evidence for the existence of so-called exophthalmos-producing substances, which included TSH and TSH-like factors (18,32,51,83). There is also some unconfirmed evidence that TSH subfragments, in association with an "abnormal serum immunoglobulin," may play a role in the pathogenesis of Graves' ophthalmopathy (7,40,41,107–110). Against this is the finding that the serum TSH level is very low in patients with associated hyperthyroidism (65). Moreover, Kourides and co-workers (43) found no increase in the level of circulating TSH subunits, and ophthalmopathy has occurred in a patient following total hypophysectomy (27), an event that seems to exclude the possibility of a major role for pituitary factors. In addition, using orbital antigen-directed MCAb, we failed to show any effect of TSH on MCAb binding to their corresponding antigens in human lacrimal gland, orbital connective tissue, eye muscle, or guinea pig harderian gland (99). As is discussed below, we have identified a soluble eye-muscle-derived antigen and corresponding circulating autoantibodies in patients with Graves' ophthalmopathy. Reactivity of serum from patients with Graves' ophthalmopathy and this antigen *in vitro* was not influenced by addition of TSH over a concentration range of 0 to 250 mU/ml (99). However, because we have not tested "exophthalmogenic factors" or TSH subfragments (e.g., as prepared by enzyme digestion of TSH), we cannot exclude a role of a pituitary TSH-like factor, although we believe such a possibility to be unlikely.

Third, orbital tissues and thyroid gland may share antigens; that is, ophthalmopathy and hyperthyroidism would be features of the same disease (Graves' disease), their variable association being due to the variable expression of cross-reacting antibodies or other mediators of the autoimmune reaction.

The association of ophthalmopathy and hyperthyroidism is well recognized. Ophthalmopathy has also been described in association with Hashimoto's thyroiditis (49,61,66,67,85,113) and idiopathic hypothyroidism (9,17,26,58). The response of ophthalmopathy to treatment of the hyperthyroidism is variable. Some workers claim that the eye disease improves after total thyroidectomy (11,105), whereas others think that it may get worse after radioactive iodine treatment (20,34,45,64,68) or partial thyroidectomy (31,82,90). A possible explanation for this assumes a role for thyroid antigens or their antibodies. Thus antibodies (e.g., LATS) and their complexes or antigens may be produced in excess after radioiodine treatment, or they may be depleted after surgical removal of the antigen. Worsening of eye disease when patients become hypothyroid following treatment has been well described (1,32,37). In most cases, however, the disease seems to run a course independent of the thyroid disorder.

Early workers considered that ophthalmopathy, hyperthyroidism, and pretibial myxedema were all manifestations of Graves' disease, and that LATS probably caused all three features by cross-reactivity with shared antigens in the thyroid, skin, and orbit (16,36,47,56). Indeed, some (16,56) pointed to a relationship between the presence and severity of ophthalmopathy and serum LATS level to strengthen this hypothesis. Others (85,88,96), however, demonstrated independence of hyperthyroidism and ophthalmopathy, whereas thyroid-stimulating antibodies (LATS, LATS-P, and human thyroid adenyl cyclase stimulator) are found in only a small proportion of patients with ophthalmic Graves' disease (49,85,88,96,101). Moreover, retro-orbital tissue does not neutralize the biologic activity of LATS (79), which suggests that the LATS antigen does not reside in orbital tissue. One study showed that there was no relation between ophthalmopathy and the serum level of thyroid-stimulating antibodies, as measured with a radioreceptor assay—these antibodies being present in 17 of 25 patients with past or present hyperthyroidism but in only 1 of 10 patients who did not have evidence of thyroid disease (96). The lack of correlation between the antibody level and the severity or duration of the eye disease further indicated the lack of a relation between ophthalmopathy and TSH-receptor antibodies.

In retrospect it is likely that the prevalence and levels of LATS in the serum are related to the severity of Graves' disease as patients with ophthalmopathy tend also to have hyperthyroidism and in some cases pretibial myxedema. Indeed, the presence of LATS has correlated best with the presence of pretibial myxedema (35,70). On the other hand, it is clear that there is some association between thyroid disease and the development of ophthalmopathy. Although a role of TSH subfragments or thyroid-derived thyroglobulin or immune complexes could explain this association, for reasons we have outlined this view is unlikely to be confirmed. One possible mechanism for the association is suggested from work in which an effect of thyroid hormone excess or deficiency on lymphocyte function was demonstrated (93,95). Thus in patients with the prerequisite genetic background, hyper- or hypothyroidism may precipitate a second autoimmune disorder (ophthalmopathy). This could also explain the response of the eye disease to treatment of the associated thyroid disorder.

The possibility of thyroid-orbital cross-reacting antigens (as the cause for the association) has not been excluded. Indeed, Kriss and colleagues (*personal communication*, 1982) produced at least one MCAb which shows cross-reactivity between thyroid membranes and eye muscle membranes, and we are presently evaluating two similar cross-reacting mouse monoclonal antibodies and a very recently produced human EBV-infected lymphocyte colony secreting antibodies against an antigen in human eye muscle, skeletal muscle, and thyroid.

Fourth, evidence is accumulating that Graves' ophthalmopathy is an organ-specific autoimmune disorder in which putative orbital antigens in eye muscle, and possibly lacrimal tissue and orbital connective tissue, are the targets for autosensitized T, B, and/or K cells (52,61,69,97,98). This mechanism does not per se exclude nonspecific or associated effects of TSH-like factors or thyroid-derived factors (other than thyroglobulin).

As described above, in Graves' ophthalmopathy there is marked infiltration of the eye muscles, orbital connective tissues, and adjacent tissues with immunocompetent cells (48,72,84). It is not known whether such cells are mediating humoral immunity [B (bone marrow)-derived lymphocytes], cell-mediated immunity [T (thymus)-derived lymphocytes], or antibody-dependent cytotoxicity [K (killer) cells]. Although the infiltration of target tissues with immunocompetent cells is not specific, it certainly suggests an immunologic basis to the disease.

Orbital autoantigens have not been well defined. The best candidates seem to be antigens that reside in the eye muscle, orbital connective tissue, or lacrimal tissue. The putative antigens may be membranous, cell-surface, or soluble. In guinea pigs and some other experimental animals the orbital connective tissue is largely replaced by the harderian gland, a lubricating gland that has an acinar structure. In humans, however, the connective tissue is loose and poorly defined and, as determined using monoclonal antibodies, does not seem to contain harderian-gland-equivalent antigens (Kuroki and Wall, *unpublished observations*). That the eye muscles are primary targets for the immunologic reaction in Graves' ophthalmopathy is suggested by several pieces of evidence. First, the eye muscles are markedly swollen, as shown by computed tomography (CT) scan and ultrasound in most patients with ophthalmopathy studied during the early phase of the disease, possibly reflecting the effect of "growth-stimulating antibodies" similar to those shown to cause goiter in some forms of chronic thyroiditis (21,22). Second, as discussed above, Gamblin and colleagues (28,29) demonstrated eye muscle dysfunction in most patients with Graves' ophthalmopathy as determined by tonometry on upward gaze. Third, eye muscle weakness associated with double vision is a frequent and often prominent clinical finding. Fourth, lymphocytic infiltration of the eye muscle is invariably found when the muscle is examined histologically. Although the widespread distribution of the inflammatory reaction in orbital connective tissue, lacrimal gland, conjunctiva, and orbital subcutaneous tissues (32,83,97) may be secondary to eye muscle reactions, representing a "spillover" reaction, additional autoimmune reactions in these tissues is a possibility as orbital tissue inflammation, in the absence of eye muscle swelling or dysfunction, is occasionally seen.

Antibodies against orbital antigens had not, until recently, been convincingly demonstrated, although in a few studies (106,111) an "abnormal immunoglobulin" from the serum of patients with ophthalmopathy caused disease when injected into experimental animals. Moreover, Singh and McKenzie (80) showed that an immunoglobulin in the serum of nine of 15 patients with ophthalmopathy enhanced the uptake of ^{35}S-sulfate by the mouse harderian gland. Furthermore, Dandona and El Kabir (14,15) showed an effect of exophthalmic serum on the weight of the guinea pig harderian gland, and antibodies against an extract of guinea pig harderian gland have been found in experimental eye disease by means of a hemagglutination test (71). Fakhri and Hobbs (23) detected antibodies that cooperated with normal lymphocytes in the serum of some patients with ophthalmopathy.

We examined the serum of patients with Graves' ophthalmopathy for orbital antibodies using a tanned-cell hemagglutination test and indirect immunofluorescence (33). In the former, soluble and membrane fractions of human lacrimal tissue and eye muscle, bovine lacrimal tissue, eye muscle, and connective tissue, and guinea pig harderian gland were used as antigen; tanned sheep red blood cells were coated with optimal concentrations of these fractions. In the immunofluorescence test the substrates used were human lacrimal gland and eye muscle, bovine lacrimal gland, eye muscle, and connective tissue, and guinea pig harderian gland. Low titers of antibodies were demonstrated by both techniques in the serum of a few of the patients and in a similar proportion of the healthy subjects and patients with Graves' hyperthyroidism but no ophthalmopathy; the differences were not significant for any fraction or tissue.

In our present studies we are attempting to identify human eye muscle antigens using Ig prepared from patients with Graves' ophthalmopathy and monoclonal antibodies. Using as probe a monoclonal antibody reactive against an antigen in crude human eye muscle cytosol, we have identified a soluble eye-muscle-derived autoantigen, and corresponding circulating autoantibodies, in the majority of patients with active Graves' ophthalmopathy. Thus when crude eye muscle cytosol was chromatographed on Sephadex G-200 superfine (pH 7.4), and 3.7-ml aliquots were tested for reactivity with the MCAb, a peak of reactivity was found to coincide with the major protein peak (Fig. 3). At an antigen concentration of 100 ng/ml, a clear difference between patients with Graves' ophthalmopathy and normal subjects was shown (Fig. 4). Taking the normal range as the mean $\pm$ 2 SD for normals, antibodies were found in 75% of patients with active Graves' ophthalmopathy, in no patient with Graves' disease without clinical eye involvement, and only rarely in patients with Hashimoto's thyroiditis or subacute thyroiditis (38).

Serial estimates of the antibodies were performed in 24 patients with eye disease, including eight who were treated with cyclophosphamide (50 to 150 mg/day for 4 months), and three

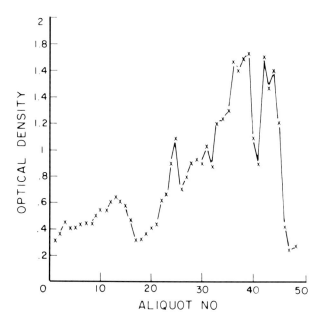

FIG. 3. Reactivity determined using an enzyme-linked immunosorbent assay of a monoclonal antibody against human eye muscle with "human eye-muscle-derived soluble antigen." Crude human eye muscle cytosol was fractionated by Sephadex G-200 chromatography. Aliquots (3.7 ml) were collected, freeze-dried, reconstituted to 0.8 ml in phosphate-buffered saline, and incubated with antibody overnight at 4°C. Results are expressed as optical density at 410 nm.

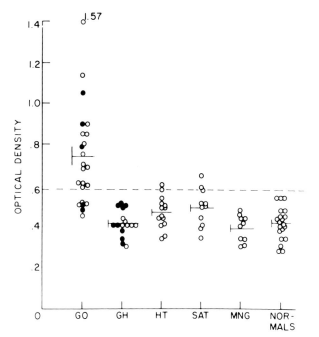

FIG. 4. Serum antibodies against a soluble antigen obtained from human eye muscle. They were measured using an enzyme-linked immunosorbent assay in patients with: active Graves' ophthalmopathy *(GO)* (●, ophthalmic Graves' disease); Graves' hyperthyroidism without eye disease *(GH)* (○, hyperthyroid; ●, euthyroid; ◒ , hypothyroid); Hashimoto's thyroiditis *(HT)*; subacute thyroiditis *(SAT)*; multinodular goiter *(MNG)*; and age/sex-matched normal subjects. Serum dilution was 1:100. Results are expressed as optical density at 410 nm. Horizontal lines represent means (± SE). Broken line (at 0.58) represents the upper limit of normal (mean ± 2 SD for normals). (From ref. 38.)

patients with Graves' hyperthyroidism who developed eye involvement sometime after treatment of their hyperthyroidism. The clinical severity of the eye disease was quantitated using a clinical index based on scores recommended by an American Thyroid Association Committee on classification (102,103). A score of 0 to 3 (3, severe; 2, moderate; 1, mild; 0, absent) was assigned to each of the following: proptosis >18 mm in one or both eyes, conjunctival injection, epiphora, chemosis, periorbital swelling, and eye muscle malfunction.

No patient had corneal ulceration or loss of vision. In all cases the orbital inflammation was active at the time of study.

Improvement (assessed at 6 months), either spontaneously or in association with cyclophosphamide treatment, was assessed as: (a) marked, if there were no signs of inflammation, reduced proptosis, and improved (and stable) eye muscle function; (b) moderate, if the inflammation was much less but still present, with or without reduced proptosis, with stable and improved eye muscle function; (c) mild, if the inflammation was only marginally less with or without a decrease in proptosis and with no significant improvement in eye muscle function; or (d) nil.

Initial antibody levels were correlated with levels of thyroid antibodies and TSH receptor antibodies. There were no significant correlations between eye muscle antibody levels and the antithyroglobulin antibody titer ($r = 0.186$, $p = $ NS), the thyroid cytoplasmic antibody titer ($r = 0.432$, $p = $ NS), or levels of TSH receptor antibodies ($r = 0.369$, $p = $ NS). There was, however, a significant positive correlation between levels of eye muscle antibody and the severity of eye disease, assessed as a clinical index ($r = 0.529$, $p < 0.01$). When tested repeatedly for up to 18 months, levels remained the same in 13, increased in four, and decreased in seven of the 24 patients tested serially. However, in patients who showed a marked or moderate improvement during the first 6 months levels tended to fall, whereas in those who did not improve levels tended to increase with mean ($\pm$ SE) optical density at the onset and at 6 months of 0.95 (± 0.15) and 0.83 (± 0.13) ($p < 0.05$), and 0.71 (± 0.15) and 0.81 (± 0.15) ($p < 0.05$), respectively. By 12 months, levels in patients who were treated with cyclophosphamide for a 4-month period tended to have decreased more than in patients who did not receive such treatment, reflecting the slightly higher levels, initially, in patients with more severe disease, although the differences were not significant for either group.

Serum levels of antibodies were also measured serially in three patients with Graves' disease who developed ophthalmopathy sometime after treatment of the hyperthyroidism. Detectable levels of antibodies against the eye-muscle-derived antigen were demonstrated in all three patients at the time they were hyperthyroid but had no signs of eye disease. Levels increased after the onset of eye disease in one of the three patients and tended to fluctuate over a 10- to 20-month period in two.

When a $100,000 \times g$ human eye muscle membrane pellet was incubated with serum from patients with Graves' ophthalmopathy and normal subjects, absorbance values were found to be very high for both patients and normals. Background, without serum, was also very high. When pure IgG, instead of serum, was used, the same high readings resulted and no difference could be demonstrated between patients and normals.

In order to further study the nature of this presumably nonspecific response, we set up all possible negative controls, eliminating one reagent at a time. A high background response, which was independent of the source of serum or IgG, was shown to be due to a reaction between human eye muscle membranes and the enzyme-conjugated antiserum, irrespective of the source of the serum or IgG. A possible reason for the observed high readings, which could obscure a specific antibody–antigen reaction in patients with Graves' ophthalmopathy, was the presence of blood-derived IgG in the membrane preparation. Using solubilized membrane proteins, it is possible to completely remove contaminating immunoglobulins. However, when eye muscle membranes, solubilized with a variety of detergents, were used as antigen and incubated with IgG prepared from patients and normal subjects, we were again unable to demonstrate differences between the two groups. We next used membrane proteins solubilized with a new zwitterionic detergent, "CHAPSO" (3-[3-cholamido-propyl-

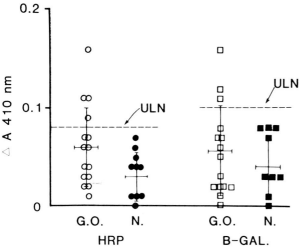

FIG. 5. Serum levels of antibodies against a "CHAPSO-solubilized eye muscle membrane antigen" in patients with Graves' ophthalmopathy assessed using an enzyme-linked immunosorbent assay. Results are expressed as optical density at 410 nm. *ULN* = upper limit of normal (mean ± 2 SD for normals). *B-Gal* = β-galactosidase. *HRP* = horseradish peroxidase. *G.O.* = Graves' ophthalmopathy. *N.* = normals.

dimethylammoniol]-1-[2-hydroxy-1-propanosulfonate]-2H$_2$O), decontaminated of blood-derived IgG by incubating with protein A Sepharose. In this case, using horseradish-peroxidase-conjugated antisera, positive reactions were found in a few patients with Graves' ophthalmopathy (Fig. 5). These findings have been confirmed in more recent tests. Most patients with positive tests had active Graves' ophthalmopathy of recent onset. Patients with negative tests had, generally, mild ophthalmopathy or severe but "burnout" disease. In addition, we have been successful in establishing: (a) a human hybridoma producing an antibody against an eye muscle membrane antigen; and (b) a colony of EBV-infected human lymphocytes producing an antibody against human eye muscle, skeletal muscle, and thyroid membrane antigens.

Sera from patients with active Graves' ophthalmopathy do not contain circulating autoantibodies against: (a) major muscle proteins (actin, myosin, actomyosin); (b) structural proteins (collagen, fibronectin); or (c) glycosaminoglycans (hyaluronic acid, chondroitin sulfate) (Kuroki and Wall, *unpublished observations*).

Although antibodies may be good markers of the autoimmune process, the mechanism for the eye muscle damage is likely to be cell-mediated, involving either K cells (in association with cell-surface-directed antibodies) or T cells. The cytotoxic effect of circulating autoantibodies can be evaluated using as targets dispersed, viable, eye muscle cells labeled with ^{51}Cr. We have developed such assays for assessing the role of thyroid cell cytotoxicity in Hashimoto's thyroiditis and Graves' hyperthyroidism (5,6), and Blau et al. (4) described methods to clone eye muscle cells obtained at surgery or autopsy, allowing the production of large numbers of muscle cells in continuous cell culture for use as a standard target. We are presently attempting to clone human eye muscle cells and develop cytotoxicity assays by modifying the thyroid cell system for use with eye muscle.

Immune complexes have not been detected in the serum of patients with euthyroid Graves' disease [although thyroglobulin–antithyroglobulin complexes are found in patients with associated thyroid disease (10)], and neither r-globulins nor complement has been demonstrated in the orbital tissues of the few patients in whom biopsies or autopsies have been performed (54).

There is also considerable evidence for a role of cell-mediated reactions against orbital antigens, although purified antigens have not been used. Cell-mediated immunity is measured indirectly by the production of lymphokines [particularly macrophage migration inhibition factor (MIF)] and by the transformation of peripheral blood lymphocytes, which measures DNA production. The recently developed leukocyte adherence inhibition test may measure a lymphokine or a cytophilic antibody (53). Several groups (52,60,61) have demonstrated the production of macrophage MIF in response to crude orbital extracts in patients with ophthalmopathy. It has been more difficult, however, to demonstrate the transformation of peripheral blood lymphocytes in response to orbital extracts, although one group of investigators detected significant transformation in response to soluble and membrane fractions of human lacrimal extracts in about one-third of patients with Graves' ophthalmopathy (97). This may be because of differences in sensitivity of the two tests or, more likely, failure to use appropriate antigen concentrations, as determined by dose-response studies, in the transformation tests. In one study significant leukocyte adherence inhibition in response to orbital or lacrimal extracts was not demonstrated in patients with Graves' ophthalmopathy (98).

Serum IgG, IgM, and IgA levels in patients with hyperthyroidism (with or without ophthalmopathy) are usually normal. Studies of patients with ophthalmopathy alone have not been carried out, but their immunoglobulin levels are also expected to be normal. There is often a family or personal history of hyperthyroidism, ophthalmopathy, Hashimoto's thyroiditis, or other autoimmune disorders in patients with Graves' disease (with or without ophthalmopathy). There is also a slightly increased prevalence of Addison's disease, pernicious anemia, rheumatoid arthritis, and diabetes in these patients (91), although these associations have not been documented for patients with ophthalmopathy alone.

Eye disease has been produced experimentally only in guinea pigs immunized with autologous harderian gland extract (71). Proptosis and infiltration of the orbital tissues with lymphocytes and plasma cells developed in association with high titers of hemagglutinating antibodies against harderian gland extract. There have been no other reports of an experimental model.

Although abnormal blood mononuclear cell counts are expected only in patients with widespread autoimmune disorders, e.g., systemic lupus erythematosus, decreased blood counts of "activated" T-lymphocytes (92) [cells thought to be associated with ongoing cell-mediated immune reactions (112)] despite normal total T lymphocyte counts, have been found in about 50% of patients with Graves' ophthalmopathy, an observation which was recently confirmed by Sergott and colleagues (78).

Finally, an association between ophthalmopathy and human leukocyte antigens (HLA) status has been shown by Schernthaner and associates (77), who found an increased frequency of HLA-Dw3 in patients with Graves' ophthalmopathy, although this was not confirmed by two other groups (3,24). Stenszky et al. (86) showed an increased prevalence of HLA-Bw35, in combination with HLA-B8, in patients with ophthalmopathy, as well as a slightly increased prevalence of HLA-B8 (alone) and HLA-DR$_7$ in these patients, suggesting that ophthalmopathy and hyperthyroidism may be separate disorders, a hypothesis which the author favors.

CONCLUSION

Although it is becoming clear that Graves' ophthalmopathy is an organ-specific autoimmune disorder with target autoantigens and corresponding circulating autoantibodies, much work is necessary to elucidate the nature of the antigens and the pathogenetic and clinical significance of the antibodies. Moreover, the likelihood that orbital tissue damage is mediated by T or K cell reactions needs to be studied. The mechanism for the association with thyroid disease is still unexplained. Recent findings from the author's laboratory on monoclonal antibodies reactive with antigens in orbital and thyroid tissues certainly raises the possibility that eye muscle autoimmunity and thyroiditis (including hyperthyroidism) may be linked because of a shared antigen(s). Although the disorders are not invariably associated, possibly because of variable expression of cross-reactivity of orbital and thyroid antibodies, this does support those workers who believe ophthalmopathy and Graves' hyperthyroidism to be closely related. Confirmation of the existence of cross-reacting antibodies, particularly if shown to be cytotoxic to target cells, would be of great importance in our understanding of the autoimmune process.

REFERENCES

1. Aranow, H., Jr., and Day, R. M. (1965): Management of thyrotoxicosis in patients with ophthalmopathy: antithyroid regimen determined primarily by ocular manifestations. *J. Clin. Endocrinol. Metab.*, 25:1–10.
2. Asboe-Hansen, G., and Iversen, K. (1951): Influence of thyrotrophic hormone on connective tissue: pathogenic significance of mucopolysaccharides in experimental exophthalmos. *Acta Endocrinol. (Copenh.)*, 8:90–96.
3. Bech, K., Lumholtz, B., Nerup, J., Thomsen, M., Platz, P., Ryder, L. P., Svejgaard, A., Siersbaek-Nielsen, K., Hansen, J. M., and Larsen, J. H. (1977): HLA antigens in Graves' disease. *Acta Endocrinol. (Copenh.)*, 86:510–516.
4. Blau, H. M., Kaplan, I., Tao, T. W., and Kriss, J. (1983): Thyroglobulin-independent cell-mediated cytotoxicity of human eye muscle cells in tissue culture by lymphocytes of a patient with Graves' ophthalmopathy. *Life Sci.*, 32:45–53.
5. Bogner, H., Schleusener, H., and Wall, J. R. (1983): Cell mediated cytotoxicity against thyroid cells in autoimmune thyroid diseases. In: *Proc. 59th Meeting of the American Thyroid Association, New Orleans, October 1983* (abstract).
6. Bogner, U., and Wall, J. R. (1984): Antibody-dependent and cell cytotoxicity against human thyroid cells in Hashimoto's thyroiditis. *Clin. Res.*, 32:262A (abstract).
7. Bolonkin, D., Tate, R. L., Luber, J. H., and Kohn, L. D. (1975): Experimental exophthalmos-binding of thyrotropin and an exophthalmogenic factor derived from thyrotropin to retro-orbital tissue plasma membranes. *J. Biol. Chem.*, 250:6516–6521.
8. Brohee, D., Delespesse, G., and Bonnyns, M. (1978): Circulating immune complexes in thyroid disease. *Ann. Endocrinol. (Paris)*, 39:20A (abstract).
9. Brownlie, B. E. W., Newton, O. A. G., and Sing, S. P. (1975): Ophthalmopathy associated with primary hypothyroidism. *Acta Endocrinol. (Copenh.)*, 79:691–699.
10. Calder, E. A., Penhale, W. J., Barnes, E. W., and Irvine, W. J. (1974): Evidence for circulating immune complexes in thyroid disease. *Br. Med. J.*, 2:30–31.
11. Catz, B., and Perzik, E. S. (1965): Subtotal surgical ablation of the thyroid, malignant exophthalmos and its relation to remnant thyroid. In: *Current Topics in Thyroid Research*, edited by C. Cassano and M. Andreoli, pp. 1183–1186. Academic Press, New York.
12. Chopra, I. J., Solomon, D. H., Chopra, U., Yoshihara, E., Terasaki, P. I., and Smith, F. (1977): Abnormalities in thyroid function in relatives of patients with Graves' disease and Hashimoto's thyroiditis: lack of correlation with inheritance of HLA-B8. *J. Clin. Endocrinol. Metab.*, 45:45–54.
13. Cupini, C., Mariotte, S., Del Nirno, U., Antonelli, A., and Pinchera, A. (1983): Humoral markers of Graves' ophthalmopathy. *Ann. Endocrinol. (Paris)*, 44.
14. Dandona, P. (1974): Ph.D. thesis, University of Oxford.
15. Dandona, P., and El Kabir, D. J. (1970): The effect of injections of exophthalmic sera on the harderian gland of the guinea pig. *Clin. Sci.*, 38:2 (abstract).
16. Day, R. M. (1978): Hyperthyroidism: clinical manifestations of eye changes. In: *The Thyroid: A Fundamental and Clinical Text*, 4th ed., edited by S. C. Werner and S. H. Ingbar, pp. 663–670. Harper & Row, New York.
17. Dean, G. W. (1968): Ophthalmopathy and hypothyroidism. *Wis. Med. J.*, 67:547–549.
18. Dobyns, B. M., and Steelman, S. L. (1953): The thyroid stimulating hormone of the anterior pituitary as distinct from exophthalmos producing substance. *Endocrinology*, 52:705–711.
19. Donaldson, S. S., Bagshaw, M. A., and Kriss, J. P. (1973): Supervoltage orbital radiotherapy for Graves' ophthalmopathy. *J. Clin. Endocrinol. Metab.*, 37:276–285.
20. Doniach, D. (1982): Autoimmune endocrine exophthalmos. *Lancet*, 2:1378–1379 (editorial).
21. Drexhage, H. A., Bottazzo, G. F., Bitensky, L., Chayen, J., and Doniach, D. (1981): Thyroid growth-blocking antibodies in primary myxedema. *Nature*, 289:594–596.
22. Drexhage, H. A., Bottazzo, G. F., Doniach, D., Bitensky, L., and Chayen, J. (1980): Evidence for thyroid growth-stimulating immunoglobulins in some goitrous thyroid diseases. *Lancet*, 2:287–292.

23. Fakhri, O., and Hobbs, J. R. (1972): Detection of antibodies which can cooperate with lymphocytes. *Lancet*, 2:403–406.

24. Farid, N. R., Sampson, L., Noel, E. P., Barnard, J. M., Mandeville, R., Larsen, B., Marshall, W. H., and Carter, N. D. (1979): A study of human leukocyte D locus related antigens in Graves' disease. *J. Clin. Invest.*, 63:108–113.

25. Forrester, J. V., Sutherland, G. R., and McDougall, I. R. (1977): Dysthyroid ophthalmopathy: orbital evaluation with B-scan ultrasonography. *J. Clin. Endocrinol. Metab.*, 45:221–224.

26. Fox, R. A., and Schwartz, T. B. (1967): Infiltrative ophthalmopathy and primary hypothyroidism. *Ann. Intern. Med.*, 67:377–379.

27. Furth, E. D., Becker, D. V., Ray, B. S., and Kane, J. W. (1962): Appearance of unilateral infiltrative exophthalmos of Graves' disease after the successful treatment of the same process in the contralateral eye by apparently total surgical hypophysectomy. *J. Clin. Endocrinol. Metab.*, 22:518–524.

28. Gamblin, G. T., Galentine, P., Harper, D. G., Chernow, B., and Eil, C. (1983): Screening for elevated intraocular pressure (IOP) on upgaze in thyroid disease. In: *Proc. 59th Meeting of the American Thyroid Association, New England* (abstract).

29. Gamblin, G. T., Harper, D. G., Galentine, P., Buck, D. R., Chernow, B., and Eil, C. (1983): Prevalence of increase intraocular pressure in Graves' disease—evidence of frequent subclinical ophthalmopathy. *N. Engl. J. Med.*, 308:420.

30. Hall, R., Ford, J., and Manson, N. (1967): Ophthalmic Graves' disease. In: *Thyrotoxicosis: Proceedings of an International Symposium, Edinburgh, May 1967*, edited by W. J. Irvine, pp. 210–220. Livingstone, Edinburgh.

31. Hamilton, R. D., Mayberry, W. E., McConahey, W. M., and Hansen, K. C. (1967): Ophthalmopathy of Graves' disease: a comparison between patients treated surgically and patients treated with radioiodide. *Mayo Clin. Proc.*, 42:812–818.

32. Harvard, C. W. H. (1972): Endocrine exophthalmos. *Br. Med. J.*, 1:360–363.

33. Henderson, J., and Wall, J. R. (1981): Failure of hemagglutination and immunofluorescence methods to detect serum orbital antibodies in patients with Graves' ophthalmopathy. *Clin. Endocrinol. (Oxf.)*, 14:153–158.

34. Hetzel, B. S., Mason, E. L., and Wang, H. K. (1968): Studies of serum long-acting thyroid stimulator (LATS) in relation to exophthalmos after therapy for thyrotoxicosis. *Australas. Ann. Med.*, 17:307–311.

35. Hetzel, B. S., and Wall, J. R. (1969): Pretibial myxoedema. *Aust. J. Dermatol.*, 10:18–25.

36. Hoffman, M. J., and Hetzel, B. S. (1966): The clinical significance of plasma thyroid-stimulating activity in hyperthyroidism. *Australas. Ann. Med.*, 15:204–209.

37. Ingbar, S. H. (1968): Large doses of radioiodine in the treatment of thyrotoxicosis. (E). *N. Engl. J. Med.*, 279:1395–1396.

38. Kodama, K., Sikorska, H., Bandy-Dafoe, P., Bayly, R., and Wall, J. R. (1982): Demonstration of a circulating autoantibody against a soluble eye muscle antigen in Graves' ophthalmopathy. *Lancet*, 2:1353–1356.

39. Kodama, K., Sikorska, H., Bayly, R., Bandy-Dafoe, P., and Wall, J. R. (1984): Use of monoclonal antibodies to investigate possible role of thyroglobulin in the pathogenesis of Graves' ophthalmopathy. *J. Clin. Endocrinol. Metab.*, 59:67–73.

40. Kohn, L. D., and Winand, R. J. (1971): Relationship of thyrotropin to exophthalmos-producing substance: formation of an exophthalmos-producing substance by pepsin digestion of pituitary glycoproteins containing both thyrotropic and exophthalmogenic activity. *J. Biol. Chem.*, 246:6570–6575.

41. Kohn, L. D., and Winand, R. J. (1974): Experimental exophthalmos: alterations of normal hormone-receptor interactions in the pathogenesis of a disease. *Isr. J. Med. Sci.*, 10:1348–1363.

42. Konishi, J., Herman, M. M., and Kriss, J. P. (1974): Binding of thyroglobulin and thyroglobulin-antithyroglobulin immune complex to extraocular muscle membrane. *Endocrinology*, 95:434–446.

43. Kourides, I. A., Weintraub, B. D., Ridgway, E. C., and Maloof, F. (1975): Pituitary secretion of free alpha and beta subunit of human thyrotropin in patients with thyroid disorders. *J. Clin. Endocrinol. Metab.*, 40:872–885.

44. Kriss, J. P. (1970): Radioisotope thyroid lymphography in patients with Graves' disease. *J. Clin. Endocrinol. Metab.*, 31:315–323.

45. Kriss, J. P., Konishi, J., and Herman, M. (1975): Studies on the pathogenesis of Graves' ophthalmopathy (with some related observations regarding therapy). *Recent Prog. Horm. Res.*, 31:533–566.

46. Kriss, J. P., and Medhi, S. Q. (1979): Cell-mediated lysis of lipid vesicles containing eye muscle protein—implications regarding pathogenesis of Graves' ophthalmopathy. *Proc. Natl. Acad. Sci. USA*, 76:2003–2007.

47. Kriss, J. P., Pleshakov, V., Rosenblum, A. L., Holderness, M., Sharp, G., and Utiger, R. (1967): Studies of the pathogenesis of the ophthalmopathy of Graves' disease. *J. Clin. Endocrinol. Metab.*, 27:582–593.

48. Kroll, A. J., and Kuwabara, T. (1966): Dysthyroid ocular myopathy: anatomy, histology, and electron microscopy. *Arch. Ophthalmol.*, 76:244–257.

49. Liddle, G. W., Heyssel, R. M., and McKenzie, J. M. (1965): Graves' disease without hyperthyroidism. *Am. J. Med.*, 30:845–848.

50. Lipman, L. M., Green, D. E., Snyder, N. J., Nelson, J. C., and Solomon, D. H. (1967): Relationship of long-acting thyroid stimulator to the clinical features and course of Graves' disease. *Am. J. Med.*, 43:486–498.

51. Ludwig, A. W., Boas, N. F., and Soffer, L. J. (1950): Role of mucopolysaccharides in pathogenesis of experimental exophthalmos. *Proc. Soc. Exp. Biol. Med.*, 73:137–140.
52. Mahieu, P., and Winand, R. (1972): Demonstration of delayed hypersensitivity to retrobulbar and thyroid tissues in human exophthalmos. *J. Clin. Endocrinol. Metab.*, 34:1090–1092.
53. Maluish, A., and Halliday, W. J. (1974): Cell-mediated immunity and specific serum factors in human cancer: the leukocyte adherence inhibition test. *J. Natl. Cancer Inst.*, 52:1415–1420.
54. McGill, D. A., and Asper, S. P., Jr. (1962): Endocrine exophthalmos: a review and a report on autoantibody studies. *N. Engl. J. Med.*, 267:133–140.
55. McKenzie, J. M. (1965): Review: pathogenesis of Graves' disease: role of the long-acting thyroid stimulator. *J. Clin. Endocrinol. Metab.*, 25:424–461.
56. McKenzie, J. M. (1968): Humoral factors in the pathogenesis of Graves' disease. *Physiol. Rev.*, 48:252–310.
57. McKenzie, J. M., and McCullagh, E. P. (1968): Observations against a causal relationship between long-acting thyroid stimulator and ophthalmopathy in Graves' disease. *J. Clin. Endocrinol. Metab.*, 28:1177–1182.
58. Michaelson, E. D., and Young, R. L. (1970): Hypothyroidism with Graves' disease. *JAMA*, 211:1351–1354.
59. Milgrom, F., and Witebsky, E. (1962): Autoantibodies and autoimmune diseases. *JAMA*, 181:706–716.
60. Mullin, B. R., Levinson, R. E., Friedman, A., Henson, D. E., Winand, R. J., and Kohn, L. D. (1977): Delayed hypersensitivity in Graves' disease and exophthalmos—identification of thyroglobulin in human orbital muscle. *Endocrinology*, 100:351–366.
61. Munro, R. E., Lamki, L., Row, V. V., and Volpé, R. (1973): Cell-mediated immunity in the exophthalmos of Graves' disease as demonstrated by the migration inhibition factor (MIF) test. *J. Clin. Endocrinol. Metab.*, 37:286–292.
62. Naffziger, H. C. (1931): Progressive exophthalmos following thyroidectomy: its pathology and treatment. *Ann. Surg.*, 94:582–586.
63. Naffziger, H. C. (1933): Pathologic changes in the orbit in progressive exophthalmos with special reference to alterations in the extra-ocular muscles and the optic disks. *Arch. Ophthalmol.*, 9:1–12.
64. Naffziger, H. C., and Jones, O. W., Jr. (1932): Surgical treatment of progressive exophthalmos following thyroidectomy. *JAMA*, 99:638–642.
65. Odell, W. D., Wilber, J. F., and Utiger, R. D. (1967): Studies of thyrotropin physiology by means of radioimmunoassay. *Recent Prog. Horm. Res.*, 23:47–85.
66. O'Donnell, J., Trokoudes, K., Silverberg, J., Row, V., and Volpé, R. (1978): Thyrotropin displacement activity of serum immunoglobulins from patients with Graves' disease. *J. Clin. Endocrinol. Metab.*, 46:770–777.
67. Ormston, B. J., Alexander, L., Evered, D. C., Clark, F., Bird, T., Appleton, T., and Hall, R. (1973): Thyrotrophin response to thyrotrophin-releasing hormone in ophthalmic Graves' disease: correlation with other aspects of thyroid function, thyroid suppressibility and activity of eye signs. *Clin. Endocrinol. (Oxf.)*, 2:369–376.
68. Pequegnat, E. P., Mayberry, W. E., McConahey, W. M., and Wyse, E. P. (1967): Large doses of radioiodine in Graves' disease: effect on ophthalmopathy and long-acting thyroid stimulator. *Mayo Clin. Proc.*, 42:802–811.
69. Pimstone, B. L., Hoffenberg, R., and Black, E. (1964): Parallel assays of thyrotrophin, long-acting thyroid stimulator and exophthalmos-producing substance in endocrine exophthalmos and pretibial myxedema. *J. Clin. Endocrinol. Metab.*, 24:976–982.
70. Pinchera, A., Pinchera, M. G., and Stanbury, J. B. (1965): Thyrotropin and long-acting thyroid stimulator assays in thyroid disease. *J. Clin. Endocrinol. Metab.*, 25:189–208.
71. Pisarev, M. A., Altschuler, N., and Davidson, T. A. (1968): Immune exophthalmos due to harderian gland antigen. *Endocrinology*, 83:903–906.
72. Riley, F. C. (1972): Orbital pathology in Graves' disease. *Mayo Clin. Proc.*, 47:975–979.
73. Rundle, F. F., Finlay-Jones, L. R., and Noad, K. B. (1953): Malignant exophthalmos: a quantitative analysis of the orbital tissues. *Australas. Ann. Med.*, 2:128–135.
74. Rundle, F. F., and Pochin, E. E. (1944): The orbital tissues in thyrotoxicosis: a quantitative analysis relating to exophthalmos. *Clin. Sci.*, 5:51–74.
75. Rundle, F. F., and Wilson, C. W. (1945): Asymmetry of exophthalmos in orbital tumour and Graves' disease. *Lancet*, 1:51–52.
76. Ruszynak, I., Foldi, M., and Szabo, G. (1967): In: *Lymphatics and Lymph Circulation; Physiology and Pathology*, 2nd ed., edited by L. Youlton, pp. 187–194. Pergamon, Oxford.
77. Schernthaner, G., Ludwig, H., Mayr, W. R., and Hofer, R. (1977): Genetic heterogeneity in thyrotoxicosis patients with and without endocrine ophthalmopathy. *Diabetes Metab.*, 3:189–192.
78. Sergott, R. C., Felberg, N. T., Savino, P. J., Blizzard, J. J., and Schatz, N. J. (1979): E-rosette formation in Graves' ophthalmopathy. *Invest. Ophthalmol. Vis. Sci.*, 18:1245–1251.
79. Shillinglaw, J., and Utiger, R. D. (1968): Failure of retro-orbital tissue to neutralize the biological activity of the long-acting thyroid stimulator. *J. Clin. Endocrinol. Metab.*, 28:1069–1070.
80. Singh, S. P., and McKenzie, J. M. (1969): Effects of thyrotrophin on ^{35}S-sulfate uptake by mouse harderian gland. *Endocrinology*, 85:952–955.
81. Sisson, J. C., Kothary, P., and Kirchick, H. (1973): The effects of lymphocytes, sera, and long-acting thyroid

stimulator from patients with Graves' disease on retrobulbar fibroblasts. *J. Clin. Endocrinol. Metab.*, 37:17–24.

82. Sloan, L. W. (1951): Surgical treatment of hyperthyroidism. *N.Y. J. Med.*, 51:2897–2902.

83. Smelser, G. K. (1936): Experimental production of exophthalmos resembling that found in Graves' disease. *Proc. Soc. Exp. Biol. Med.*, 35:128–130.

84. Smelser, G. K. (1937): A comparative study of experimental and clinical exophthalmos. *Am. J. Ophthalmol.*, 20:1189–1203.

85. Solomon, D. H., Chopra, I. J., Chopra, U., and Smith, F. J. (1977): Identification of subgroups of euthyroid Graves' ophthalmopathy. *N. Engl. J. Med.*, 296:181–186.

86. Stenszky, V., Kozma, L., Balazo, C. S., and Farid, N. R. (1983): HLA-DR associations with Graves' disease in Eastern Hungary. *Clin. Invest. Med.*, 6:181–184.

87. Tamai, H., Nakagawa, T., Ohsako, N., Fukino, O., Takahashi, H., Matsuzurka, F., Kuma, K., and Nagataki, S. (1980): Changes in thyroid functions in patients with euthyroid Graves' disease. *J. Clin. Endocrinol. Metab.*, 50:108–112.

88. Teng, C. S., Smith, B. R., Clayton, B., Evered, D. C., Clark, F., and Hall, R. (1977): Thyroid-stimulating immunoglobulins in ophthalmic Graves' disease. *Clin. Endocrinol. (Oxf.)*, 6:207–211.

89. Tengroth, B. (1964): Histological studies of orbital tissues in a case of endocrine exophthalmos before and after remission. *Acta Ophthalmol. (Copenh.)*, 42:588–591.

90. Thomas, H. M., Jr., and Woods, A. C. (1936): Progressive exophthalmos following thyroidectomy. *Bull. Johns Hopkins Hosp.*, 59:99–113.

91. Volpé, R. (1977): The role of autoimmunity in hypoendocrine and hyperendocrine function with special emphasis on autoimmune thyroid disease. *Ann. Intern. Med.*, 87:86–99.

92. Wall, J. R., Gray, B., and Greenwood, D. M. (1977): Total and "activated" peripheral blood T-lymphocytes in patients with thyroid disorders. *Acta Endocrinol. (Copenh.)*, 85:753–759.

93. Wall, J. R., Joyner, D. M., Ryan, E. A., and Wren, S. F. G. (1979): Effect of experimental hyper- and hypothyroidism on B and T lymphocyte reactivity to bacterial, fungal and tissue antigens. In: *Proceedings of the Serono Symposium on Autoimmune Aspects of Endocrine Disorders, Pisa, Italy, April 1979*, vol. 33, edited by A. Pinchera, D. Doniach, G. F. Fenzi, and L. Baschieri, pp. 215–219. Academic Press, New York.

94. Wall, J. R., Odgers, R. J., and Hetzel, B. S. (1973): Immunological studies of the eye changes of thyrotoxicosis. *Aust. N. Z. J. Med.*, 3:162–168.

95. Wall, J. R., and Ryan, E. A. (1980): Effect of experimental hyper- and hypothyroidism on immune reactivity. In: *Proceedings of the 8th International Thyroid Congress, Sydney, Australia, February 3–8*, edited by J. R. Stockitt and S. Nagataki, pp. 781–784. Australian Academy of Science, Canberra.

96. Wall, J. R., Strakosch, C. R., Fang, S. L., Ingbar, S. H., and Braverman, L. E. (1979): Thyroid binding antibodies and other immunological abnormalities in patients with Graves' ophthalmopathy: effect of treatment with cyclophosphamide. *Clin. Endocrinol. (Oxf.)*, 10:79–91.

97. Wall, J. R., Trewin, A., Fang, S. L., Ingbar, S. H., and Braverman, L. E. (1978): Studies on immunoreactivity to human lacrimal gland fractions in patients with ophthalmic Graves' disease. *J. Endocrinol. Invest.*, 1:253–258.

98. Wall, J. R., Walters, B. A., and Grant, C. (1979): Leukocyte adherence inhibition in response to human orbital and lacrimal extracts in patients with Graves' ophthalmopathy. *J. Endocrinol. Invest.*, 2:375–378.

99. Waring, S., Kodama, K., Sikorska, H., and Wall, J. R. (1983): TSH and orbital antibodies. *Lancet*, 2:224–225.

100. Wegelius, O., Naumann, J., and Brunish, R. (1959): Uptake of ^{35}S-labelled sulfate in the harderian and the ventral lacrimal glands of the guinea pig during stimulation with ophthalmotrophic pituitary agents: a new assay method for the ophthalmotrophic activity in thyrotropin preparations. *Acta Endocrinol. (Copenh.)*, 30:53–60.

101. Werner, S. C. (1955): Euthyroid patients with early eye signs of Graves' disease: their responses to L-triiodothyronine and thyrotropin. *Am. J. Med.*, 18:608–612.

102. Werner, S. C. (1969): Classification of the eye changes in Graves' disease (C). *J. Clin. Endocrinol. Metab.*, 29:982–984.

103. Werner, S. C. (1977): Modification of the classification of the eye changes in Graves' disease: recommendations of the Ad Hoc Committee of the American Thyroid Association (C). *J. Clin. Endocrinol. Metab.*, 44:203–204.

104. Werner, S. C., Coleman, J., and Franzen, L. A. (1974): Ultrasonographic evidence of a consistent orbital involvement in Graves' disease. *N. Engl. J. Med.*, 290:1447–1450.

105. White, I. L. (1979): Total thyroid ablation: a prerequisite to orbital decompression for Graves' disease ophthalmopathy. *Laryngoscope*, 84:1869–1875.

106. Winand, R. (1971): Endocrinologie et immunologie. In: *Rapports de la XIème Réunion des Endocrinologistes de Langue Française. Les Adénomes Hypophysaires Secrétants: Endocrinopathies et Immunologie*, edited by H. Van Cauwenberg and A. Luyck, pp. 309–315. Masson, Paris.

107. Winand, R. J., and Kohn, L. D. (1970): Relationship of thyrotropin to exophthalmic-producing substance: purification of homogeneous glycoproteins containing both activities from [^{3}H]-labeled pituitary extracts. *J. Biol. Chem.*, 245:967–975.

108. Winand, R. J., and Kohn, L. D. (1972): Pathogenesis of human and experimental exophthalmos. In: *Proceedings of the Fourth International Congress of Endocrinology, Washington, D. C., June 18–24*, edited by R. O. Scow, F. G. J. Ebling, and I. W. Henderson, pp. 1150–1155. Excerpta Medica, Amsterdam.

109. Winand, R. J., and Kohn, L. D. (1972): The binding of [³H] thyrotropin and ³H-labelled exophthalmogenic factor by plasma membranes of retro-orbital tissue. *Proc. Natl. Acad. Sci. USA*, 69:1711–1715.

110. Winand, R. J., and Kohn, L. D. (1975): Stimulation of adenylate cyclase activity in retro-orbital tissue membranes by thyrotropin and an exophthalmogenic factor derived from thyrotropin. *J. Biol. Chem.*, 250:6522–6526.

111. Winand, R. J., Salmon, J., and Lambert, P. H. (1971): Characterization of the exophthalmic factor isolated from the serum of patients with malignant exophthalmos. In: *Further Advances in Thyroid Research*, edited by K. Fellinger and R. Hofer, pp. 583–593. Verlage der Wiener Mediz Akad, Vienna.

112. Wybran, J., and Fundenberg, H. H. (1973): Thymus-derived rosette-forming cells in various human disease states: cancer, lymphoma, bacterial and viral infections and other diseases. *J. Clin. Invest.*, 52:1026–1032.

113. Wyse, E. P., McConahey, W. M., Woolner, L. B., Scholz, D. A., and Kearns, T. P. (1968): Ophthalmopathy without hyperthyroidism in patients with histologic Hashimoto's thyroiditis. *J. Clin. Endocrinol. Metab.*, 28:1623–1629.

114. Yamamoto, K., Itoh, K., Yoshida, S., Saito, K., Sakamoto, Y., Matsuda, A., Saito, T., and Kuzuya, T. (1979): A quantitative analysis of orbital soft tissue in Graves' disease based on B-mode ultrasonography. *Endocrinol. Jpn.*, 26:255–261.

115. Zakarija, M., McKenzie, J. M., and Banovac, K. (1980): Clinical significance of assay of thyroid-stimulating antibody in Graves' disease. *Ann. Intern. Med.*, 93:28–32.

The Eye and Orbit in Thyroid Disease, edited by
C. A. Gorman et al. Raven Press, New York 1984.

Graves' Disease and Myasthenia Gravis

*Michael J. Garlepp and †Roger L. Dawkins

†*Departments of Clinical Immunology, Royal Perth Hospital and The Queen Elizabeth II Medical
Centre, and* *†*University of Western Australia, Perth, Western Australia 6001*

The association between myasthenia gravis (MG) and thyroid disease, particularly Graves' disease, has been known for many years. Approximately 5% of patients with MG are said to develop Graves' disease, although a lesser percentage of those with thyrotoxicosis (0.2%) subsequently develop MG (27,33). The two diseases have much in common. Both are mediated by autoantibodies to membrane receptors, and they share certain immunogenetic features, e.g., HLA and Gm associations. In this chapter we review these similarities after discussing the pathogenesis of MG and then explore the overlap between the two diseases.

MYASTHENIA GRAVIS

MG is a disease of skeletal muscle characterized by excessive muscle fatigability which can be reversed by administration of anticholinesterase. In 1960 Simpson postulated an autoimmune etiology for MG (32). This hypothesis was based, in part, on the frequent co-occurrence of thyroid disease and thyroid autoantibodies in patients with MG. Subsequently it has been demonstrated that the vast majority (>90%) of patients with generalized adult-onset MG possess an autoantibody which is responsible for the clinical features of the disease (22). This autoantibody reacts with the nicotinic acetylcholine receptor (AChR) of skeletal muscle. Most information regarding the structure of the nicotinic AChR has come from the study of AChR purified from the electric organs of *Torpedo* spp. or *Electrophorus* spp. The AChR is a pentamer of molecular weight 250,000. The subunits are present in a molar stoichiometry $\alpha_2\beta\gamma\delta$ and have molecular weights of 40,000, 50,000, 60,000, and 65,000, respectively (23). Purification of mammalian AChR has provided evidence for subunits of similar size (25). Together these subunits make up the ACh binding site and the ion channel which opens after ACh attachment, resulting in depolarization of the muscle membrane.

Patients with generalized MG have been shown to have a decreased number of AChR at their motor end-plates (11), and electron microscopic studies have shown the motor end-plates to be simplified with decreased junctional folds and widened synaptic space. Furthermore, immunoglobulin and complement have been demonstrated to be present on the postsynaptic membrane using ultrastructural techniques (10).

The most commonly used assay for anti-AChR is that described by Lindstrom (22). The specificity and high affinity of α-bungarotoxin (α-neurotoxin from *Bungarus multicinctus*) for the AChR allows it to be tagged in a crude muscle extract by means of radiolabeled toxin. Anti-AChR may then be detected by means of a radioimmunoassay (16,22).

The mechanism of action of anti-AChR has yet to be clarified. Four possible mechanisms are generally considered, and each has gained some experimental support (1,7):

1. Directly blocking access of ACh to AChR could result in the defect in neuromuscular transmission seen in MG. Some patients do possess anti-AChR capable of blocking AChR, although these autoantibodies seem to be in the minority.

2. A further mechanism is that of antigenic modulation. Here anti-AChR directed at antigenic determinants peripheral to the ACh binding site cross-link adjacent AChR, causing aggregation, internalization, and an increase in degradation rate. This results in a decrease in available AChR at the motor end-plate.

3. Complement may be important in bringing about damage to the postsynaptic membrane with a resultant loss of AChR. Depletion of C3 or C4 in rats or mice reduced the pathogenic effect of passively transferred anti-AChR (21,35), although the absence of C5 had no effect (35).

4. Anti-AChR bound to receptor might also impair function by preventing a conformational change normally induced by ACh binding and so prevent depolarization of the postsynaptic membrane (1).

Whatever the mechanism of action of anti-AChR, several pieces of evidence indicate that it has a primary role in disease pathogenesis:

1. Present in majority of patients with generalized MG.
2. Titer fluctuates with disease activity in the individual patient.
3. Therapy which reduces anti-AChR titer is effective treatment.
4. Passive transfer (transplacental or to mice) produces disease.
5. Presence of anti-AChR in D-penicillamine-induced MG.
6. Presence of anti-AChR in idiopathic canine MG.
7. Anti-AChR responsible for disease signs in experimental autoimmune MG.
8. Monoclonal experimental anti-AChR produces signs of experimental autoimmune MG.

The utility of the assay for anti-AChR as an aid in the diagnosis of MG is beyond doubt. However, attention must be paid to several points when interpreting the results. The assay used to measure anti-AChR is critical. Assays using heterologous antigen or detecting blocking anti-AChR are less sensitive than those using human AChR as antigen.

One should be aware of the clinical subgroup of MG under consideration (Fig. 1). Patients classified as juvenile or congenital MG (disease onset at < 12 years of age) may have disease mediated by anti-AChR, but the majority have myasthenia of diverse etiology, which is probably not autoimmune in origin (9). Patients with mild generalized MG may have ocular muscle involvement which progresses to generalized weakness with a rise in anti-AChR titer. In some cases, however, disease remains restricted to the ocular muscles. Anti-AChR is rare in such patients. The autoantibody profiles and the HLA association in restricted ocular MG differ from those in generalized MG, and the disease may be mediated by an autoantibody directed at ocular muscle which is not detected by the current anti-AChR assay (see below). Thus the standard assay is less useful in these conditions. The relationship between restricted ocular MG, generalized MG, and thyrotoxicosis is depicted in Fig. 2. Although clearly an oversimplification, at least these relationships can be tested.

The clinician should be aware of the occasional apparent "false-positive" result in some patients with systemic lupus erythematosus (SLE), thyrotoxicosis, or thymoma. We believe that such patients have subclinical or latent MG and that subsequent elevation of anti-AChR titer above their particular "threshold" results in the development of overt disease (4,16).

Antibodies to the contractile components of skeletal muscle may also be seen in MG. These antistriational antibodies are related to the presence of a thymoma in MG (28). Their pathogenic role is unknown.

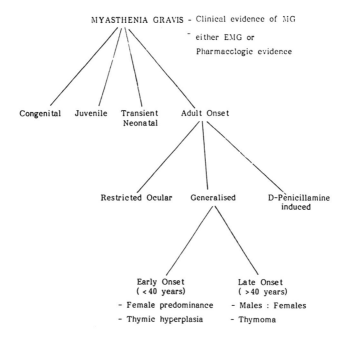

FIG. 1. Subgroups of MG. D-Penicillamine-induced MG may present with ocular or generalized muscle involvement but is almost invariably anti-AChR-positive. Several forms of congenital and juvenile myasthenia have been described. Transient neonatal MG is mediated by anti-AChR after placental transfer.

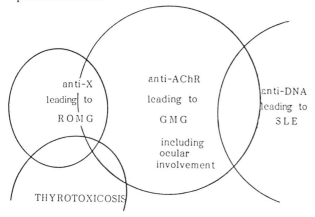

FIG. 2. Oversimplified model of the possible relationships among: generalized MG *(GMG)* mediated by anti-AChR, which can affect peripheral and extraocular muscle; restricted ocular MG *(ROMG)*, possibly mediated by a separate autoantibody *(anti-X)* which has little if any effect on peripheral muscle; systemic lupus erythematosus *(SLE)*; and Graves' disease. The relationships of subtypes of Graves' disease are not shown.

SIMILARITIES BETWEEN MG AND GRAVES' DISEASE

Autoantibodies

A comparison of anti-AChR and antibodies to the thyrotropin (thyroid-stimulating hormone; TSH) receptor (anti-TSHR) is shown in Table 1. Both autoantibodies are capable of bringing about their effect by binding to antigenic determinants peripheral to the hormone binding site. Both have been shown to vary in their degree of cross-reactivity with xenogeneic receptors when various patients are compared (18,38). In the case of anti-AChR this variation in specificity probably reflects reactivity with different antigenic determinants on

TABLE 1. *Comparison of Anti-AChR and anti-TSHR*

Characteristic	Anti-AChR	Anti-TSHR
Immunoglobulin class	IgG	IgG
Specificity varies among patients resulting in:		
Variation in xenogeneic cross-reactivity	+	+
Individual threshold titers	+	+
Sequential titers reflect fluctuations in disease activity	+	+
Causes transient disease in neonate	+	+
May block hormone binding	+	+
May be trophic	?	+
May be stimulatory	?	+

the AChR and determines its effectivensss in the induction of motor end-plate damage and muscle weakness.

Fine specificity may also determine whether thyrotropin receptor binding antibodies stimulate thyroid hormone production, stimulate thyroid growth, or prevent access of TSH to its receptor (8,24). The specificity may determine the disease manifestations in any particular patient.

The titers of these autoantibodies cannot be used to predict disease severity between patients. Within the one patient, however, fluctuations in titer reflect disease activity so that anti-AChR measurement may be used to monitor MG in an individual patient (16). The same is true in Graves' disease. Successful therapy results in a fall in anti-TSHR titer, and persistence of the autoantibody has been used as an indicator of subsequent relapse (6,12).

Immunogenetics

In Caucasians it has been clear for several years that HLA B8 is associated with a subgroup of patients with MG who develop disease before 40 years of age, have thymic hyperplasia and high titers of anti-AChR, and are predominantly female. This association has since been shown to reflect an association with the supratype A1,B8,C4AQ0, C4B1,BfS,DR3 (5).

Several reports have implicated HLA B8 with Graves' disease in Caucasians, but it has now been demonstrated that DR3 is more strongly associated with Graves' disease than is HLA B8 (12), and, as with MG, the association of B8,DR3 is with early onset of disease. It is likely that further investigation will reveal the strongest association with the above-mentioned supratype. The demonstration of reduced C4 concentrations in HLA B8-positive patients with Graves' disease probably reflects the presence of the C4A null allele (34).

In both diseases HLA B8 has also been associated with a suppressor cell defect (2,39). Such a defect may be important in conferring susceptibility to relapse in Graves' disease patients with DR3 (12,30) as well as the high anti-AChR titers and fluctuating disease course in patients with MG who have HLA B8,DR3.

As mentioned above, MG is a heterogeneous disease. HLA Bw35 and DR1 are associated with D-penicillamine-induced MG (14), whereas DR5 is increased in purely ocular MG (Garlepp, *unpublished observations*).

Graves' disease is also immunogenetically heterogeneous. HLA DR3 has been associated with ophthalmopathy and the presence of anti-TSHR (12,30), whereas DR5 was associated with the absence of both of these features (30). HLA Bw35 has also been associated with severe Graves' ophthalmopathy (31).

In other races different HLA associations have been reported. In Chinese individuals with Graves' disease the association is with HLA Bw46 (3). No comparable study has been completed in Chinese MG, although a small study of Thai Chinese patients with MG revealed a small increase in B8 and possibly in Bw46 (13). In Japanese Graves' disease HLA Bw35, Dw12, and DR5 have been reported to be increased (12,36). It is of interest that Kawa et al. (19) reported a decrease in Bw52 and an increase in Bw51 in Japanese Graves' disease. A similar disturbance in the distribution of these antigens was observed in Japanese MG (13).

The immunogenetic similarities extend to the Gm system. In Japanese, phenotypes containing G1m(2) have been shown to be increased in both diseases (26). In Caucasians no particular phenotype seems to be associated with MG per se, but the presence of the homozygous phenotype Gm(3;5) does influence the development of anti-AChR and antistriational antibodies (17). Farid et al. (12) reported an increased prevalence of phenotypes containing G1m(3) and G3m(5) in patients with Graves' disease; 100% of this patient group had phenotypes containing G1m(3) and G3m(5) compared with 80% of a control population. Our own data do not support this 100% association. Whether any association exists between particular phenotypes and autoantibodies is unknown. In a study of multiple-case families Uno et al. (36) showed that genes linked to both HLA and Gm influence the development of Graves' disease. In different families, however, the Gm haplotype differed.

Thymus

Approximately 90% of patients with MG have some thymic involvement. Sixty percent have thymic hyperplasia or an abundance of germinal centers. In Graves' disease also there is a frequent occurrence of thymic hyperplasia and germinal center formation. The significance of the thymic hyperplasia in the pathogenesis of these diseases remains to be determined.

Co-occurrence of Graves' Disease and MG

Clearly, thyroid disease, including thyrotoxicosis, frequently occurs in patients with generalized MG. Subclinical MG may be present well before the development of clinically obvious MG. Abnormal electromyographic results characteristic of MG (29) and anti-AChR (16) have been demonstrated in patients with thyrotoxicosis who subsequently developed MG.

Analysis of the co-occurrence of thyroid disease with MG at the Eighth International Histocompatibility Workshop revealed that thyrotoxicosis was much more frequently associated with ocular MG than with generalized MG. This association was also reflected in the autoantibody profiles of the two forms of MG (15). Ocular MG had a very high frequency of thyroid autoantibodies (40%), although a relatively low frequency of antinuclear antibodies (6%) compared to generalized MG (12% and 27%, respectively). Patients with ocular MG rarely had antistriational antibodies. Thus it seemed that ocular MG was qualitatively different from generalized MG, was probably an autoimmune disease, and was mediated by an autoantibody to muscle antigen which was yet to be identified. We predicted that this autoantibody, reactive with extraocular neuromuscular junctions, will be demonstrated in some patients with generalized MG, some patients with thyrotoxicosis, and all patients with MG restricted to extraocular muscles (Fig. 2). Indeed, some evidence is accumulating for the existence of antigens unique to extraocular muscle (20). It has also been reported that sera from patients with ocular MG react preferentially with AChR extracted from extraocular muscle (37). Such reports require confirmation.

The condition of euthyroid Graves' ophthalmopathy reflects this situation. Most patients were negative for anti-TSHR, and when they were detected the autoantibodies differed in specificity compared to those in patients with untreated active Graves' disease (6).

CONCLUSION

The genetic relationship between MG and Graves' disease is quite clear. As well as a common HLA and Gm association, there is a familial aggregation of the diseases, patients with Graves' disease often having relatives with MG or vice versa (33). It is likely that a genetically determined immunoregulatory defect confers susceptibility to the induction of the autoantibodies to membrane receptors seen in these diseases. Whether anti-AChR or anti-TSHR develops is determined by other genetic factors or environmental factors. This seems to be the case in D-penicillamine-induced MG.

The development of either ocular MG or Graves' ophthalmopathy may in turn be genetically determined. Both ocular diseases do seem to be genetically and immunologically distinct. They are likely to be immunologically mediated and to be part of an overlapping group of diseases which in the past have been broadly classified as Graves' disease and MG.

REFERENCES

1. Albuquerque, E. X., Warnick, J. E., Mayer, R. F., Eldefrawi, A. T., and Eldefrawi, M. E. (1981): Recent advances in the molecular mechanisms of human and animal models of myasthenia gravis. *Ann. N.Y. Acad. Sci.*, 377:496–518.
2. Balazs, C., Stenszky, V., Szerze, P., Kozma, L., and Leovey, A. (1979): Connection between HLA-B8 antigen and suppressor T cell activity in Graves' disease. *Transplant. Proc.*, 11:1314.
3. Chan, S. H., Yeo, P. P. B., Cheah, J. S., and Pin, L. (1982): Thyroid disease—Chinese. In: *Immunogenetics in Rheumatology*, edited by R. L. Dawkins, F. T. Christiansen, and P. J. Zilko, pp. 272–274. Excerpta Medica, Amsterdam.
4. Dawkins, R. L. (1983): Muscle disorders. In: *Immunology in Medicine*, edited by E. J. Holborow and W. G. Reeves, pp. 439–465. Academic Press, London.
5. Dawkins, R. L., Christiansen, F. T., Kay, P. H., Garlepp, M. J., McCluskey, J., Hollingsworth, P. N., and Zilko, P. J. (1983): Disease associations with complotypes, supratypes and haplotypes. *Immunol. Rev.*, 70:5–22.
6. De Baets, M., Elewaut, A., Dacremont, G., and Vermeulen, A. (1982): Autoantibodies to the thyrotropin receptor and their significance in autoimmune thyroid disease. In: *Immunological Analysis: Recent Progress in Diagnostic Laboratory Immunology*, edited by E. M. Nakamura, W. Dito, and E. S. Tucker, pp. 37–51. Masson, New York.
7. Drachman, D. B. (1981): The biology of myasthenia gravis. *Annu. Rev. Neurosci.*, 4:195–225.
8. Drexhage, H. A., Botazzo, G. F., Bitensky, L., Chayen, J., and Doniach, D. (1981): Thyroid growth blocking antibodies in primary myxoedema. *Nature*, 289:594–596.
9. Engel, A. G., Lambert, E. H., Mulder, D. M., Gomez, M. R., Whitaker, J. N., Hart, Z., and Sahashi, K. (1981): Recently recognised congenital myasthenic syndromes. *Ann. N.Y. Acad. Sci.*, 377:614–639.
10. Engel, A. G., Sahashi, K., and Fumagalli, G. (1981): The immunopathology of acquired myasthenia gravis. *Ann. N.Y. Acad. Sci.*, 377:158–174.
11. Famborough, D. M., Drachman, D. B., and Satyamurti, S. (1973): Neuromuscular junction in myasthenia gravis: decreased acetylcholine receptors. *Science*, 182:293–295.
12. Farid, N. R. (1981): Graves' disease. In: *HLA in Endocrine and Metabolic Disease*, edited by N. R. Farid, pp. 85–143. Academic Press, New York.
13. Garlepp, M. J., Christiansen, F. T., Dawkins, R. L., Chiewsilp, P., and Takata, H. (1982): Myasthenia gravis. In: *Immunogenetics in Rheumatology*, edited by R. L. Dawkins, F. T. Christiansen, and P. J. Zilko, pp. 259–263. Excerpta Medica, Amsterdam.
14. Garlepp, M. J., Dawkins, R. L., and Christiansen, F. T. (1983): HLA antigens and acetylcholine receptor antibodies in D-penicillamine induced myasthenia gravis. *Br. Med. J.*, 286:338–340.
15. Garlepp, M. J., Dawkins, R. L., Christiansen, F. T., Lawton, J., Luciani, G., McLeod, J., Bradley, J., Genkins,

G., and Teng, C. S. (1981): Autoimmunity in ocular and generalised myasthenia gravis. *J. Neuroimmunol.*, 1:325–332.

16. Garlepp, M. J., Kay, P., and Dawkins, R. L. (1982): The diagnostic significance of autoantibodies to the acetylcholine receptor. *J. Neuroimmunol.*, 3:337–350.

17. Garlepp, M. J., Kay, P., and Dawkins, R. L. (1984): Immunoglobulin allotype association with autoantibodies in myasthenia gravis. *Disease Markers (in press)*.

18. Garlepp, M. J., Kay, P. H., Dawkins, R. C., Bucknall, R., and Kemp, A. (1981): Cross reactivity of anti-acetylcholine receptor autoantibodies. *Muscle Nerve*, 4:282–286.

19. Kawa, A., Nakamura, S., Kono, Y., Maeda, Y., and Kanehisa, T. (1979): A negative association of HLA Bw52 with Graves' disease and insulin-dependent diabetes with juvenile onset among Japanese population. *Experientia*, 35:547–548.

20. Kodama, K., Sikorska, H., Bandy-Dafoe, P., Bayly, R., and Wall, J. R. (1982): Demonstration of a circulating autoantibody against a soluble eye-muscle antigen in Graves' ophthalmopathy. *Lancet*, 2:1353–1356.

21. Lennon, V. A., and Lambert, E. H. (1981): Monoclonal autoantibodies to acetylcholine receptors: evidence for a dominant idiotype and requirement of complement for pathogenicity. *Ann. N.Y. Acad. Sci.*, 377:77–96.

22. Lindstrom, J. (1977): An assay for antibodies to human acetylcholine receptor in serum from patients with myasthenia gravis. *Clin. Immunol. Immunopathol.*, 7:36–43.

23. Lindstrom, J. (1979): Autoimmune response to acetylcholine receptors in myasthenia gravis and its animal model. *Adv. Immunol.*, 27:1–50.

24. Matsurra, N., Yamada, Y., Nohara, Y., Konishi, J., Kasagi, K., Endo, K., Kojima, H., and Wataya, K. (1980): Familial neonatal transient hypothyroidism due to maternal TSH-binding inhibitor immunoglobulins. *N. Engl. J. Med.*, 393:738–741.

25. Momoi, M. Y., and Lennon, V. A. (1982): Purification and biochemical characterisation of nicotinic acetylcholine receptors of human muscle. *J. Biol. Chem.*, 257:12757–12764.

26. Nakao, Y., Matsumoto, H., Miyazaki, T., Nishitani, H., Takatsuki, K., Kasukawa, R., Nakayama, S., Izumi, S., Fujita, T., and Tsuji, K. (1980): IgG heavy chain allotypes (Gm) in autoimmune diseases. *Clin. Exp. Immunol.*, 42:20–26.

27. Osserman, K. E., Tsairis, P., and Weiner, L. B. (1967): Myasthenia gravis and thyroid disease—clinical and immunological correlation. *J. Mt. Sinai Hosp.*, 34:469–483.

28. Peers, J., McDonald, B., and Dawkins, R. L. (1977): The reactivity of the antistriational antibodies associated with thymoma and myasthenia gravis. *Clin. Exp. Immunol.*, 27:66–73.

29. Puvanendran, K., Cheah, J. S., Naganathan, N., Yeo, P. P. B., and Wong, P. K. (1979): Neuromuscular transmission in thyrotoxicosis. *J. Neurol. Sci.*, 43:47–57.

30. Schleusener, H., Schernthaner, G., Mayr, W. T., Kotulla, P., Bogner, U., Finke, R., Meinhold, H., Koppenhagen, K., and Wenzel, K. W. (1983): HLA-DR3 and HLA-DR5 associated thyrotoxicosis—two different types of toxic diffuse goiter. *J. Clin. Endocrinol. Metab.*, 56:781–785.

31. Sergott, R., Felberg, N. T., Savino, P. J., Blizzard, J. J., Schatz, N. J., and Sanford, C. A. (1983): Association of HLA antigen Bw35 with severe Graves' ophthalmopathy. *Invest. Ophthalmol. Vis. Sci.*, 24:124–127.

32. Simpson, J. A. (1960): Myasthenia gravis: a new hypothesis. *Scott. Med. J.*, 5:419–436.

33. Simpson, J. A. (1968): The correlations between myasthenia gravis and disorders of the thyroid gland. In: *Research in Muscular Dystrophy. Proceedings of the Fourth Symposium*, pp. 31–34. Pitman, London.

34. Tom, W., and Farid, N. T. (1981): Reduced C4 in HLA-B8 positive patients with Graves' disease. *Hum. Hered.*, 31:227–231.

35. Toyka, K. V., Drachman, D. B., Griffin, D. E., Pestronk, A., Winkelstein, J. A., Fishbeck, K. H., and Kao, I. (1977): Myasthenia gravis: study of humoral immune mechanisms by passive transfer to mice. *N. Engl. J. Med.*, 296:125–131.

36. Uno, H., Sasazuki, T., Tamai, H., and Matsumoto, H. (1981): Two major genes, linked to HLA and Gm, control susceptibility to Graves' disease. *Nature*, 292:768–770.

37. Vincent, A., and Newsom-Davis, J. (1980): Anti-acetylcholine receptor antibodies. *J. Neurol. Neurosurg. Psychiatry*, 43:590–600.

38. Zakarija, M., and McKenzie, J. M. (1978): Zoological specificity of human thyroid-stimulating antibody. *J. Clin. Endocrinol. Metab.*, 47:249–254.

39. Zilko, P. J., Dawkins, R. L., Holmes, K., and Witt, C. (1979): Genetic control of suppressor lymphocyte function in myasthenia gravis: relationship of impaired suppressor function to HLA B8/DRw3 and cold-reactive lymphocytotoxic antibodies. *Clin. Immunol. Immunopathol.*, 14:222–230.

The Eye and Orbit in Thyroid Disease, edited by
C. A. Gorman et al. Raven Press, New York 1984.

Clinical Presentations of Graves' Ophthalmopathy

Ian D. Hay

*Division of Endocrinology and Department of Internal Medicine, Mayo Clinic,
Rochester, Minnesota 55905*

The third part of this volume deals with the clinical and laboratory evaluation of the patient with Graves' ophthalmopathy. The present chapter considers current classifications of the orbital changes in Graves' disease and describes the wide variety of eye and orbital signs which may be seen in this disease. The four chapters which immediately follow describe in further detail those ancillary techniques which may be usefully employed by the neuro-ophthalmologist to supplement the information obtained by the primary physician from the initial eye examination. The principles underlying the formulation of a clinical diagnosis are considered in this chapter; for a detailed description of thyroid function testing and orbital imaging, the reader is referred to chapters by Brennan and Gorman, by Forbes and by Ossoinig, *this volume*. Ophthalmic diseases, which may be confused with Graves' orbitopathy, receive mention in this chapter; however, the differential diagnosis of Graves' ophthalmopathy is given more detailed consideration in the chapter by Waller and Jacobson, *this volume*.

CLASSIFICATION OF ORBITAL CHANGES

The first formal classification of the eye changes of Graves' disease was devised in 1969 by a special committee of the American Thyroid Association (ATA) chaired by Dr. Sidney C. Werner (42). The classification was initially presented in both an abridged and a detailed form. The abridged form summarized the six classes which had been devised, the first letter of the definition of each class constituting the mnemonic *NO SPECS*. The detailed classification provided specific criteria for grading the signs within each class and identified the activity of the orbital process as "active, static, or inactive."

TABLE 1. *Abridged classification of eye changes in
Graves' disease*

Class	Definition
0	*No physical signs or symptoms*
1	*Only signs, no symptoms (signs limited to upper lid retraction, stare, and lid lag)*
2	*Soft-tissue involvement (symptoms and signs)*
3	*Proptosis*
4	*Extraocular muscle movement*
5	*Corneal involvement*
6	*Sight loss (optic nerve involvement)*

From Werner (43).

TABLE 2. *Detailed classification of eye changes of Graves' disease*

Grade	Suggestions for grading
Class 0	No physical signs or symptoms
Class 1	Only signs (signs limited to upper lid retraction, stare, and lid lag)
Class 2	Soft-tissue involvement with symptoms and signs
0	Absent
a	Minimal
b	Moderate
c	Marked
Class 3	Proptosis 3 mm or more in excess of upper normal limits, with or without symptoms
0	Absent
a	3- to 4-mm increase over upper normal
b	5- to 7-mm increase
c	8 mm or more increase
Class 4	Extraocular muscle involvement (usually with diplopia, other symptoms, and other signs)
0	Absent
a	Limitation of motion of extreme gaze
b	Evident restriction of motion
c	Fixation of globe or globes
Class 5	Corneal involvement (primarily due to lagophthalmos)
0	Absent
a	Stippling of cornea
b	Ulceration
c	Clouding, necrosis, perforation
Class 6	Sight loss (due to optic nerve involvement)
0	Absent
a	Disc pallor or choking, or visual field defect; vision 20/20 to 20/60
b	Same, but vision 20/70 to 20/200
c	Blindness; i.e., failure to perceive light, vision <20/200

From Werner (43).

In 1977 an Ad Hoc Committee of the ATA, again chaired by Werner, published several modifications to the original classification (43). As before, the classification had two forms: the abridged (Table 1) and the detailed (Table 2). Although the original six classes were retained, changes were made in the criteria for classes 1 and 3. It was emphasized that progression of disease need not be sequential through each of the classes. Also, it was noted that the amount of myopia and/or racial differences in orbital depth could influence the measured normal upper limits of proptosis.

In 1981 Van Dyk suggested a further modification to the ATA classification which he hoped would permit "greater clinical specificity" in the description of patients with orbital Graves' disease. He advised the return of criteria for grading patients in class 2 (soft tissue involvement) and urged that symptoms be excluded from the definition. His proposed modification to the detailed classification of class 2 orbital changes listed six soft tissue signs, the first letter of each forming the mnemonic *RELIEF*.

*R*esistance to retrodisplacement of eye
*E*dema of conjuntiva/caruncle
*L*acrimal gland enlargement
*I*njection to conjunctiva, focal or diffuse
*E*dema of lids
*F*ullness of lids

In 1982 Feldon and Unsold (12), from the University of Southern California, described a simple classification of Graves' ophthalmopathy based entirely on the evaluation of seven

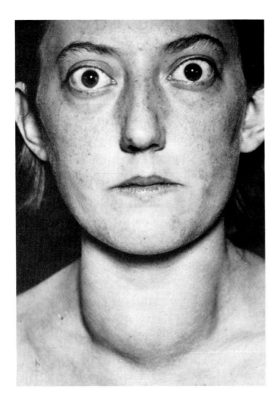

FIG. 1. Typical facies and neck of patient with hyperthyroidism due to Graves' disease. Note class 1 eye changes and symmetrical diffuse thyroid enlargement.

clinical signs: proptosis, lid retraction, lid lag, horizontal oculomotor dysfunction, vertical oculomotor dysfunction, optic nerve involvement, and periorbital edema. These signs were judged as mild, moderate, or severe based on "strict semiquantitative clinical criteria," and the patients in their studies (12,13) were said to be "categorized easily" into three classes on the basis of the overall clinical severity of disease. Probably it is too early to discern if such a simple schema will be found to be as clinically useful as the older, more complex modified ATA classification (43).

Involvement of Lids: ATA Class 1

In class 1 of the ATA classification, patients with Graves' ophthalmopathy have eye signs limited to upper lid retraction, stare, and lid lag (Fig. 1). These signs, although considered by Werner (44) as "little more than a cosmetic blemish," may provide a major source of concern and anxiety to the affected patient (33). In class 1 involvement the patients have a characteristic "startled" appearance, or "stare," because the upper lid on one or both sides is retracted, thereby exposing the superior corneoscleral limbus (Fig. 2). When the eyes pursue a slowly downward-moving target, the lid (or both lids) "lag" behind. The presence of both lid retraction (Dalrymple's sign) and lid lag (Von Graefe's sign), even when subtle, is considered highly suggestive of Graves' ophthalmopathy but is by no means pathognomonic (33).

Retraction of the upper lids has been described as the most characteristic ocular sign of Graves' disease (4), and it is said to occur in at least 50% of patients with ophthalmopathy (10). However, it may also be seen with other causes of hyperthyroidism, e.g., toxic

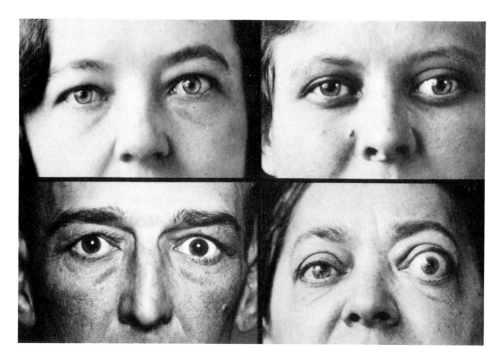

FIG. 2. Varying degrees of left upper lid retraction in four patients with unilateral/asymmetrical Graves' orbitopathy. Three have class 1 changes, but proptosis in excess of 22 mm on the lower right grades that patient as class 3.

multinodular goiter, hyperfunctioning autonomous nodules, subacute thyroiditis, and thyrotoxicosis factitia (21).

For years, based on Claude Bernard's experimental production of lid lag in animals, excessive sympathetic nervous system activity was uncritically accepted as the mechanism responsible for lid retraction in Graves' disease (33). The retraction was attributed principally to overstimulation of Müller's muscle, a small sympathetically innervated muscle which arises from the undersurface of the levator palpebrae and inserts on the superior border of the upper tarsus (24). Evidence for sympathetic overactivity was inferred from the knowledge that propranolol (a β-blocker), when used systemically, could produce a ptotic effect on the upper lid, and that the topical administration of the postganglionic blocker guanethidine resulted in a significant lowering of the retracted eyelid in the majority of thyrotoxic patients with eyelid retraction (24).

Recently, however, it has been clinically observed that there are many instances of eyelid retraction for which the sympathetic overactivity theory is an inadequate explanation. Principal among these observations are the facts that: (a) the retraction is not abolished by cervical sympathectomy (31); (b) many retracted eyelids fail to drop toward normal with guanethidine (24); (c) eyelid retraction may be present in the eumetabolic or hypometabolic patient (24); and (d) retraction persists with sleep, general anesthesia, and retrobulbar anesthesia (29). The fact that unilateral lid retraction is so common makes a sympathetic overactivity extremely unlikely. Also, if the lashes or lid margin are grasped and an attempt is made to draw the retracted lid downward, resistance is often encountered, another observation suggesting a mechanical restriction of the levator muscle rather than excess sympathetic tone (33).

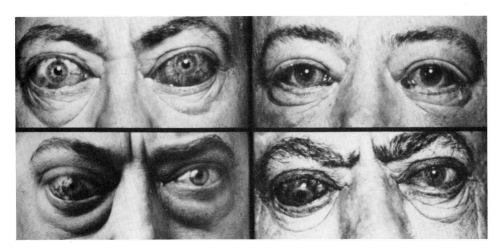

FIG. 3. Conjunctival injection in class 2. Associated features demonstrable include lid retraction *(upper left)*, enlargement of caruncles *(upper right)*, orbital fat protrusion *(lower left)*, and right inferior rectus muscle restriction *(lower right)*.

On the basis of the results of high-resolution ultrasonic (34,35) and computed tomographic (CT) scans (11,39) of the orbit, it is being increasingly accepted that thyroid orbitopathy is a diffuse process resulting in a panmyositis affecting all muscles of the orbit simultaneously (24). From these findings it can be inferred that the same process of inflammation, thickening, and ultimate fibrosis which affects the recti and oblique muscles in class 4 involvement may also involve the levator and Müller's muscle in the upper eyelid and cause restricted movement and contraction, resulting in a pharmacologically irreversible elevation of the upper eyelid (24). Such a mechanism would provide a more acceptable explanation than sympathetic overactivity for the fairly frequent finding of eyelid retraction in those euthyroid patients who present with no thyrotoxic history or those who develop eye signs many years after successful ablative therapy for hyperthyroidism.

Soft Tissue Involvement: ATA Class 2

Classes 2 to 6 of the ATA classification represent the severe eye changes with a potentially serious prognosis, formerly called "infiltrative," "progressive," or "malignant" (42). It is said that approximately half of patients with Graves' ophthalmopathy fall within this overall category (4), which is characterized by a consistent enlargement of extraocular muscles, resulting in an increase in orbital contents, a "tight orbit," and an increase in orbital pressure (11,38). The edema resulting from the swollen extraocular muscles coupled with the increased orbital pressure probably cause a "slowdown of the normally precarious removal of the fluids in the interstitial space," a process to which venous stasis, resulting from compression of apical veins by enlarged muscles, also probably contributes (39).

In the 1969 ATA statement, class 2 symptoms were described as excessive lacrimation, a "sandy" sensation, retrobulbar discomfort, and photophobia (42). Relevant signs included edema of conjunctivae and lids, conjunctival injection, fullness of lids (often with orbital fat extrusion), palpable lacrimal glands, and swollen extraocular muscle palpable laterally beneath the lower lids (Figs. 3 to 6). In Van Dyk's opinion, the inclusion of symptoms in class 2 was a mistake (40). In his proposed modification (see p. 129), criteria for inclusion

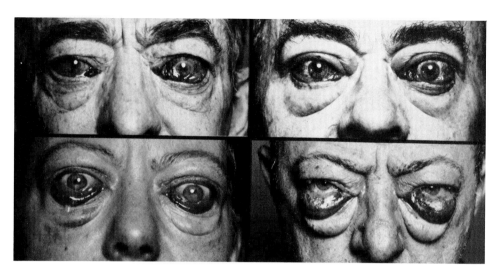

FIG. 4. Variable chemosis in class 2c. Caruncular prolapse and diffuse conjunctival injection are present in both of the upper examples. Bilateral conjunctival prolapse and periorbital edema are prominent features of the two lower examples, particularly that on the lower right.

were limited to six signs remembered by the mnemonic RELIEF and described in full below.

Resistance to retrodisplacement of the eye into the orbit results because the orbit is infiltrated and waterlogged. In contrast to the normal orbit, which allows about 5 mm of backward displacement of the eyes, the orbit involved by the Graves' process provides variable resistance to retrodisplacement, and forward bulging of the orbital septum is rarely visible on pushing against the globe.

Edema of the conjunctiva and the caruncle, referred to as chemosis, may be represented only by a small fold of redundant conjunctiva hanging over the mucocutaneous junction of the lower lid (Fig. 3). However, with more marked involvement, there may be frank prolapse of the conjunctiva across the lower lid, a prolapse in which the caruncle usually participates (Fig. 4).

Lacrimal gland enlargement may rarely be palpable but more often is seen as a contrast-enhancing superolateral mass on orbital CT scan. Infiltration of the gland causes enlargement, which is made more prominent by the gland's involvement in the generalized anterior movement of orbital structures.

Injection of the conjunctiva may occur in the presence or absence of chemosis (Fig. 3). When conjunctival edema is minimal, an intense focal hyperemia may be seen outlining and overlying the swollen horizontal rectus tendons, sometimes extending anterior to the insertion of the tendon toward the limbus (Plate I, color plates, see p. 136). When gross chemosis is present the conjunctivae are diffusely hyperemic and the presence at the lateral canthus of large, tortuous, purplish vascular loops with overlying chemosis (Plates I and II, color plates) is considered highly characteristic of Graves' ophthalmopathy (17).

Edema and *fullness* of lids may occur separately, but sometimes the signs are not precisely separable (Figs. 5, 6, and Plate II). It is probable that lid fullness is caused by edema, infiltration, or fat extrusion behind the orbital septum, whereas lid edema reflects fluid anterior to the septum, just under the skin and orbicularis muscle (40).

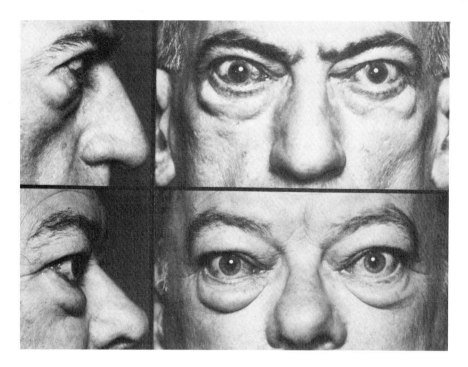

FIG. 5. Comparison of orbital fat prolapse *(upper)* and periorbital edema *(lower)* in two patients who also demonstrate lid retraction and conjunctival injection. Note the discrete fat protrusion temporally and the dependent nature of the lower lid edema, best demonstrated in the lateral view of the right orbit.

Proptosis: ATA Class 3

It has been said that the position of the globe in the orbit is comparable to that of an egg in an egg cup (17). Padding the bottom of the cup causes the egg to sit higher, whereas if the egg is prevented from rising the pressure behind it increases. In Graves' disease a still unidentified pathogen or its mediator induces swelling, infiltration, and later fibrosis with eventual muscular contractures. Within the unyielding confines of the bony orbit the swollen retrobulbar tissues tend to push the eye forward. Proptosis, in this context, is "nature's decompression" (18).

In the 1977 modification of the ATA classification, patients with proptosis up to 22 mm (2 mm above the Caucasian normal) were placed in class 1 (43). Those with proptosis in excess of 22 mm, even without symptoms, were placed in class 3. It was recognized that for Japanese and black Americans the upper normal values for proptosis were, respectively, 18 and 22 mm. Because of these ethnic variations in the proptosis baseline, the grading (a, b, or c) for class 3 was changed from being based on the actual millimeters of forward protrusion of the eye to a grade based on the extent to which the proptosis reading exceeded normal (Table 2).

It has been estimated that about 20 to 25% of patients with Graves' disease develop proptosis (6,10). Eye findings are typically bilateral (Plate I), although the severity of involvement may differ significantly between the two eyes (7,8,11). Occasionally patients present with unilateral signs (Fig. 2) and symptoms (28). In Graves' disease, however, an asymmetry in exophthalmos rarely exceeds 6 mm (20,32). Sometimes advance of exoph-

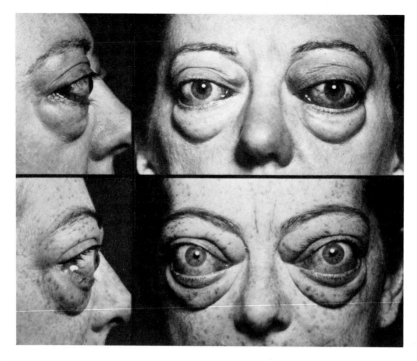

FIG. 6. Two patients with periorbital fullness probably due to a combination of orbital fat prolapse and edema. Both also demonstrate bilateral proptosis, lid retraction, and conjunctival injection.

thalmos is so rapid that the lids cannot be closed over the eyes (Figs. 8 and Plate II). When the lids are shut, there is incomplete closure of the palpebral fissure (lagophthalmos), and this can result in exposure and injury to the bulbar conjunctiva and cornea (4).

It is widely recognized that Graves' ophthalmopathy can account for 15 to 28% of all cases of unilateral exophthalmos (17). In spite of what may seem to be a unilateral process, pathologic involvement of the intraorbital contents does occur bilaterally, and this can be confirmed by ultrasonography or computed tomography (11,34,38,39,45). It is this bilateral involvement that provides an important clinical clue to differentiating "unilateral" Graves' ophthalmopathy from an orbital mass lesion (31).

Normally, the globes sink back 1 to 3 mm into the orbits when the recumbent position is assumed (22). In Graves' ophthalmopathy the normal retrodisplacement of the globes is absent bilaterally, even though only one eye might seem proptotic. By contrast, if a mass lesion is present, the proptotic eye may not retropulse but the opposite "normal" eye relaxes back into the orbit.

Extraocular Muscle Involvement: ATA Class 4

Based on a study in which over 200 orbits of patients with Graves' disease were scanned by high-resolution CT, Trokel and Jakobiec (39) concluded that the extraocular muscles are the most consistently involved focus of disease in Graves' orbitopathy, an observation which has been substantiated by histopathologic evaluation of both biopsy and autopsy tissue (3). Clinically and radiologically, the range of abnormality varies from minimal enlargement of a few muscles in patients with class 1 disease to enormous enlargement of multiple muscles in class 4 disease (39). In the initial stages of disease the enlarged muscles maintain the

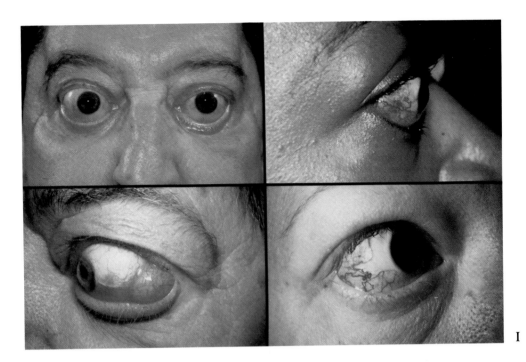

I

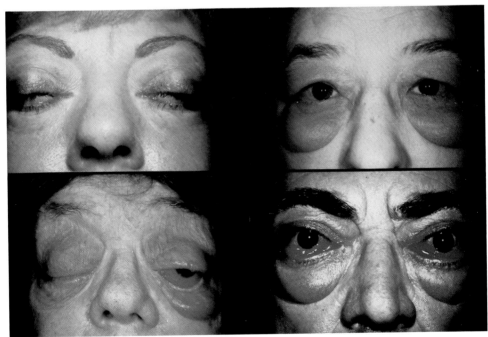

II

Color plates for *Endocrine Ophthalmopathy: Differential Diagnosis* by Robert R. Waller and David H. Jacobson, pp. 213–219. (See legend opposite p. 137.)

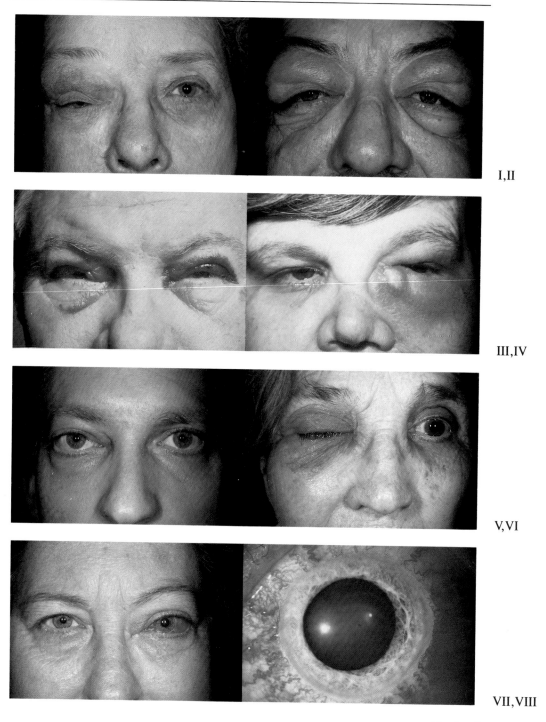

I,II

III,IV

V,VI

VII,VIII

(Continued)

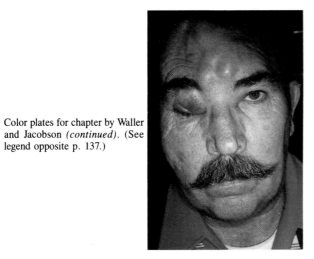
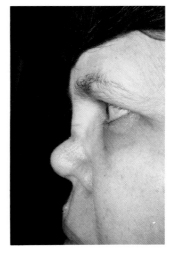

Color plates for chapter by Waller and Jacobson *(continued)*. (See legend opposite p. 137.)

IX,X

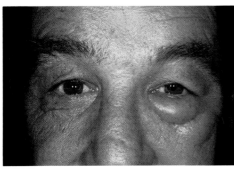
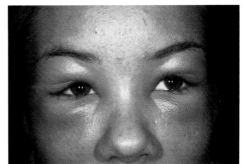

XI,XII

Color plates for *Transantral Orbital Decompression* by Lawrence W. DeSanto, pp. 231–251. (See legend opposite p. 137.)

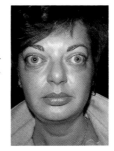
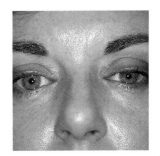

I,II

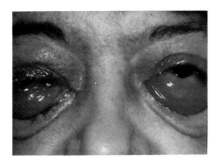
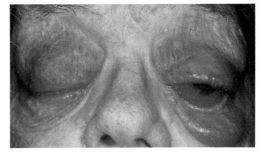

III,IV

Legends to Plates I and II from chapter by Ian D. Hay, pp. 129–142.

Plate I. Eyes in the *upper left* panel show bilateral asymmetrical lid retraction and exophthalmos. In the *upper right* panel, conjunctival injection and edema are present, overlying the anterior insertion of the lateral rectus muscle. The lower eyes demonstrate *(on right)* visibly enlarged insertions of extraocular muscles and *(on left)* striking orbital prolapse.

Plate II. Bilateral lagophthalmos and marked lid edema are demonstrated in the *upper left and right* panels, respectively. Lower eyes demonstrate *(on left)* unilateral and *(on right)* bilateral prolapsed, edematous, injected conjunctivae, as well as lower lid edema and *(on left)* asymmetrical bilateral lagophthalmos.

Legends to Plates I–XII from chapter by Robert R. Waller and David H. Jacobson, pp. 213–219.

Plate I. Unilateral orbital pseudotumor (biopsy-proved). Note the eyelid edema and erythema, superior orbital mass, and globe displacement.

Plate II. Sarcoidosis. Note the dramatic eyelid edema. Masses were palpable in the region of both lacrimal glands.

Plate III. Amyloidosis. Note the bilateral periorbital edema and erythema with an infiltrative process involving the lids.

Plate IV. Wegener's granulomatosis. Note the nasal lacrimal duct obstruction and saddle-nose deformity.

Plate V. Contiguous sinus disease. Edema, erythema, and globe displacement of the right eye. Previous ethmoidectomy scar is apparent on the right.

Plate VI. Metastatic melanoma. Note the unilateral inflammatory signs.

Plate VII. Low-flow dural shunt. Note the episcleral vessel tortuosity and proptosis of the left eye.

Plate VIII. Close-up photograph of the patient depicted in *Plate VII.*

Plate IX. Lymphoma (biopsy-proved). Note the superior nasal orbital mass and paraorbital involvement.

Plate X. Lateral view of patient depicted in *Plate IV.*

Plate XI. Patient with infected plastic implant for blowout fracture of the left orbit. Palpation of the inferior orbital rim revealed an extruding implant.

Plate XII. Mononucleosis. Note the brawny finger edema not unlike Graves' disease.

Legends to Plates I–IV from chapter by Lawrence W. DeSanto, pp. 231–251.

Plates I and II. *Plate I:* Preoperative transantral decompression (June, 1976). *Plate II:* Postoperative (September, 1977). The patient has undergone transantral orbital decompression, recession of inferior and medial rectus muscles, and Müller's muscle muotomy.

Plates III and IV. Two patients who illustrate the severe congestive changes of Graves' ophthalmopathy.

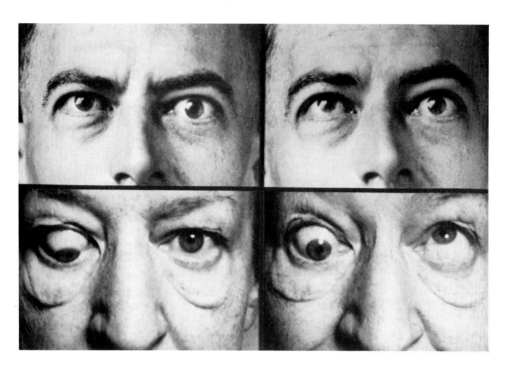

FIG. 7. Class 4 eye changes due to inferior rectus muscle restriction. In the upper (class 4a) example, there is left hypotropia, especially marked when the patient attempts upgaze. In the lower (class 4b) example, there is evident restriction of motion due to "tethering" of the right inferior rectus muscle.

ability to contract, but later they become fibrotic and are unable to relax. These fibrotic extraocular muscles restrict mobility by a "tethering" action and present as an apparent underaction of the antagonist muscle. In severe and massive involvement of the muscles, the ability to contract may be lost and the resultant restriction in motion may eventually result in class 4c changes with fixation of the position of the globe.

Patients with clinically significant extraocular muscle involvement usually complain of intermittent or slowly progressive vertical or oblique diplopia (33). Occasionally, especially during acutely active inflammatory phases, they may complain of a mild painful "pulling" sensation on attempted upgaze. As inflammation subsides, the ophthalmoplegia is usually not accompanied by pain, except perhaps for a foreign body sensation. A useful physical finding is enlargement and injection of the extraocular muscle insertions, often seen through the conjunctiva (Plate I). Proptosis at this stage is variable, and minimal amounts of proptosis (class 2) may coexist with marked limitation of ocular motility (33).

Of the six extraocular muscles, the four recti muscles are particularly involved in the restrictive process. Clinical involvement is most common in the inferior rectus (60 to 70%), less frequent in the medial rectus (25%), and uncommon (10%) in the superior rectus (35). The lateral recti are seldom involved (9). Quantification of extraocular muscle enlargement by CT scanning has recently allowed the demonstration of a regular increase in total extraocular muscle volume with increasing ophthalmopathy (13). Although in a study of eight patients with variably severe Graves' ophthalmopathy inferior rectus enlargement was apparent in all patients, only medial and lateral rectus muscle volumes increased in propor-

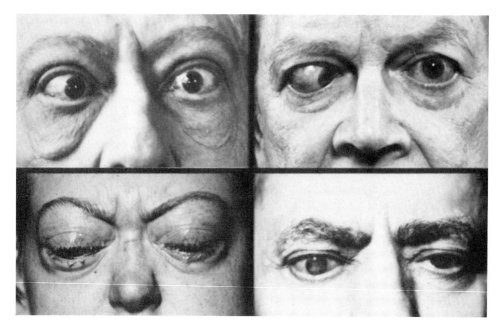

FIG. 8. Upper eyes demonstrate right medial rectus muscle restriction of moderate (4b) and marked (4c) degree. Lagophthalmos is shown on the lower left, and the class 5c change of leukoma (corneal scarring) is demonstrable *(lower right)* in the eye of the patient who 9 months earlier had the inferior rectus muscle restriction shown in Fig. 3.

tion to the severity of clinical disease (13). Because the horizontally acting muscles contribute significantly to apical optic nerve compression (26), it was suggested that horizontal eye muscle dysfunction in Graves' ophthalmopathy may be an ominous clinical sign (13).

In the typical patient with class 4 changes, the inferior rectus muscle is first affected, resulting in an early limitation of upgaze (Fig. 7). A decrease in lateral movements occurs later (Fig. 8), and downward movement is impaired less frequently. Because innervation to the muscles of both eyes is equal (Hering's law), attempts to observe an object with the more severely involved eye can result in increased innervation being sent to both eyes, and as a consequence there may be "overshoot" of the less severely affected eye (4).

It is generally agreed that the inferior extraocular muscles suffer more severe involvement than the others. Hodes and co-workers (24) suggested three possible explanations for the observed inferior muscle dominance in the restrictive process. First, they suggested that because twice as many muscles, with far more complex actions, are involved in vertical eye movements than in horizontal eye movements, one might anticipate, based on numbers alone, a predominace of vertical muscle symptomatology. Second, unlike the horizontal muscles, the vertical muscles are paired and they cross one another within the orbit. The inferior crossing is possibly more prone to reactive adhesions because unlike the superior crossing, which occurs between a muscle and a tendon, the inferior one occurs between two muscles with a consequent larger area of surface contact. Finally, they point out that horizontal fusional vergence is considerably greater than vertical fusional vergence, thereby allowing an individual to compensate for deficits in horizontal eye movements.

Clinically, the restrictive extraocular muscle involvement of Graves' ophthalmopathy should be differentiated from other neurologic entities, e.g., neurogenic palsy and myasthenia gravis, which may complicate thyrotoxicosis. Toward this end, the forced duction test is indispensable (31). In this test the examiner determines if there is mechanical resistance by actually taking hold of the globe and attempting to move it in the direction that the patient cannot (33). The presence of a positive test, implying restrictive phenomena, is almost diagnostic of orbital disease and usually excludes neurogenic disease (31), except in those cases of longstanding ocular deviation where there may be secondary muscular contractions (33).

When a patient with extraocular muscle involvement turns the eye upward, restrictive tethering of the enlarged extraocular muscles, especially the inferior recti, pressing against the globe raises the intraocular pressure (19). This is of diagnostic significance, as a rise in intraocular pressure of >4 mm Hg in moving from one gaze position to another is pathognomonic of restrictive orbital disease (46). Gamblin et al. (15) showed that of 55 Graves' patients without proptosis who had either no eye signs (classes 0 through 1) or mild signs of soft tissue involvement (class 2a), 36 (65%) had an elevated intraocular pressure on upgaze in one or both eyes. All 25 patients with severe eye disease (classes 3 through 5) had an abnormal elevation on upgaze in at least one eye. All seven patients with Graves' disease and unilateral proptosis demonstrated positional pressure elevation not only in the proptotic eye but also in the contralateral nonprotruding eye. Thus, like the test of globe retrodisplacement in recumbency (22) described under class 3 changes, the measurement of intraocular pressures by applanation tonometry may be helpful clinically in establishing bilateral orbital involvement in those patients who present initially with a unilateral proptosis, a concept which is further discussed in the chapter by Gamblin et al., *this volume.*

Corneal Involvement: ATA Class 5

In Graves' ophthalmopathy corneal exposure is thought to result in drying of the ocular surface (4,31). Corneal exposure has been attributed to upper lid retraction, exophthalmos, lagophthalmos, inability to elevate the eyes, and a decreased blink rate (4,31,33,44). Five factors, potentially associated with corneal exposure in Graves' disease, were evaluated to determine which ones were associated with ocular surface damage (16). Analysis revealed that only increased palpebral fissure width and increased blink rate were significant predictors of ocular surface damage, as measured by rose Bengal staining. None of the other factors generally considered important in corneal exposure (exophthalmos, lid lag, lagophthalmos) was significantly correlated with ocular surface damage. It is therefore now believed that increased palpebral fissure width accelerates tear film evaporation, allowing an increase in tear film osmolarity with resultant ocular surface damage and a secondary increase in blink rate (16).

Patients with class 5 disease and ocular surface symptoms may complain of excess tearing (81%), a gritty or sandy sensation (45%), burning (45%), or a foreign body sensation (23%) (16). In the ATA classification (42), minimal involvement is characterized by corneal stippling, moderate by corneal ulceration, and marked by clouding, necrosis, and perforation (Fig. 8). When ulcers occur, they are usually located in the central cornea (33), and if they become secondarily infected (e.g., with *Pseudomonas aeruginosa*), globe perforation may occur with resultant loss of the eye (4).

Optic Nerve Involvement: ATA Class 6

Visual loss due to optic neuropathy is infrequent in Graves' ophthalmopathy (4,26). When present in one or both eyes, it may result in a progressive decrease of visual acuity, impairment of color vision, an afferent papillary defect, optic disc congestion or atrophy, and visual field defects (26). In 1933 Naffziger first suggested that optic neuropathy in Graves' disease could be caused by compression of the optic nerve at the orbital apex, where the swollen muscle bellies of the extraocular muscles converge at the annulus of Zinn (30). Recently the ability of high-resolution CT scanners to resolve structures at the orbital apex has allowed the demonstration that dysthyroid optic neuropathy is consistently associated with substantially enlarged extraocular muscles at the orbital apex in tight juxtaposition to the optic nerve (26,39). The consequent apical compression may result in optic neuropathy by direct pressure on the nerve or its blood supply (26). The results of fluorescein angiography and orbital venography in 20 patients with class 6 changes suggest that increased intraorbital pressure exerts a profound effect on visual function through interference with first the orbital and then, later, the ocular circulation (1).

In most patients with class 6 disease the optic nerve involvement is bilateral, although the two eyes may not necessarily be affected simultaneously or to the same extent (5,26). In 24 to 31% of cases the presentation is limited to one eye (5,6,26,37). Congestive signs and symptoms almost always precede visual loss, which may be gradual or rapidly progressive (33,37). On funduscopic examination the optic discs appear normal in 40%, whereas in about one-third hyperemia or frank papilledema may be seen (26). In neglected cases with irreversible visual loss, optic atrophy with disc pallor may be present (4,33). Chorioretinal striae may be an additional funduscopic finding (14). The appearance of the optic disc, unless optic atrophy is severe, does not correlate with visual acuity nor does it predict the potential for recovery of vision with treatment (33). The optic neuropathy of Graves' disease is considered in greater detail in the chapter by Younge, *this volume.*

Visual symptoms of dysthyroid optic neuropathy (DON) are often variable and inconsistent, ranging from a normal visual acuity of 20/20 (class 6a) to a sharp decrease to an acuity of <20/200 (class 6c) with failure to perceive light (26,42). Color vision, as tested by Ishihara pseudoisochromatic plates, may be normal but in a majority of patients is affected to a variable extent (26). Proptosis, as measured by Hertel exophthalmometry, can vary from a minimum of 18 mm (class 1) to a maximum of 30 mm (class 3). Afferent papillary responses are found to be defective in most cases of DON, but in a minority they are retained (26).

The most consistent physical finding in DON is a change in the visual field, as indicated by Goldmann perimetry (26). Field changes described include enlargement of the blind spot, central or paracentral scotomas, or an irregular contraction of the field (26). In a large series of patients with DON, Trobe found central scotomas in 94%, arcuate or altitudinal defects in the inferior or superior field in 72%, and a generalized constriction of the field in 25% (36). The most common perimetric finding was a combination of a central scotoma (with reduced acuity) and an inferior arcuate nerve fiber bundle defect (33,36).

FORMULATION OF CLINICAL DIAGNOSIS

When hyperthyroid patients exhibit simultaneously and bilaterally most or all of the characteristic findings of Graves' ophthalmopathy, the diagnosis is straightforward, and specialized diagnostic tests are unnecessary. When a history of hyperthyroidism is absent and the eye findings are few, subtle in expression, or monocular, one may encounter considerable diagnostic difficulty. When the eye findings are not diagnostic, clinicians seek evidence that thyroid function is abnormal or that thyroid regulation is disordered. If such evidence is found, the clinician presumes to link it with diagnostically nonspecific eye findings to conclude that the observed eye changes are caused by Graves' ophthalmopathy (17). Clearly, patients with disordered thyroid function or regulation sometimes have unrelated eye disorders (2,23,27). Conversely, some patients with endocrine ophthalmopathy have no demonstrable change in thyroid control or function (41). Nevertheless, when considering a diagnosis of Graves' ophthalmopathy, one seeks to establish that the eye findings are at least consistent with that diagnosis, that thyroid function or regulation is somehow disordered, and that conditions such as orbital tumors which may mimic Graves' eye disease have been adequately excluded. (See Waller and Jacobson, *this volume*, for further details of differential diagnoses.)

The individual eye changes described in Graves' ophthalmopathy vary considerably in specificity (17). The concurrence of bilateral lid retraction with proptosis and ophthalmoplegia is quite diagnostic, whereas the isolated occurrence of periorbital edema, chemosis, conjunctival injection, proptosis, or extraocular muscle dysfunction in one eye is nonspecific (19). Although no single finding is pathognomonic, certain patterns can be considered diagnostic. When all the major clinical and laboratory features of Graves' disease are present, the diagnosis is ensured. However, as is considered further in the chapter by Waller and Jacobson, *this volume*, on differential diagnosis, the involvement in isolation of the eyelids, muscles, or optic nerves always leaves the diagnosis open to question (25).

REFERENCES

1. Cant, J. S., and Wilson, T. M. (1974): The ocular and orbital circulations in dysthyroid ophthalmopathy. *Trans. Ophthalmol. Soc. U.K.*, 94:416–429.
2. Cohen, J. S. (1973): Optic neuropathy of Graves' disease, hyperthyroidism and ocular myasthenia gravis. *Arch. Ophthalmol.*, 90:131–134.
3. Daicker, B. (1979): The histologic substrate of the extraocular muscle thickening seen in dysthyroid orbitopathy. *Klin. Monatsbl. Augenheilkd.*, 174:843–847.
4. Day, R. M. (1978): Eye changes of hyperthyroidism: clinical manifestations. In: *The Thyroid*, 4th ed., edited by S. C. Werner and S. H. Ingbar, pp. 663–670. Harper & Row, New York.
5. Day, R. M., and Carroll, F. D. (1962): Optic nerve involvement associated with thyroid dysfunction. *Arch. Ophthalmol.*, 67:289–294.
6. DeSanto, L. W. (1980): The total rehabilitation of Graves' ophthalmopathy. *Laryngoscope*, 90:1652–1678.
7. Drescher, E. P., and Benedict, W. L. (1950): Asymmetric exophthalmos. *Arch. Ophthalmol.*, 44:104–128.
8. Duke-Elder, S., and MacFaul, P. (1974): *System of Ophthalmology*, Vol. 9, pp. 935–968. Mosby, St. Louis.
9. Dyer, J. A. (1976): The oculorotatory muscles in Graves' disease. *Trans. Ophthalmol. Soc.*, 74:425–456.
10. Eden, K. C., and Trotter, W. R. (1942): Lid-retraction in toxic diffuse goitre. *Lancet*, 2:385–386.
11. Enzmann, D., Marshall, W. H., Rosenthal, A. R., and Kriss, J. P. (1976): Computed tomography in Graves' ophthalmopathy. *Radiology*, 118:615–620.
12. Feldon, S. E., and Unsold, R. (1982): Graves' ophthalmopathy evaluated by infrared eye-movement recordings. *Arch. Ophthalmol.*, 100:324–328.
13. Feldon, S. E., and Weiner, J. M. (1982): Clinical significance of extraocular muscle volumes in Graves' ophthalmopathy: a quantitative computed tomographic study. *Arch. Ophthalmol.*, 100:1266–1269.
14. Frisen, L. (1979): Chorioretinal folds. In: *Topics in Neuro-Ophthalmology*, edited by H. S. Thompson, pp. 75–77. Williams & Wilkins, Baltimore.
15. Gamblin, G. T., Harper, D. G., Galentine, P., Buck, D. R., Chernow, B., and Eil, C. (1983): Prevalence of increased intraocular pressure in Graves' disease—evidence of frequent subclinical ophthalmopathy. *N. Engl. J. Med.*, 308:420–424.
16. Gilbard, J. P., and Farris, R. L. (1983): Ocular surface drying and tear film osmolarity in thyroid eye disease. *Acta Ophthalmol. (Copenh.)*, 61:108–116.
17. Gorman, C. A. (1978): The presentation and management of endocrine ophthalmopathy. *Clin. Endocrinol. Metab.*, 7:67–96.
18. Gorman, C. A. (1983): Ophthalmopathy of Graves' disease. *N. Engl. J. Med.*, 308:453–454.
19. Gorman, C. A. (1984): Extrathyroidal manifestations of Graves' disease. In: *The Thyroid*, 5th ed., edited by S. Ingbar and L. Braverman. Lippincott, Philadelphia. (In press.)
20. Hall, R., Kirkham, K., Doniach, D., and El Kabir, D. (1970): Ophthalmic Graves' disease, diagnosis, and pathogenesis. *Lancet*, 1:375–378.
21. Hamburger, J. I., and Sugar, H. S. (1972): What the internist should know about the ophthalmopathy of Graves' disease. *Arch. Intern. Med.*, 129:131–139.

22. Hauer, J. (1969): Additional clinical sign of "unilateral" endocrine exophthalmos. *Br. J. Ophthalmol.*, 53:210–211.
23. Henderson, J. W. (1973): *Orbital Tumors.* Saunders, Philadelphia.
24. Hodes, B. L., Frazee, L., and Szmyd, S. (1979): Thyroid orbitopathy: an update. *Ophthalmol. Surg.*, 10:25–33.
25. Jacobson, D. H., and Gorman, C. A. (1984): Endocrine ophthalmopathy: current ideas concerning etiology, pathogenesis, and treatment. *Endocrine Rev.*, 5:200–220.
26. Kennerdel, J. S., Rosenbaum, A. E., and El-Hoshy, M. (1981): Apical optic nerve compression of dysthyroid optic neuropathy on computed tomography. *Arch. Ophthalmol.*, 99:807–809.
27. Lavergne, G. (1975): Pitfalls in the diagnosis of endocrine exophthalmopathy. *Mod. Probl. Ophthalmol.*, 14:421–429.
28. Lawton, N. F. (1979): Exclusion of dysthyroid eye disease as a cause of unilateral proptosis. *Trans. Ophthalmol. Soc. U.K.*, 99:226–228.
29. McLean, J. M., and Norton, E. W. D. (1958): Unilateral lid retraction without exophthalmos. *Arch. Ophthalmol.*, 61:681–686.
30. Naffziger, H. C. (1933): Pathologic changes in the orbit in progressive exophthalmos: with special reference to alterations in the extraocular muscles and the optic disks. *Arch. Ophthalmol.*, 91:1–6.
31. Perlmutter, J. C., Burde, R. M., Gado, M., and Roper-Hall, G. (1977): Endocrine ophthalmopathy: a disease wearing many masks. In: *Neuro-ophthalmology: Symposium of the University of Miami and the Bascom Palmer Eye Institute*, Vol. 9, edited by J. S. Glaser, pp. 160–176. Mosby, St. Louis.
32. Rundle, F. F., and Wilson, C. W. (1945): Asymmetry of exophthalmos in orbital tumor and Graves' disease. *Lancet*, 1:151–153.
33. Sergott, R. C., and Glaser, J. S. (1981): Graves' ophthalmopathy: a clinical and immunological review. *Surv. Ophthalmol.*, 26:1–21.
34. Shammas, H. J. F., Minckler, D. S., and Ogden, C. (1980): Ultrasound in early thyroid orbitopathy. *Arch. Ophthalmol.*, 98:277–279.
35. Smith, J. L. (1972): Recent advances in therapy of thyroid eye disease. In: *Neuro-ophthalmology: Symposium of the University of Miami and the Bascom Palmer Eye Institute*, Vol. 6, edited by J. L. Smith, pp. 1–10. Mosby, St. Louis.
36. Trobe, J. D. (1981): Optic nerve involvement in dysthyroidism. *Ophthalmology*, 88:488–492.
37. Trobe, J. D., Glaser, J. S., and Laflamme, P. (1978): Dysthyroid optic neuropathy: clinical profile and rationale for management. *Arch. Ophthalmol.*, 96:1199–1209.
38. Trokel, S. L., and Hilal, S. K. (1980): Submillimeter resolution CT scanning of orbital disease. *Ophthalmology*, 87:412–417.
39. Trokel, S. L., and Jakobiec, F. A. (1981): Correlation of CT scanning and pathologic features of ophthalmic Graves' disease. *Ophthalmology*, 88:553–564.
40. Van Dyk, H. J. L. (1981): Orbital Graves' disease: a modification of the "no specs" classification. *Ophthalmology*, 88:479–483.
41. Volpé, R. (1981): Studies of the immunological aspects of thyroid disease. *Monogr. Endocrinol.*, 20:85–111.
42. Werner, S. C. (1969): Classification of the eye changes of Graves' disease. *J. Clin. Endocrinol. Metab.*, 29:982–984.
43. Werner, S. C. (1977): Modification of the classification of the eye changes of Graves' disease: recommendations of the Ad Hoc Committee of the American Thyroid Association. *J. Clin. Endocrinol. Metab.*, 44:203–209.
44. Werner, S. C. (1978): Eye changes of hyperthyroidism: introduction. In: *The Thyroid*, 4th ed., edited by S. C. Werner and S. H. Ingbar, pp. 655–659. Harper & Row, New York.
45. Werner, S. C., Coleman, D. J., and Franzen, L. A. (1974): Ultrasonographic evidence of a consistent orbital involvement in Graves' disease. *N. Engl. J. Med.*, 290:1447–1450.
46. Zappia, R. J., Winkelman, J. Z., and Gay, A. J. (1971): Intraocular pressure changes in normal subjects and the adhesive muscle syndrome. *Am. J. Ophthalmol.*, 71:880–884.

The Eye and Orbit in Thyroid Disease, edited by
C. A. Gorman et al. Raven Press, New York 1984.

Eye Examination Techniques in Graves' Ophthalmopathy

Brian R. Younge

Department of Ophthalmology, Mayo Clinic, Rochester, Minnesota 55905

The highly variable modes of presentation encountered in Graves' ophthalmopathy frequently lead to misdiagnosis early in the disease. The disorder can cause external eye symptoms related to tearing, proptosis, soft tissue swelling, cosmetic changes, and discomfort that ranges from a burning sensation to deep orbital discomfort to excruciating pain around the outside of the eye. It can produce alterations in vision (by affecting the tear film), choroidal folds, choked discs, and compressive optic neuropathy as well as diplopia of all sorts due to muscle imbalance. It can cause lid retraction or ptosis, and sometimes both. Finally, this disorder is as perplexing to the examiner as it is to the patient because we have yet to find the cause, much less the definitive cure. We are often left with "soothing drops and soothing words" as our mainstay of treatment until something drastic must be done.

Ocular symptoms may precede or follow the diagnosis and treatment of hyperthyroidism (4). The findings include periorbital puffiness, a staring appearance, tearing and irritation, and a variable amount of exophthalmos that often starts unilaterally (Fig. 1). As the symptoms progress, the eyes become red, the vessels over the muscle insertions become plethoric, the bulbar conjunctiva becomes edematous, and very often diplopia develops in certain positions of gaze. It is usually late in the disorder that vision is compromised due to corneal breakdown or optic neuropathy, both of which are reversible in their early stages.

EXAMINATION OF THE EYE

A thorough and complete eye examination includes the usual measurements of best corrected vision, pupillary responses, ocular rotations, confrontation fields, flashlight inspection of the external eye and adnexa, ophthalmoscopic examination, and measurement of intraocular tensions. Then some special observations are made that pertain to the Graves' disease patient; these are described below.

Vision and Pupils

Hyperopia may be induced by pressure of swollen orbital tissues on the back of the globe, often hinted at by relatively poor near-vision; pinhole acuity may help improve the vision in the presence of tear film or corneal abnormalities not corrected by refraction. Before the pupils are dilated, a relative afferent pupil defect may be found with careful testing, indicating asymmetrical optic nerve compromise (see "Optic Neuropathy," below); such a finding may be lacking if both eyes have similar optic neuropathy. Thus the cause of reduced vision must be determined: refractive error, abnormal tear film or corneal drying, retinal distortion by choroidal folds, or optic neuropathy.

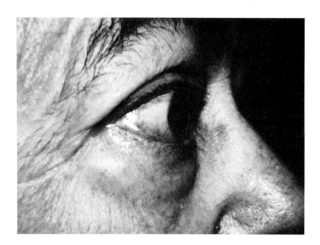

FIG. 1. Lateral profile of a patient with early orbitopathy, showing lid retraction, periorbital puffiness, mild chemosis, and moderate exophthalmos.

Ocular Motility

The range of eye movements is often compromised, particularly in up and out positions, and this may be most obvious upon comparing the two eyes in extremes of versions. Very few disorders affect the inferior rectus muscle as consistently as does Graves' disease, and one must think of the limitations of movement as being due to restriction rather than paresis, although both can occur, as in patients with both Graves' disease and myasthenia gravis. A

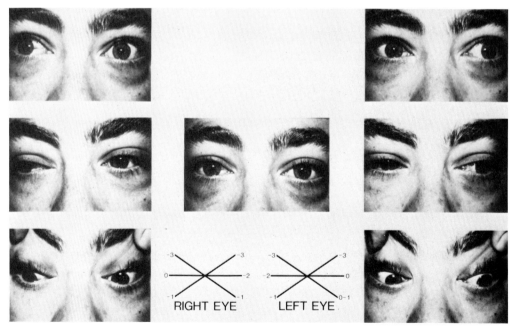

FIG. 2. Eyes in the cardinal positions of gaze—straight ahead, right and left, and oblique (up and down; right and left)—in a young man with early orbitopathy. The grading system used to quantitate the range of eye movement is shown by line diagram. 0, normal; − 1, mild limitation; − 2, moderate limitation; − 3, moderately severe limitation; − 4, complete limitation.

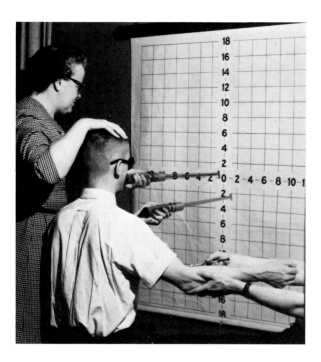

FIG. 3. Lancaster red–green test. Examiner aims the green light; patient aims the red light in an attempt to cover the position of green light. Because the patient wears a red lens over his right eye and a green lens over his left eye, the position of the red light indicates the position that the right eye sees—in this case ~2 prism diopters down and out related to the left eye. To test the left eye, the patient and examiner exchange lights. (From ref. 6a, by permission.)

simple diagram of the cardinal positions is useful for following the patient, with the limitation of movement graded from 0 to − 4 (Fig. 2).

Measurement of the position of one eye relative to the other in the cardinal positions of gaze is most easily done with the Lancaster red–green test. In this instance, the patient has a red lens over his right eye and a green lens over his left. The examiner controls a red or green light and gives the patient the other colored light. The right eye can see only the red light through the red lens, and the left can see only the green. The patient then aims his light to correspond to positions the examiner indicates on the screen with the other light. In this way the direction of each eye is shown by the position of the lights (Fig. 3). The separation of the two eyes is recorded (in prism diopters) for future comparisons.

A forced duction test may be useful to test limitation of eye movements, but this is stressful to a patient with red eyes, puffy lids, and tearing. An alternative is to measure the intraocular pressures in slight downward gaze and then in extreme upward and outward gaze. This is easily done with the hand-held Perkins applanation tonometer (Fig. 4) or the Makay–Marg instrument. An increase of more than 4 to 5 mm Hg is indicative of tethering of the globe by the opposing inferior rectus muscle. It is not unusual for the pressure to increase from normal (10 to 20 mm Hg) to nearly 40 mm Hg in this test.

External Eye

In addition to obvious periorbital edema and gross exophthalmos, one should look for the dilated vessels that often appear at the insertions of the lateral and sometimes the medial rectus muscles. This is quite common and rather characteristic of Graves' disease. The orbits should be palpated for the resistance to retropulsion of the globe. This may be asymmetrical, depending on the stage of the disorder. Failure of the globe to recede at least 1 mm into the orbit on measurements with the exophthalmometer on the patient in the

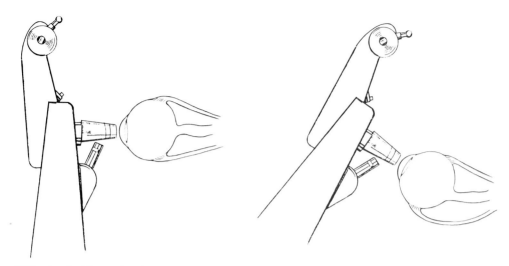

FIG. 4. Perkins applanation tonometry. **Left:** In primary position, slight downward gaze. **Right:** In upward gaze, pressure increases because of "tethering" effect of a tight inferior rectus muscle (shown as rather loose here, the normally related muscle).

reclining position also is a sign of expanded orbital soft tissue. Although exophthalmometry is not an accurate means of measuring exophthalmos, it is a useful procedure when done with care, especially if repeated by the same examiner under similar circumstances with the same instrument.

I prefer to use the Hertel instrument because the optics of the mirror system prevent significant error by parallax (Fig. 5). It is important to fit the reference pieces comfortably and correctly against the lateral orbital rim so that the same base measurement is used in the future. Examination of the eyelids is covered in detail in the chapter by Waller on eyelid malpositions in Graves' ophthalmopathy, *this volume*. Basically, one needs to note the width of the palpebral fissure, the position of the upper lid relative to the superior limbus (e.g., 2 mm above), and the presence of lid lag as the patient follows a target into downward gaze. One occasionally sees ptosis as a manifestation of Graves' disease, and ocular myasthenia can accompany this disorder, producing strange eye findings (Fig. 6). Many eponyms are used for external eye signs which are varied and often confusing (Table 1). Imagine this case history being told among students of Graves' disease:

> A 24-year-old developed Basedow's disease and within 2 years came down with Parry's disease that started with Dalrymple's sign and Enroth's sign. Her von Graefe's sign was also present, but Griffith's sign was not. The globe lag of Means was accompanied by Joffroy's sign, but soon thereafter Sainton's sign became manifest. As the patient contemplated her fate, Stellwag's sign gave way to Rosenbach's sign because the patient closed her eyes gently, tremulous all over, including the blinking lids. The examiner could no longer see the Knies sign, or Cowen's or Loewi's, but they are less important.

Ophthalmoscopy

In the majority of cases the ophthalmoscopic examination gives normal results, although on occasion there are some surprises. Disc edema (Fig. 7) identical in appearance to that of papilledema secondary to increased intracranial pressure can occur, and this can seriously compromise vision if left untreated too long. Choroidal folds—horizontal lines across the posterior pole of the eye (Fig. 7)—may result from the orbital pressure; after reversal of the

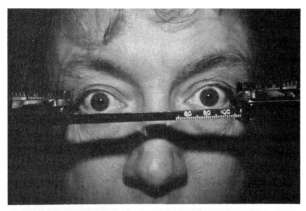

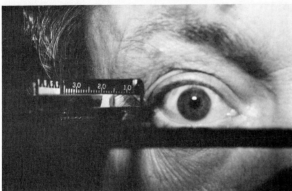

FIG. 5. Top: Hertel exophthalmometry. Note the position of the scale over the apex of the cornea in the mirror. Right eye measures 16.5 mm, left eye 16.0 mm. **Bottom:** Magnified view, showing scale and cornea. The effect of parallax is minimal because these images are in the same plane.

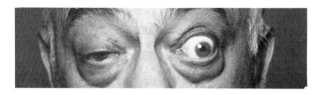

FIG. 6. Patient with Graves' disease and myasthenia gravis. Eyelids would retract alternately, or sometimes synchronously, and then become ptotic. When the right upper lid is retracted, the left becomes ptotic and the left eye goes down and out.

underlying disorder, these may persist as pigment lines even though the folds themselves resolve (1). Such folds may distort vision and decrease visual acuity. Often the clarity of the media is considerably impaired because of exposure keratopathy, and one is well advised to use the indirect ophthalmoscope for a better overview of the fundus.

OPTIC NEUROPATHY

Relevant Anatomy

The optic nerve courses 25 mm within the orbit, curving gently in an S-shape en route to the optic canal. It is closely surrounded in its posterior part by the muscle cone. If one considers the orbit to be essentially a closed space with a firm anterior wall ("orbital septum"), as tissue within this closed space becomes thickened to the point that the orbital septum becomes tight the optic nerve is stretched out and pressure within the orbit increases and is transmitted to all the tissues equally (hydraulic principle). At this point, an attempt

TABLE 1. *Eponyms for external eye signs*

Eponym	Definition
Ballet's sign	Complete immobility of globe without internal ophthalmoplegia
Boston's sign	Jerky, uneven downward movement of lid on downward gaze, not corresponding to eye
Dalrymple's sign	Staring appearance
Enroth's sign	Fullness of lids due to edema
Gifford's sign	Difficulty in everting upper lid
Griffiths' sign	Lagging of lower lid on upward gaze
Jellinek's sign	Inconstant pigmentation of lids
Joffroy's sign	Absence of forehead creases on upward gaze
Kocher's sign	Spasmodic increase in lid retraction with intense fixation
Means' globe lag	More rapid movement of lid in upward gaze compared to globe movement
Möbius' sign	Difficulty converging
Rosenbach's sign	Trembling of lids on gentle closure
Sainton's sign	Contraction of frontalis after levator has ceased
Stellwag's sign	Infrequent, incomplete blinking
Suker's sign	Inability to hold fixation in extreme lateral gaze
von Graefe's sign	Lid lag

to retropulse the globes is met with considerable resistance. In addition to the hydrostatic pressure, the tightness of the tissues in the posterior cone region is further increased by the proximity of the narrowing orbital walls and the thickened muscles. Orbital decompression reduces the orbital pressure, and thus there is a reasonable explanation for reversible compressive optic neuropathy—reversible even though decompression may not actually

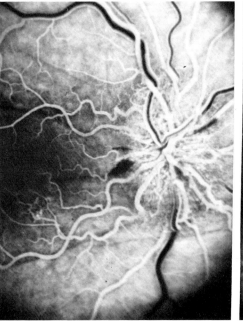
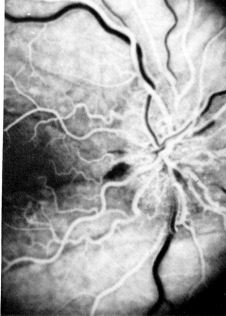

FIG. 7. Fluorescence angiography in a patient with a choroidal fold across the posterior pole. Patient also has papilledema (view by converging the eyes to see in stereo).

involve the region of the optic canal. The type of visual deficit that results from such compression affects color vision and acuity and produces optic nerve-type field defects (see below).

Relative Afferent Pupil Defect

As with any disorder that affects optic nerve transmission, Graves' disease can compromise the optic nerve sufficiently to affect the afferent loop of the pupillary light reflex pathway. Although often bilateral, an asymmetry may show up in the swinging flashlight test as a relative afferent pupil defect. This is important because it is one of the few objective signs that the observer can elicit and is independent of the clarity of the media, the refractive error, and the degree of the proptosis. The examiner should ensure that he knows the technique of this simple test.

Visual Fields

Perimetry is often difficult in the patient with Graves' disease, largely because of the inability to maintain comfortable straight-ahead gaze in many instances and also because of the chronic irritation of the exposed globe. It is important to have the patient refracted correctly because there is a general tendency to hypermetropia in many of these patients due to the increased retrobulbar pressure, sometimes associated with choroidal folds. Tangent screen examinations are perhaps the most satisfactory for the patient because the head can be comfortably positioned. The usual effect of severe Graves' disease on the visual fields is generalized depression, although there may be localized defects of arcuate form or unusual paracentral or central scotomas. Blind-spot enlargement occurs in those with disc edema. Irregular defects are common, but all of these defects are of the optic nerve type (Figs. 8 and 9). True glaucomatous defects are rare and occur with about the same frequency as in the general population (unpublished data from the Mayo Clinic series reported by DeSanto). Nonetheless, it is common to see patients being treated with antiglaucoma medications largely because intraocular pressure may be increased even in the straight-ahead position; in slight downward gaze the pressure is more likely to be normal.

Visual field defects are usually seen in conjunction with impaired perception of pseudoisochromatic color plates, decreased central visual acuity, prolongation of latency in visual evoked potentials, and, in asymmetrical involvement, a relative afferent pupil defect. These findings indicate optic nerve compromise. For the most part these defects are reversible after orbital decompression, similar to the reversible bitemporal hemianopia of pituitary tumors. There are favorable responses to other modalities of treatment, and sometimes improvement occurs with the evolution of the disorder over time. If one could pick out those cases that would behave in such a manner, it would be easy to know which patients should undergo decompression.

Static perimetry shows similar defects whether performed manually or by an automated perimeter, with the whole of the field being depressed in threshold values compared to normal (Fig. 10). Central values may be depressed in the presence of normal acuity, as they are in other mild optic neuropathies, e.g., the optic neuritis of multiple sclerosis. As our experience with the automated static perimeters develops, we are seeing the defects perhaps differently than we saw them on standard kinetic perimetry. In these examples, kinetic perimetry would have shown only a relative depression manifested by shrinking isopters with the small targets.

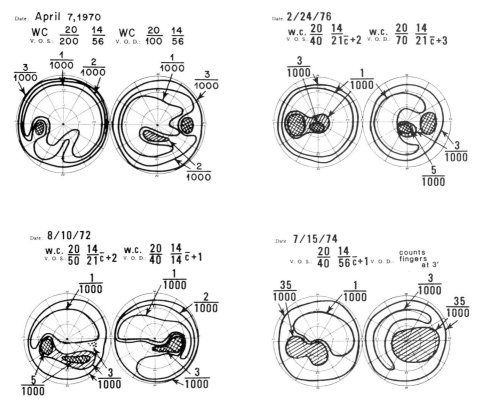

FIG. 8. Tangent screen examinations. **Top left:** Depression generally, more so superiorly right and inferiorly left, with a paracentral scotoma right. **Top right:** Relative central scotomas with mildly depressed vision. **Bottom left:** Similar defects, inferior arc-like. **Bottom right:** Dense central defect in right eye; relative defect in left eye.

The results of judiciously applied orbital decompression are dramatic and predictable in more than 85 to 90% patients who have optic neuropathy and reduced vision (Fig. 11). In those with severe loss of vision, the time to recovery may be considerably prolonged, but usually there is some immediate improvement followed by gradual further recovery. Of the 72 patients in DeSanto's study who had optic nerve involvement, 32 had received steroids, a few had been treated with radiation, and some had undergone other forms of decompression including transfrontal craniotomy. All of these patients improved, with one exception who had been treated with orbital irradiation (6,000 rads). Only three among this series had glaucoma, one with an arcuate defect. All eight patients who had had choked discs recovered; the edema subsided rapidly postoperatively.

Some comments about other treatment modalities are warranted because orbital surgery is not readily available in all areas, and there is considerable pressure to use low-dose radiation treatment or other lesser surgical procedures the ophthalmologist may be able to perform himself. Ravin et al. (6) described treatment of 37 patients with x-ray irradiation; nine had optic neuropathy. These nine exhibited the most dramatic response to treatment in that series, only one requiring further steroids and decompression. Trobe et al. (8) reported improvement of vision (two lines or more) and fields in 21 patients after using steroids as the first treatment, supervoltage irradiation as the second, and orbital decompression as the last resort. They noted improvement in 50% of those treated by irradiation. Some of these

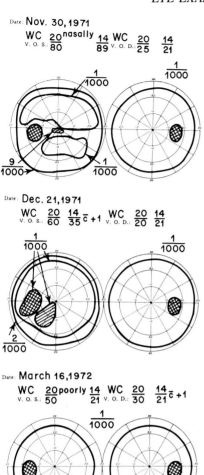

Date: Nov. 30, 1971

Date: Dec. 21, 1971

Date: March 16, 1972

FIG. 9. Fields showing gradual improvement after decompression.

then underwent operation. One of their patients who had been treated with steroids, irradiation, and decompression from above later underwent decompression transantrally at our institution.

We have decompressed an additional 14 patients who were radiation-treatment failures from other institutions and all but one improved considerably (3). The one who did not had received 6,000 rads to the orbits, and optic atrophy had already begun to develop along with cataracts and neovascularization. Kriss et al. (5) reported good to excellent results of radiation treatment given to 141 patients (71% of the 121 that were followed); only four went on to orbital decompression. Unfortunately, these investigators did not separate those with optic neuropathy, and it was difficult to distinguish those who might have had spontaneous remission from those who had received radiation. Teng et al. (7) evaluated 20 patients who had moderately severe Graves' disease, but none of these had optic neuropathy; they were not impressed with the results of radiation treatment. Covington et al. (2) reported good results after treatment of seven patients, four of whom had optic neuropathy.

None of these reports adequately discussed the long-term effects and risks of radiation treatment. Most of the patients with Graves' ophthalmopathy are 40 to 50 years old. Their

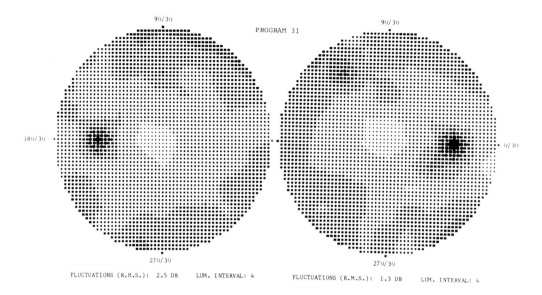

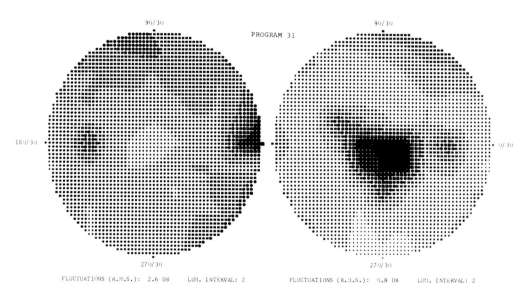

FIG. 10. Computer-assisted perimetry. Gray scale printout representing central 30° of visual field. Dark areas are seen poorly; light areas are seen well. **Top:** Patient with mild optic neuropathy of Graves' disease. Right eye (20/40) has mild generalized depression; left eye (20/20) is normal. **Bottom:** Patient with more severe optic neuropathy of Graves' disease. Note the large central scotoma in the right eye and mild general depression in the left eye.

disorder is not malignant, and it is for the most part self-limiting. To subject such patients with nonmalignant disease to a potentially carcinogenic agent seems inappropriate.

In our series we were able to restore vision to normal or near-normal in 90% of cases (Fig. 11), and fields were improved substantially in 85%. Although this is not the ideal treatment of this disorder because it entails the risk of surgical intervention—perhaps several

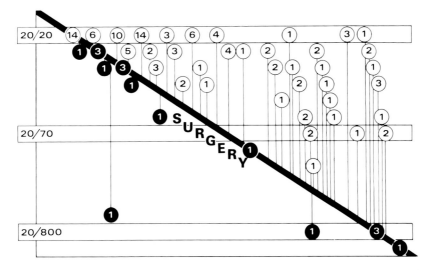

FIG. 11. Results of surgical decompression: effect on visual acuity. The dark diagonal bar represents initial vision; lines to circles represent postoperative change in acuity. Numbers in the circles are the numbers of eyes so changed. Note that very few eyes became worse. Most improved, some from very poor vision preoperatively. (From ref. 3.)

times—to rehabilitate the patient, we have been pleased with the results overall, particularly as the number of cases increases. It seems to us that the use of ionizing radiation might entail risks as yet undetermined in young individuals. Because our approach is producing rapid improvement with a high probability of substantial improvement, we have not hesitated to recommend decompression for those with optic neuropathy. Surgical risks are acceptable when the surgeon is experienced. The risks with a well-done decompression are fewer than those inherent in long-term, high-dose steroid therapy. Fortunately, we may see the end of this disorder within the decade and no longer will be needing surgical treatment for these patients. Knowledge of the definitive cause, and thus the cure, is close at hand.

REFERENCES

1. Bullock, J. D., and Waller, R. R. (1978): Choroidal folding in orbital disease. In: *Proceedings of the 3rd International Symposium on Orbital Disorders: Amsterdam, September 5–7, 1977*, edited by The Orbital Centre of the Amsterdam University Eye Hospital, The Netherlands Ophthalmic Research Institute, The Netherlands Ophthalmological Society, and The New York Eye and Ear Infirmary, pp. 483–488. Dr. W. Junk bv Publishers, Boston.
2. Covington, E. E., Lobes, L., and Sudarsanam, A. (1977): Radiation therapy for exophthalmos: report of seven cases. *Radiology*, 122:797–799.
3. DeSanto, L. W. (1980): The total rehabilitation of Graves' ophthalmopathy. *Laryngoscope*, 90:1652–1678.
4. Gorman, C. A. (1983): Temporal relationship between onset of Graves' ophthalmopathy and diagnosis of thyrotoxicosis. *Mayo Clin. Proc.*, 58:515–519.
5. Kriss, J. P., McDougall, I. R., and Donaldson, S. S. (1981): Graves' ophthalmopathy: hypothesis of its pathogenesis and result of treatment by supervoltage orbital radiotherapy. In: *Thyroid University Case Reports*, Vol. 3, No. 3. Parke-Davis, Morris Plains, New Jersey.
6. Ravin, J. G., Sisson, J. C., and Knapp, W. T. (1975): Orbital radiation for the ocular changes of Graves' disease. *Am. J. Ophthalmol.*, 79:285–288.
6a. Retzlaff, J. A., Kearns, T. P., Howard, F. M., Jr., Cronin, M. L. (1969): Lancaster red-green test in evaluation of edrophonium effect in myasthenia gravis. *J. Ophthamol.*, 67:13.
7. Teng, C. S., Crombie, A. L., Hall, R., and Ross, W. M. (1980): An evaluation of supervoltage orbital irradiation for Graves' ophthalmopathy. *Clin. Endocrinol. (Oxf.)*, 13:545–551.
8. Trobe, J. D., Glaser, J. S., and Laflamme, P. (1978): Dysthyroid optic neuropathy: clinical profile and rationale for management. *Arch. Ophthalmol.*, 96:1199–1209.

The Eye and Orbit in Thyroid Disease, edited by
C. A. Gorman et al. Raven Press, New York 1984.

Intraocular Pressure and Thyroid Disease

*George T. Gamblin, **Paul G. Galentine III, and †Charles Eil

*Portsmouth Naval Hospital, Portsmouth, Virginia 23708; and Departments of **Ophthalmology
and †Endocrinology, Bethesda Naval Hospital, Bethesda, Maryland 20814*

The existence of a relationship between intraocular pressure and thyroid disease was
suggested as long ago as 1901 when Brailey and Eyre (4) first alleged that glaucoma
occurred more frequently in hyperthyroid subjects than in the normal population. Subsequently, numerous reports, often contradictory, were devoted to this topic. Much of the
confusion surrounding this issue has resulted from the failure to appreciate, until relatively
recently, the importance of eye posture when measuring intraocular pressure.

It is now well recognized that patients with thyroid exophthalmos frequently exhibit
transient positional changes in intraocular pressure (5,7,8,14,27,36,42,48,53), especially on
upgaze. This probably reflects compression of the globe by the opposing inelastic extraocular
muscle. In addition, abnormal intraocular pressure elevations on upgaze have been detected
in many patients with Graves' disease without exophthalmos (14,27), indicative of apparent
subclinical ophthalmopathy. In view of these findings, it has been suggested that the measurement of intraocular pressure may be useful clinically in the evaluation of Graves'
ophthalmopathy.

In this chapter we review what is currently known of the relationship between thyroid
dysfunction and intraocular pressure. Although the association between thyroid disease and
nonpositional intraocular pressure changes is discussed, we focus primarily on the positional
changes in intraocular pressure because of its greater relevance to thyroid-related orbital
disease. Before proceeding further, however, the reader should first have some understanding
of ocular hydrodynamics and the methods available for assessing intraocular tension.

AQUEOUS HUMOR CIRCULATION

Under normal conditions, intraocular pressure is between 10 and 22 mm Hg and is
dependent on the rate of aqueous humor formation and resistance to outflow from the eye.
The total volume of aqueous is 125 μl with approximately 80% occupying the anterior
chamber and 20% in the posterior chamber. Aqueous is constantly produced by the epithelium of the ciliary body (Fig. 1) at a rate of 2 to 3 μl/min by a process which involves
diffusion, ultrafiltration, and active transport. From the posterior chamber, the fluid passes
through the pupil into the anterior chamber where it flows peripherally. At the irido-corneal-
scleral angle, the aqueous is filtered by the trabeculum and passes into Schlemm's canal
where it is ultimately conducted into the venous system. Most of the resistance to aqueous
outflow resides in the trabecular meshwork (41).

MEASUREMENT OF INTRAOCULAR PRESSURE

The measurement of intraocular pressure can be accomplished by either manometry or
tonometry. Manometry involves placing a cannula in the anterior chamber of the eye and is

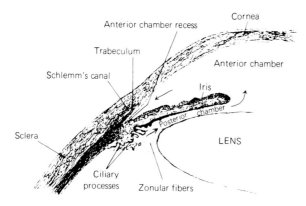

FIG. 1. Flow of aqueous humor. (From ref. 45a.)

the only method that measures intraocular pressure directly. It is the most accurate method of measurement, but because it is invasive and attended with certain morbidity its use is restricted to laboratory animals.

With tonometry, intraocular pressure can be determined indirectly by measuring the force required to deform the surface of the eye, either by applanation or indentation. Indentation tonometry, which predates the applanation technique, relies on the principle that the depth of indentation produced by a given force in a fluid-filled compartment is related to the internal pressure. Instruments designed on this principle were available as early as the mid-nineteenth century. The only instrument of this type in widespread use today is the Shiotz tonometer (38) introduced in 1905. Indentation tonometry suffers from several methodological flaws (to be discussed below) and, as a result, is less accurate than any of the applanation tonometers currently available. However, because of its simplicity, portability, and low cost, the Shiotz tonometer has enjoyed widespread use primarily as a screening tool for glaucoma by the general practitioner (52).

Applanation tonometry is based on the principle that the pressure within a sphere can be determined by the force required to applanate (or flatten) a known area on its surface. (Pressure is defined mathematically, by $p = f/a$ where p is the internal pressure, f is the force applied, and a is the area over which the force acts.) It can be performed by measuring either the force required to applanate a fixed area or by measuring the area flattened by a fixed force (31).

Three complicating factors can affect the accuracy of tonometry: (a) corneal elasticity; (b) tear meniscus attraction; and (c) aqueous displacement. Corneal elasticity refers to the corneal resistance to deformation which must be overcome during tonometry; this force elevates the pressure reading obtained. Tear meniscus attraction is the force produced by the surface tension of tears, which tends to pull the tonometer head toward the cornea and thus would lower the reading obtained for intraocular pressure. Finally, deformation of the cornea displaces fluid which transiently produces a falsely high intraocular pressure reading (31).

Unfortunately, both indentation (Shiotz) and fixed-force applanation tonometers (Maklokov, Halberg, and Inglima-Posner) fail to correct for these factors (31,39). Furthermore, because all are hand-held, inadvertent tilting of the tonometer head may result in eccentric corneal contact and thus lead to an erroneous measurement.

Applanation tonometry using a fixed area represents the most accurate clinical method available for measuring intraocular pressure. An instrument of this kind was first developed by Fick during the late nineteenth century (12) and was later refined by Goldmann (15).

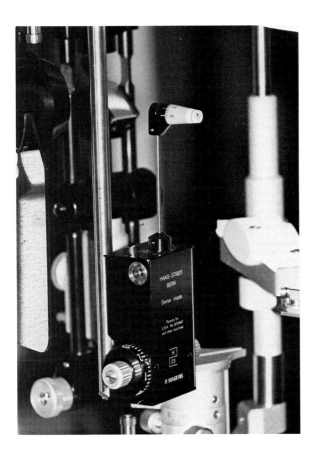

FIG. 2. Goldmann applanation tonometer.

The latter tonometer, which bears Goldmann's name and has become the standard tonometer in use today, determines intraocular pressure by measuring the force required to flatten a fixed circular area on the cornea 3.06 mm in diameter. For this area the opposing forces of corneal elasticity and tear meniscus attraction are balanced and the displacement of aqueous is negligible (0.5 μl, or a pressure increase of 3%) (16,17,31). Thus all the potential sources of artifact in the measurement of intraocular pressure are minimized.

The measurement is obtained by using a cylinder of the required diameter mounted on an arm that is advanced by means of a spring-loaded knob. This spring controls the amount of force applied by the applanating cylinder, and this can be read from a scale on the knob (Fig. 2). The Goldmann instrument relies on an optical means to determine the endpoint in pressure measurement. This endpoint is determined in the following manner. The tonometer is mounted on a slit lamp biomicroscope (Fig. 3). A fluorescent dye is placed in the eye in order to aid in the visualization of the endpoint. When the corneal surface is flattened beneath the applanator, the tear film which has been forced off the corneal surface forms a meniscus around the edge of the applanator. If one views this through a clear plastic applanator under blue light, a ring of fluorescence is seen. However, if two prisms are placed in the cylinder and appropriately positioned, this image is split into two semicircles (mires). The prisms can then be adjusted so that the two mires are optically separated by 3.06 mm. When the flattened surface of the cornea is that of a circle with the same diameter, the images barely touch (Fig. 4). Vernier acuity can then be utilized to identify the endpoint.

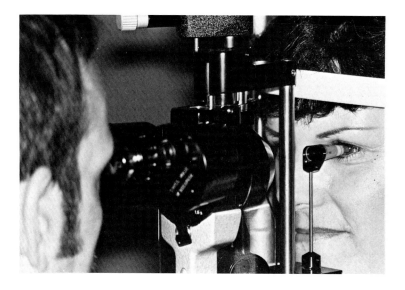

FIG. 3. Demonstration of applanation tonometry. Note that a slit-lamp biomicroscope is used to determine the endpoint.

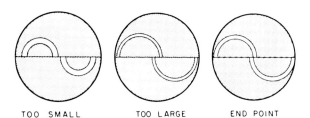

TOO SMALL   TOO LARGE   END POINT

FIG. 4. Appearance of mires through the slit-lamp biomicroscope when performing applanation tonometry. (From ref. 22a.)

The Draeger and Perkins (34) tonometers are portable hand-held instruments which utilize the same principle as the Goldmann applanation tonometer. Some ophthalmologists believe that these tonometers more accurately follow the curve of the cornea when positional changes of intraocular pressure are being measured (28). However, the instruments share the same inaccuracy inherent in all hand-held tonometers described above. Their major advantage is their portability, allowing applanation tonometry to be performed at the bedside or in the operating room where a Goldmann unit cannot be utilized (10).

Elevated intraocular pressure may result from increased aqueous production or increased resistance to outflow. The relative contribution of each of these variables can be approximated by tonography (not to be confused with tonometry), which is performed by recording the change in intraocular pressure over time in response to the application of a weight. Tonography employs an indentation tonometer with an electronic recording device. This technique is based on the formula derived from Grant (19); $V/Pt = C$, where V is the change in volume of the globe, P the change of pressure within the eye, t the time, and C the "coefficient of aqueous outflow." The validity of this measuring device has been challenged because indentation of the eye induces changes in aqueous formation and blood flow. However, apparently these effects negate each other to a large extent, as tonography results have been shown to compare favorably with perfusion studies of the eye (6,23). Tonography seems to be the most practical method for studying ocular hydrodynamics in human subjects.

NONPOSITIONAL INTRAOCULAR PRESSURE CHANGES
IN THYROID DISEASE

In view of the well-recognized hemodynamic effects of thyroid hormone excess or deficiency in man, it would not be unreasonable to expect that thyroid disease might affect ocular hydrodynamics. Indeed, intraocular pressure changes have been described in other endocrine states, e.g., hypercortisolism (1,3,24,26,35), acromegaly (22), and pregnancy (33). Furthermore, because Graves' disease is frequently accompanied by swelling and inflammation of the retrobulbar soft tissues, it is easy to imagine how obstruction to aqueous outflow might increase intraocular tension.

A possible link between intraocular hypertension and thyroid disease was first appreciated by Brailey and Eyre in 1901 (4), when they reported five young women with hyperthyroidism and exophthalmos who had evidence of glaucoma by palpation. During the first half of the twentieth century, at least 25 studies examining intraocular pressure among patients with thyroid hyper- and hypofunction were published. These older studies were thoroughly reviewed by Pohjanpelto (36), who emphasized the lack of agreement on this question. It should be noted that tonometry from this era was poorly developed and predated recognition of the importance of eye posture when measuring intraocular pressure (5).

Interest in thyroid-related intraocular pressure changes was renewed during the 1960's by a retrospective study of McLenachan and Davies (29). These authors found thyroid dysfunction in 45 of 100 patients with open-angle glaucoma, including 16 with thyrotoxicosis and 16 with hypothyroidism. Becker et al. (2) noted that protein-bound iodine (PBI) levels in patients with open-angle glaucoma were significantly lower than in patients with closed-angle glaucoma. Finally, the most dramatic findings were those of Vasilieva (45), who studied 53 patients with hyperthyroidism and found that all had increased intraocular pressure which correlated directly with thyroid hormone levels. Other investigators, paying close attention to eye position when performing tonometry, have failed to corroborate these findings. In fact, Weekers and co-workers, who originally reported a high incidence of glaucoma among patients with Graves' exophthalmos (46), later retracted this claim when it was realized that intraocular tension had been measured in upgaze (47,48). Overestimation of intraocular tension resulting from upward gaze in patients with Graves' disease with (7,8,14,27,36,42,52) and without (14,27) exophthalmos has since been well documented.

Cheng and Perkins (7), in a convincing study of 155 patients with thyroid disease, found only two cases of glaucoma. This prevalence of glaucoma is no greater than that for all individuals over 40 years of age (2.0 to 2.4%) (25). There were 17 patients with exophthalmos, and all had normal intraocular pressure in the primary position. Furthermore, there was no significant difference in the mean intraocular pressures among patients who were either hyperthyroid, euthyroid, or hypothyroid at the time of the eye examination.

Pohjanpelto (36), in an elegant study which also carefully took into account direction of gaze, examined 187 patients with various thyroid disorders and found a somewhat higher prevalence of glaucoma ($\sim 6\%$) among patients with a history of hyperthyroidism; however, as a group these patients had an average intraocular pressure which was no different from normal. The prevalence of glaucoma among patients with a history of hypothyroidism was normal. Longitudinal studies in the hyperthyroid patients indicated that intraocular pressure was independent of thyroid hormone levels. Although exophthalmic subjects had minimally higher, but statistically significant, intraocular pressure readings, the prevalence of glaucoma among these patients was no greater than among hyperthyroid subjects without exophthalmos. Furthermore, there was no correlation between intraocular tension and degree of proptosis. The failure of Cheng and Perkins (7) to appreciate a higher prevalence of glaucoma among hyperthyroid patients may have been due to the younger population examined (46 years versus 52.1 years) as the incidence of glaucoma is known to increase with age. Regardless of the true incidence of glaucoma, the two studies (7,36) agreed that neither thyroid hormone levels nor orbital involvement greatly influence intraocular pressure when positional errors are excluded. It is interesting to note that tonographic studies of hyperthyroid subjects suggest a significantly higher rate of aqueous formation. However, this is countered by an increase in aqueous outflow. Both of these variables normalize with restoration of the euthyroid state (36). Thus hyperthyroidism seems to be associated with a hyperdynamic aqueous circulation but with no net change in intraocular tension.

Although glaucoma among hypothyroid patients is no more common than in the general population (7,36), some patients with both hypothyroidism and glaucoma have been reported to have dramatic improvement in intraocular pressure with the institution of thyroid hormone therapy (20,21,29,36). Tonographic studies indicate that this effect is achieved by improving aqueous outflow with little or no effect on aqueous formation (36). It seems that in some patients with a genetic predisposition for glaucoma hypothyroidism may be a precipitating factor for the initiation of intraocular hypertension. How hypothyroidism decreases aqueous outflow is unclear; however, it has been postulated that in myxedema a mucopolysaccharide is deposited in the intertrabecular spaces of the anterior chamber (29). This has yet to be demonstrated.

POSITIONAL INTRAOCULAR CHANGES IN THYROID DISEASE

The first hint that direction of gaze alters intraocular pressure in patients with thyroid exophthalmos was provided in 1918 by Wessely (51), who noted that these patients frequently exhibited great variations in intraocular pressure. However, it was not until more than 30 years later that Braley (5) recognized the true significance of this observation. He reported a patient with severe Graves' ophthalmopathy, manifested by marked proptosis, soft tissue swelling, ophthalmoplegia, and papilledema, who exhibited a 20 mm Hg rise in intraocular pressure bilaterally when the eyes were moved from the resting position (slight downgaze 5° to 10°) to the primary position (0°). This was in contrast to normal eyes, which have been shown to have a negligible rise in intraocular pressure (<2 mm Hg) with elevation (9,14,27,53). Braley attributed this finding to an inelastic opposing inferior rectus muscle which during upgaze compressed the globe and caused a transient elevation of intraocular pressure. Other investigators have since confirmed this to be a frequent finding in patients with Graves' exophthalmos (7,8,14,27,36,42,48,53).

Positional intraocular pressure changes in patients with Graves' exophthalmos, although most commonly demonstrated in upward gaze, occur in other positions of regard as well (9,27). This is not surprising as it is known that extraocular muscles other than the inferior recti are affected in Graves' ophthalmopathy. Orbital computed tomographic (CT) studies of these patients indicate that the inferior rectus is most frequently involved, followed by the medial, superior, and lateral recti (11,14). Given this information, one would then expect intraocular pressure abnormalities to be present most commonly in upgaze, followed in decreasing order by lateral gaze, downgaze, and medial gaze. However, aside from the studies mentioned earlier (9,27), few data for intraocular pressure measurements taken in these other positions in patients with Graves' eye disease have been reported.

Investigators (14,27,53) have suggested that the measurement of positional intraocular pressure changes may be clinically useful in the detection of orbital involvement in Graves'

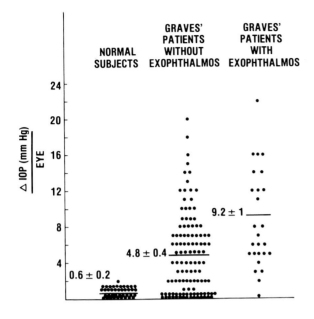

FIG. 5. Magnitude of change in intraocular pressure *(IOP)* in normal subjects and in patients with Graves' disease. (From ref. 14.)

disease as well as in monitoring the progression of ophthalmopathy. Lyons (27), in a study of 36 patients with Graves' exophthalmos, found that all demonstrated significant ($\geqslant 3$ mm Hg) intraocular pressure increases on upgaze. Additionally, of nine patients with Graves' disease with lid retraction only, four had abnormal pressure readings. We (14) examined 80 patients with Graves' disease (Fig. 5), most of whom had little or no clinical evidence of eye involvement. Exophthalmos was present in 21 (26%), and all had pressure increases on upgaze. Of the remaining 59 patients without exophthalmos, 40 (68%) had ophthalmopathy as indicated by intraocular pressure. Eight patients without exophthalmos but with abnormal intraocular pressures underwent CT which confirmed the presence of extraocular muscle enlargement (primarily inferior and medial recti) in six of these patients. The presence of intraocular pressure abnormalities in most patients without clinical eye disease is consistent with orbital ultrasonographic (50) and CT (11) studies, which also indicate frequent subclinical ophthalmopathy.

In addition to being a sensitive indicator of Graves' eye disease, the measurement of positional intraocular pressure changes may be useful clinically in monitoring the progression of ophthalmopathy and its response to therapy (49). Pressure changes seem to correlate well with severity of ophthalmopathy, as suggested by the data of Draeger and Schneider (9), who found that intraocular pressure increases on upgaze were greater in patients with exophthalmos complicated by ophthalmoplegia and soft tissue involvement than in patients with exophthalmos alone. Furthermore, positional pressure changes have been shown to be generally greater in Graves' patients with exophthalmos than in those without it (14) (Fig. 5). Longitudinal studies comparing pressure changes with severity of orbital disease would be helpful in further assessing this clinical application. It is worthwhile to note here that in cross-sectional studies we noted that the percentage of Graves' patients with ophthalmopathy (as judged by positional intraocular pressure readings) increased with the time elapsed from the diagnosis of Graves' disease and was nearly universal after 10 years (Fig. 6). From these data it seems that some degree of ophthalmopathy eventually occurs in almost all patients with Graves' disease.

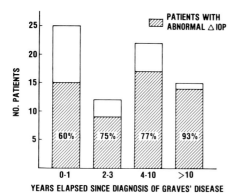

FIG. 6. Incidence of abnormal change in intraocular pressure *(IOP)* in patients with Graves' disease, according to time since diagnosis. (From ref. 14.)

It should be recognized that the presence of positional intraocular pressure changes is not specific for Graves' ophthalmopathy. Both orbital myositis and orbital fracture with inferior rectus entrapment have been shown to cause intraocular pressure increases in upgaze (53). Conceivably, any process, including primary or metastatic tumor, previous orbital surgery, or irradiation, which leads to restriction of extraocular muscle movement could cause this phenomenon. On the other hand, normal subjects (9,14,27,53) as well as patients with glaucoma, heterotropia, and ocular palsy (53) have been demonstrated to have negligible (≤2 mm Hg) rises in intraocular pressure on upgaze. There has been only one report (37) of "normal" subjects exhibiting increased intraocular pressure on upgaze; however, these patients had no thyroid evaluation and may in fact have had subclinical Graves' disease. To date we have evaluated 54 normal subjects and only one had an unexplained small pressure rise on upgaze (13,14). Thus if the above listed conditions which might restrict extraocular muscle movement can be excluded, it is reasonable to infer the presence of Graves' ophthalmopathy when there is a rise in intraocular pressure on upgaze.

Unilateral exophthalmos, especially when not associated with obvious thyroid disease, can present a difficult diagnostic dilemma where intraocular pressure measurements may be of value. Here the demonstration of bilateral orbital involvement, as indicated by intraocular pressure, would tend to support the presence of Graves' disease and to exclude processes which are usually unilateral, including orbital myositis and primary orbital tumors (44). Zappia et al. (53) studied five patients with unilateral proptosis secondary to orbital myositis and found abnormal pressure changes in the involved side only. In contrast, we have examined seven patients with Graves' disease and unilateral proptosis, and all had bilateral intraocular pressure elevations (14). These observations are consistent with the results of high-resolution orbital CT scanning, which showed that the extraocular muscles in the nonprotruding eye are frequently enlarged in patients with Graves' disease and unilateral exophathalmos (44). Although the demonstration of bilateral orbital involvement provides more support for the presence of Graves' ophthalmopathy, it should be emphasized that this finding alone is not diagnostic and should be interpreted in light of the clinical setting. Conversely, unilateral orbital involvement, although uncommon (11), may also represent Graves' ophthalmopathy.

The measurement of intraocular pressure in upgaze may also be helpful clinically in differentiating ophthalmoplegia due to Graves' disease from that occurring as a result of ocular muscle palsy. The true cause of opthalmoplegia in patients with Graves' disease without exophthalmos can easily be overlooked and erroneously attributed to extraocular muscle palsy. Patients with limited upgaze due to Graves' disease almost always exhibit pressure elevations when vertical movement is attempted (14,36,53). In contrast, patients with extraocular muscle palsy uniformly fail to raise their intraocular pressure when attempting upgaze (53). Hence this test seems to be highly reliable in distinguishing these two conditions. It should be noted that there is a higher incidence of myasthenia gravis among patients with Graves' disease (30). Thus in patients with Graves' disease, ophthalmoplegia should not automatically be assumed to result from Graves' ophthalmopathy. Conversely, limited extraocular muscle movement in a patient with myasthenia gravis may be due to concomitant Graves' ophthalmopathy.

The frequent presence of subclinical ophthalmopathy in Graves' disease, as indicated by positional intraocular pressure changes (14), orbital ultrasonography (50), and CT (11), supports the concept of a close relationship between the thyroidal and orbital components of Graves' disease and argues against the theory that Graves' ophthalmopathy represents a distinct, separate autoimmune disease (32,40). This connection has been further strengthened by the data of Tamai et al. (43), who found some evidence of subtle thyroid dysfunction (i.e., either goiter, high ^{131}I uptake, T_3 nonsuppressibility, or unresponsiveness to thyrotropin-releasing hormone) in all 57 patients with euthyroid Graves' ophthalmopathy. Furthermore, of 27 euthyroid patients followed for 6 months to 3 years, 17 became thyrotoxic. Finally, the close temporal relationship between the onset of ophthalmopathy and hyperthyroidism noted by Gorman (18) in 81% of patients with severe Graves' ophthalmopathy is additional evidence in favor of a closely related pathogenesis.

MANAGEMENT OF INTRAOCULAR HYPERTENSION IN THE PATIENT WITH GRAVES' OPHTHALMOPATHY

When confronted with a patient with elevated intraocular pressure, it is first necessary to distinguish positional from nonpositional pressure elevations. This distinction can be made by having the patient examined with the eyes in the resting position, which is normally $-5°$ to $-10°$ downgaze. In patients with severe tethering of the inferior rectus and fixed downgaze, the resting position may even be lower. The presence of elevated intraocular pressure in the resting position in patients with Graves' ophthalmopathy should be regarded as a separate, primary process unrelated to the degree of orbital involvement or hyperthyroidism (7,36). Management of this population should follow the same guidelines established for other patients with glaucoma or suspected glaucoma. In the rare patient with Graves' ophthalmopathy and glaucoma who has visual field abnormalities, one should always be aware of the possibility of optic nerve compression. In general, optic neuropathy is suggested by more central visual field defects and the lack of visual field improvement following normalization of intraocular pressure (see Gamblin, *this volume*, for further discussion of optic neuropathy.

Intraocular pressure elevations which are strictly positional in patients with Graves' ophthalmopathy do not portend the same threat to vision as do the constantly elevated pressures in the resting position. Cross-sectional studies of Graves' patients with purely positional intraocular hypertension have not demonstrated either visual field defects or cupping of the optic disc (27,36). This is not surprising as the pressure rise resulting from compression of the globe by an enlarged extraocular muscle is transient, lasting only a few seconds. Thus although the presence of positional intraocular pressure changes reflects some degree of extraocular muscle restrictions, treatment of the pressure change per se is not indicated.

SUMMARY

1. Applanation tonometry determined with a device using a fixed area provides the most accurate clinical method for estimating intraocular pressure.

2. Thyroid hormone alterations and the ophthalmopathy of Graves' disease exert little effect on intraocular pressure if the measurement is performed with the eyes in the resting position (5° to 10° downgaze).

3. Elevated intraocular pressure in upgaze is uniformly present in patients with Graves' exophthalmos.

4. Elevated intraocular pressure in upgaze is also frequently found in patients with no signs or symptoms of eye disease, consistent with subclinical ophthalmopathy.

5. The measurement of positional intraocular pressure changes may be clinically useful in the evaluation of patients with unilateral exophthalmos and with ophthalmoplegia.

6. Elevations in intraocular pressure, if present only in upgaze, do not require therapy; patients with intraocular pressure in the resting position, however, should be managed for glaucoma in the usual fashion.

7. The frequent presence of subclinical ophthalmopathy, as indicated by positional intraocular pressure changes, supports the concept of a closely related pathogenesis for the orbital and thyroidal components of Graves' disease.

8. The measurement of positional changes in intraocular pressure, heretofore regarded as a potential source of error in the diagnosis of glaucoma, may provide a useful, sensitive, and noninvasive tool for the detection of Graves' ophthalmopathy as well as a means of monitoring its progression and response to therapy.

ACKNOWLEDGMENTS

The authors are grateful to Ms. Cathy Morris for preparation of the manuscript.

This work was supported in part by funds (project CIC 81-06-1511) from the Bureau of Medicine and Surgery, Department of the Navy.

The opinions expressed herein are those of the authors and are not to be construed as reflecting the views of the Department of the Navy, the Naval Service at large, or the Department of Defense.

REFERENCES

1. Alfano, J. E. (1963): Changes in the intraocular pressure associated with systemic steroid therapy. *Am. J. Ophthalmol.*, 56:245–247.
2. Becker, B., Kolker, A. E., and Ballin, N. (1966): Thyroid function and glaucoma. *Am. J. Ophthalmol.*, 61:997–999.
3. Bernstein, H. N., and Schwartz, B. (1962): Effects of long-term systemic steroids on ocular pressure on tonographic values. *Arch. Ophthalmol.*, 68:742–753.
4. Brailey, W. A., and Eyre, J. W. H. (1901): Exophthalmic goitre with increased tension. *Ophthalmol. Rev.*, 20:147–148.
5. Braley, A. E. (1953): Malignant exophthalmos. *Am. J. Ophthalmol.*, 36:1286–1290.
6. Brubaker, R. F. (1967): Determination of episcleral venous pressure in the eye: a comparison of three methods. *Arch. Ophthalmol.*, 77:110–114.
7. Cheng, H., and Perkins, E. S. (1967): Thyroid disease and glaucoma. *Br. J. Ophthalmol.*, 51:547–553.
8. Draeger, J., and Schneider, C. (1963): Ein beitrag zur differenzierung der verlaufsfermen der endokrinen ophthalmopathie. *Klin. Monatsbl. Augenheilkd.*, 143:104–116.
9. Draeger, J., and Schneider, C. (1975): Intraocular pressure and direction of gaze in endocrine exophthalmos. *Proc. Int. Symp. Orbital Disorders, 2nd, 1973) Mod. Probl. Ophthalmol.*, 14:439–445.
10. Dunn, J. S., and Brubaker, R. F. (1973): Perkins applanation tonometer: clinical and laboratory evaluation. *Arch. Ophthalmol.*, 89:149–151.
11. Enzmann, D. R., Donaldson, S. S., and Kriss, J. P. (1979): Appearance of Graves' disease on orbital computed tomography. *J. Comput. Assist. Tomogr.*, 3:815–819.

12. Fick, A.: Ein neves ophthalmotonometer (dissertation), Wurzburg, 1888.
13. Gamblin, G. T., Galentine, P. G., Harper, D. G., Chernow, B., and Eil, C. (1983): Screening for elevated intraocular pressure (IOP) on upgaze in thyroid disease. *Endocrinol.*, 113(Suppl.):T6 (Abstr.).
14. Gamblin, G. T., Harper, D. G., Galentine, P., Buck, D. R., Chernow, B., and Eil, C. (1983): Prevalence of increased intraocular pressure in Graves' disease: evidence of frequent subclinical ophthalmopathy. *N. Engl. J. Med.*, 308:420–424.
15. Goldmann, H. (1955): Un nouveau tonomètre á applanation. *Bull. Soc. Fr. Ophthalmol.*, 67:474–478.
16. Goldmann, H., and Schmidt, T. (1957): Uber applanationstonometrie. *Ophthalmologica*, 134:221–242.
17. Goldmann, H., and Schmidt, T. (1961): Weiterer beitrag zur applantionstonometrie. *Ophthalmologica*, 141:441–456.
18. Gorman, C. A. (1983): Temporal relationship between onset of Graves' ophthalmopathy and diagnosis of thyrotoxicosis. *Mayo Clin. Proc.*, 58:515–519.
19. Grant, W. M. (1950): Tonographic method for measuring the facility and rate of outflow in human eyes. *Arch. Ophthalmol.*, 44:204–214.
20. Hertel, E. (1918): Weiterer beitrag zur lehre von augendruck. *Ber Dtsch. Ophthalmol. Ges.*, 41:57–61.
21. Hertel, E. (1920): Einiges über den augendruck und glaukom. *Klin. Monatsbl. Augenheilkd.*, 64:390–392.
22. Howard, G. M., and English, F. P. (1965): Occurrence of glaucoma in acromegalics. *Arch. Ophthalmol.*, 73:765–768.
22a. Kolker, A. E., and Hetherington, J., Jr. (1983): *Becker-Shaffer's Diagnosis and Therapy of the Glaucomas*, 5th ed., Mosby, St. Louis.
23. Kottler, M., Brubaker, R., and Macri, F. (1970): The decay kinetics of substances which leave the anterior chamber by bulk flow. *Invest. Ophthalmol.*, 9:758.
24. Lerman, S. (1963): Steroid therapy in secondary glaucoma. *Am. J. Ophthalmol.*, 56:31–33.
25. Leydhecker, W. (1960): *Glaukom, Ein Handbuch*. Springer, Berlin.
26. Linner, E. (1959): The rate of aqueous flow and the adrenals. *Trans. Ophthalmol. Soc. U.K.*, 79:27–32.
27. Lyons, D. E. (1971): Postural changes in intraocular pressure in dysthyroid exophthalmos. *Trans. Ophthalmol. Soc. U.K.*, 91:799–803.
28. Manor, R. S., Kurz, O., and Lewitus, Z. (1974): Intraocular pressure in endocrinological patients with exophthalmos. *Ophthalmologica*, 168:241–252.
29. McLenachan, J., and Davies, D. M. (1965): Glaucoma and the thyroid. *Br. J. Ophthalmol.*, 49:441–444.
30. Millikan, C. H., and Haines, S. F. (1953): Thyroid gland in relation to neuromuscular disease. *Arch. Intern. Med.*, 92:5–39.
31. Moses, R. A., editor (1975): *Adler's Physiology of the Eye*. Mosby, St. Louis.
32. Munro, R. E., Lamki, L., Row, V. V., and Volpé, R. (1973): Cell mediated immunity in the exophthalmos of Graves' disease as demonstrated by the migration inhibition factor (MIF) test. *J. Clin. Endocrinol. Metab.*, 37:286–292.
33. Patterson, G. D., and Miller, S. J. H. (1963): Hormonal influences in simple glaucoma. *Br. J. Ophthalmol.*, 47:129–137.
34. Perkins, E. S. (1965): Hand-held applanation tonometer. *Br. J. Ophthalmol.*, 49:591–593.
35. Perkins, E. S. (1965): Steroid-induced glaucoma. *Proc. R. Soc. Med.*, 58:531–533.
36. Pohjanpelto, P. (1968): The thyroid gland and intraocular pressure: tonographic study of 187 patients with thyroid disease. *Acta Ophthalmol. [Suppl.] (Copenh.)*, 97:1–70.
37. Reader, A. L., III (1982): Normal variations in intraocular pressure: on vertical gaze. *Ophthalmology*, 89:1084–1087.
38. Schiotz, H. (1924): Tonometrie. *Acta Ophthalmol. (Copenh.)*, 2:1.
39. Schmidt, T. F. A. (1974): Calibration of the Maklakoff tonometer. *Am. J. Ophthalmol.*, 77:740–746.
40. Solomon, D. H., Chopra, I. J., Chopra, U., and Smith, F. J. (1977): Identification of subgroups of euthyroid Graves; ophthalmopathy. *N. Engl. J. Med.*, 296:181–186.
41. Spaeth, G. L. (1978): Tonography and tonometry. In: *Clinical Ophthalmology*, edited by T. D. Duane, pp. 1–32. Harper & Row, Hagerstown, Maryland.
42. Strazhdina, T. D. (1968): Significance of tonometry in the differential diagnosis of malignant exophthalmos. *Vestn. Oftalmol.*, 1:54–57.
43. Tamai, H., Nakagawa, T., Ohsako, N., Fukino, O., Takahashi, H., Matsuzuka, F., Kuma, K., and Nagataki, S. (1980): Changes in thyroid functions in patients with euthyroid Graves' disease. *J. Clin. Endocrinol. Metab.*, 50:108–112.
44. Trokel, S. L., and Hilal, S. K. (1979): Recognition and differential diagnosis of enlarged extraocular muscles in computed tomography. *Am. J. Ophthalmol.*, 87:503–512.
45. Vasilieva, L. K. (1965): Disorders of the intraocular pressure regulation in endocrine diseases. *Vestn. Oftalmol.*, 78:70–77.
45a. Vaughn, D., and Asbury, T. (1983): *General Ophthalmology*, 10th ed. Lange, Los Altos, California.
46. Weekers, R., and Lavergne, G. (1958): Changes in ocular rigidity in endocrine exophthalmos. *Br. J. Ophthalmol.*, 42:680–685.
47. Weekers, R., Prijot, E., and Lavergne, G. (1959): Errors of tonometry, tonography, and rigidity measurement in certain forms of endocrine exophthalmos. *Bull. Soc. Belge Ophtalmol.*, 123:564–577.

48. Weekers, R., Prijot, E., and Lavergne, G. (1960): Mesure de la pression oculaire, de la résistance á l'écoulement de l'humeur aqueuse et de la rigidité dans les exophtalmies endocriniennes. *Ophthalmologica,* 139:382–392.

49. Weetman, A. P., McGregor, A. M., Ludgate, M., Beck, L., Mills, P. V., Lazarus, J. H., and Hall, R. (1983): Cyclosporin improves Graves' ophthalmopathy. *Lancet,* 2:486–489.

50. Werner, S. C., Coleman, D. J., and Franzen, L. A. (1974): Ultrasonographic evidence of consistent orbital involvement in Graves' disease. *N. Engl. J. Med.,* 290:1447–1450.

51. Wessely, K. (1918): Discussion of Weiterer beitrag zur lehre von augendruck. *Ber. Dtsch. Ophthalmol. Ges.,* 41:80–81.

52. Wilensky, J. T. (1980): Glaucoma. In: *Principles and Practice of Ophthalmology,* edited by G. A. Peyman, D. R. Saunders, and M. F. Goldberg, pp. 671–737, Saunders, Philadelphia.

53. Zappia, R. J., Winkelman, J. Z., and Gay, A. J. (1971): Intraocular pressure changes in normal subjects and the adhesive muscle syndrome. *Am. J. Ophthalmol.,* 71:880–883.

The Eye and Orbit in Thyroid Disease, edited by
C. A. Gorman et al. Raven Press, New York 1984.

Ocular Electromyography and Saccadic Velocity Measurements in Thyroid Eye Disease

Henry S. Metz

*Department of Ophthalmology, University of Rochester School of Medicine and Dentistry,
Rochester, New York 14642*

In 1952 Björk introduced the technique of electromyography of the extraocular muscles (1). These muscles exhibit certain anatomic, pharmacologic, and physiological characteristics which make the interpretation of the electromyogram (EMG) more hazardous than those of peripheral skeletal muscle.

EXTRAOCULAR MUSCLES

Extraocular muscle motor units differ considerably from those of peripheral skeletal musculature (3). The amplitude ranges from 20 to 600 μV (average 200 μV in primary position). They are generally diphasic or triphasic in form. The duration is short, ranging from 1 to 2 msec with an average of 1.5 msec. The firing rate is very high, up to several hundred discharges per second. This is due to the low innervation ratio, with one axon distributed to every five to 10 muscle fibers. It seems likely that this low innervation ratio permits the rapid, high-frequency firing which is responsible for the finely graded, exquisitely coordinated movements of the eyes.

Another difference between the extraocular muscles and the peripheral skeletal musculature lies in the existence of constant tonic activity in the alert state in the extraocular muscles. They fire constantly at high rates of discharge in the primary position, increasing as the eye rotates into the field of action of that muscle and diminishing as the eye rotates out of this field of action. Normal extraocular muscles do not fatigue.

EMG PATTERNS

Jampolsky (5) pointed out that the EMG does not discern relative strength and weakness of extraocular muscles, except for gross defects. The EMG changes reflect relative changes or attempted changes in eye position. The EMG does not reveal the specific function the muscle may be performing.

Paresis of moderate to severe degree is characterized by irregular or sparse recruitment, poorly sustained discharge, and loss of the interference pattern characteristically seen with effort (3). In the presence of marked paresis, the motor units are frequently decreased in amplitude with a high incidence of polyphasic and reinnervation units. Electrical silence, even in severe degrees of palsy, is relatively infrequent. Mild palsies are accompanied by profuse discharge of remaining units, constituting a nondiagnostic pattern.

In cases of pseudopalsy due to mechanical restriction of the globe, there is normal, abundant activity of the EMG, disproportionate to the failure of rotation of the globe (3).

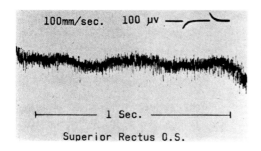

FIG. 1. EMG of the superior rectus muscle in a patient with thyroid eye disease. The tracing shows electrical activity at maximal contraction of the muscle with a myopathic pattern. (From ref. 14.)

Passive movement of the globe does not alter innervation. Electrical activity of the muscle therefore follows the effort, not the position of the eye.

The characteristic findings of myopathy are of relatively abundant, low-amplitude, high-frequency discharge. The motor unit action potential shows considerable diminution in duration. This is thought to be due to the loss of muscle fibers in the individual motor unit, which also decreases the voltage amplitude. In myopathy the neuron is apparently intact. Because of the loss of viable muscle fibers, a comparable range of movement requires a greater firing rate and recruitment of motor units. There is poor mechanical muscle capability despite apparently adequate electrical capability.

THYROID MYOPATHY

Skeletal Myopathy

The EMG findings in thyrotoxic myopathy offer no features which differentiate this disorder from other endocrine diseases or the other myopathies. Skeletal myopathy has been accepted as an integral component of the clinical picture of thyrotoxicosis. There may be complaints of generalized weakness, sometimes accompanied by objective loss of muscle power and atrophy (8). The EMG has revealed myopathic changes in many cases of thyrotoxicosis, regardless of whether obvious weakness and muscle wasting were present.

The most frequent changes noted are a shortened mean potential duration and increased polyphasia. Even at reduced strength, there is a full interference pattern. EMG findings are often recorded in these muscles, even if the histologic findings are completely normal (7,13). Pipberger and associates (12) believed that the EMG is superior to other tests in the detection of muscle changes.

Ocular Myopathy

Breinin reported EMG studies in thyroid myopathy (2). He indicated that only one of 12 patients demonstrated a pattern of myopathy, whereas a pattern of neurogenic palsy occurred in most. These were observed later in the disease and became marked in the more congestive forms of exophthalmos.

Schultz et al. (14) obtained ocular EMGs consistent with a diagnosis of primary myopathy in 10 patients with limited ocular rotations associated with thyrotoxicosis. There was reduction in the amplitude of the action potential without loss in the number of motor units as estimated from the interference pattern (Fig. 1). In none was there clear evidence of denervation. The recordings from extraocular muscles in three patients with only slight impairment of ocular motility were within normal limits. Schultz et al. concluded "that thyrotoxic ophthalmoplegia is due to a true myopathy," which is in agreement with EMG and histologic findings in thyrotoxic myopathy involving skeletal muscles.

Magora et al. (8) reported myopathic tracings in patients with thyrotoxic ophthalmoplegia. The amplitudes were low ($<$150 μV compared to normals of 340 to 460 μV), and the duration was shortened (0.5 to 1 msec compared to normal values of 1 to 1.5 msec). A full interference pattern without loss of motor units was observed.

Miller and associates (11) found normal action potentials in all of their seven patients with hypotropias associated with thyroid dysfunction. There was no evidence of paralysis or dystrophy. However, recordings were only from the superior rectus and one or more horizontal rectus muscles, not from the inferior recti. Miller et al. did conclude that because the superior recti were normal the inferior rectus contracture, found on forced-duction testing, was not secondary to superior rectus paresis.

Jensen was in agreement in his EMG study (6). He suggested that limited ocular motility in endocrine ophthalmoplegia is not caused by myopathy but by mechanical immobilization. Metz (9) noted normal EMG patterns from the vertical recti of two patients with endocrine ophthalmopathy.

Myasthenia gravis has been noted in a higher percentage of patients with thyroid disease than in the general population. The EMG findings of myasthenia may therefore be found in some patients with endocrine ophthalmopathy. Fatigue of motor units (3) followed by recovery of activity with rest helps to establish the diagnosis. Prolonged voluntary inner-vation leads to decreased frequency and amplitude of the action potentials. Following intravenous injection of Tensilon, there is activation of numerous motor units and an increase in discharge frequency. Sometimes there is subclinical improvement with Tensilon. An increase in the EMG response may be noted without an observable improvement in eye movement (5), making the test more sensitive diagnostically. The EMG shows that the muscle is pharmacologically responsive, and hence the test is positive. This response is not seen in normal muscle or other palsies. These EMG findings seem to be diagnostic for myasthenia. Magora and associates (8) found a myasthenic response in one of their eight patients with thyroid ophthalmopathy (12%). However, this series of patients is too small to draw any conclusions about the coincidence of these two conditions.

In summary, the distinctive structure of normal extraocular muscles is associated with a characteristic EMG pattern which differs from that seen in peripheral skeletal muscle in the rapid high-frequency firing and the existence of constant tonic activity in the alert state. Although a single unconfirmed report identified a pattern of neurogenic palsy in 11 of 12 patients studied in Graves' ophthalmopathy, the balance of evidence favors a myopathic process. There are numerous studies to indicate that limitation of extraocular motion in patients with Graves' disease is due to restriction of tight extraocular muscles rather than to paresis.

SACCADIC VELOCITY

Limitation of ocular rotations in thyroid eye disease is usually due to mechanical restric-tions. This can be documented with positive forced-duction test findings. Quantitative forced-duction measurements in patients with thyroid ophthalmopathy demonstrate increased stiffness (steep length–tension curve) with continued upward rotation of the globe. Following inferior rectus disinsertion and inferior rectus recession, the stiffness is diminished—the length–tension curve is flattened (10) (Fig. 2). The range of upward rotation is increased postoperatively.

Metz found that horizontal and vertical saccadic velocity measurements in 15 patients with noncongestive endocrine ophthalmopathy were normal (9). Unpublished studies on 12

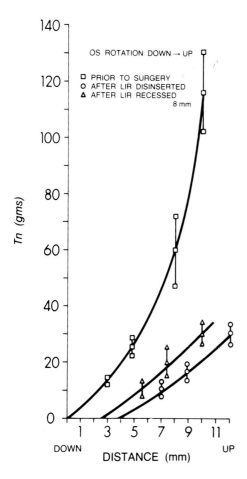

FIG. 2. Length–tension curves, with rotation of the globe upward in a patient with thyroid eye disease. The length–tension curve is steep prior to surgery and displaced upward and flattened after both disinsertion and recession of the inferior rectus muscle.

additional patients by the same investigator were similarly normal. Active force generation studies by Scott have also failed to indicate any evidence of paresis (9). Hermann (4) reported two patients with Graves' disease and inferior rectus palsy demonstrated by slowing of the downward saccade. The forced-duction test was found to be negative. However, these slow saccades are unusual, as velocities are most often rapid in restrictive ocular motility disorders.

ACKNOWLEDGMENTS

This work was supported by NEI grant EYO 3891–02 and a grant from Research to Prevent Blindness.

REFERENCES

1. Björk, A. (1952): Electrical activity of human extrinsic eye muscles. *Experientia*, 8:226–229.
2. Breinin, G. M. (1957): New aspects of ophthalmologic diagnosis. *Arch. Ophthalmol.*, 58:375–388.
3. Goodgold, J., and Eberstein, A. (1972): *Electrodiagnosis of Neuromuscular Diseases*, pp. 206–212. Williams & Wilkins, Baltimore.
4. Hermann, J. S. (1982): Paretic thyroid myopathy. *Ophthalmology*, 89:473–478.
5. Jampolsky, A. (1970): What can electromyography do for the ophthalmologist? *Invest. Ophthalmol.*, 9:570–599.
6. Jensen, S. F. (1971): Endocrine ophthalmoplegia. *Acta Ophthalmol. (Copenh.)*, 49:679–684.

7. Ludin, H. P. (1980): Myopathies. In: *Electromyography in Practice*, pp. 93–120. Thieme-Stratton, New York.
8. Magora, A., Chaco, J., and Zauberman, H. (1968): An electromyographic investigation of ophthalmoplegia in thyrotoxicosis. *Arch. Ophthalmol.*, 79:170–173.
9. Metz, H. S. (1977): Saccadic velocity studies in patients with endocrine ocular disease. *Am. J. Ophthalmol.*, 84:695–699.
10. Metz, H. S., and Cohen, G. (1982): Quantitative forced duction measurements in strabismus. In: *Proceedings of the Fourth Meeting of the International Strabismological Association, Asilomar, California (in press)*.
11. Miller, J. E., van Heuven, W., and Ward, R. (1965): Surgical correction of nystagmus associated with thyroid dysfunction. *Arch. Ophthalmol.*, 74:509–515.
12. Pipberger, H., Kulin, R., and Wegmann, T. (1955): Muscular disturbances associated with hyperthyroidism. *Schweiz. Med. Wochenschr.*, 85:390–393.
13. Puvanendran, K., Cheah, J. S., and Wong, P. K. (1977): Electromyographic study in thyrotoxic periodic paralysis. *Aust. N. Z. J. Med.*, 7:507–510.
14. Schultz, R. O., Van Allen, M. W., and Blodi, F. C. (1960): Endocrine ophthalmoplegia. *Arch. Ophthalmol.*, 63:217–225.

The Eye and Orbit in Thyroid Disease, edited by
C. A. Gorman et al. Raven Press, New York 1984.

Computerized Imaging Evaluation: CT and NMR Scanning and Computed Volume Measurement

Glenn Forbes

Department of Diagnostic Radiology, Mayo Clinic, Rochester, Minnesota 55905

Computed tomography (CT) has become the key imaging modality in diagnosing orbital lesions. As a relatively noninvasive examination, it provides a high rate of information return regarding many characteristics of orbital mass, infection, associated sinus or intracranial disease, and bony structure. Late-generation, high-resolution equipment has refined its capabilities and established CT as a preferred screening diagnostic procedure and a definitive imaging method for many orbital lesions. Confronting a clinical problem of orbital pain, proptosis, diplopia, or change in visual acuity, one may be looking for an orbital mass or, if there are known systemic or endocrine abnormalities, associated orbital pathologic infiltration. CT may enable one to exclude orbital masses with a high degree of confidence; and usually it can provide a basis for diagnosis and detailed anatomic delineation of other lesions, including tumor, inflammatory and endocrine changes, and injuries due to trauma.

For proptosis, orbital CT can differentiate numerous causes other than Graves' disease; and exclusion of other causes is one of the first concerns when imaging the potential Graves' patient. Late-generation CT has detected orbital tumors with accuracy exceeding 95% (10). Such orbital masses are commonly discrete, encapsulated, and unilateral; they are occasionally calcified, and many lend themselves to contrast enhancement (11). Also clearly discernible are paraorbital lesions that may extend into the orbit, e.g., sinus mucoceles, pyoceles, carcinoma, sphenoid ridge meningiomas, and bony dysplasias (2,8). Bone destruction, soft tissue calcification, and discrete well-defined mass outlines are findings not usually associated with endocrine ophthalmopathy.

However, there are several infiltrative orbital processes whose images can resemble or overlap the imaging spectrum of Graves' disease, and these may pose more difficult diagnostic problems. Inflammatory pseudotumor, orbital myositis, and certain forms of lymphoma may present as nondiscrete, amorphous, soft tissue densities along the margins of the muscle cone, thus giving the appearance of extraocular muscle enlargement. Findings that may help differentiate these lesions from features of true Graves' disease include scleral thickening with pseudotumor (1), anterior periorbital soft tissue edema and thickening with myositis (12), and amorphous mass and bone destruction with lymphoma (10,11). The coronal views may be very useful for further characterizing the soft tissue mass and defining its extent for differential diagnosis. This is particularly true in displaying lesions adjacent to the floor or roof of the orbit. Most Graves' patients show abnormalities in both orbits, whereas these other conditions more often are unilateral. With experience, the interpretation of high-resolution orbital CT can exclude most of even these difficult lesions and can correctly identify the uniform muscle enlargement or increased ground substance in the fat compartment, both of which are characteristically associated with Graves' disease.

TECHNIQUES

CT Scanning

High-quality orbital CT requires certain modifications from the standard head examination. These include the use of thin slices (which may even overlap) to discern small structures, a different reference angle in the axial plane, and the addition of coronal projections, which we have found extremely useful in fully evaluating orbital problems. Acceptable slices may range from 5 mm down to 1.5 mm. The thinnest cuts offer less volume-averaging and the highest resolution, but they also require more scans and thus longer scanning times. Because of collimation, however, the radiation dose to the lens is comparable, being on the order of 3 to 5 R for most orbital CT examinations (8,10).

Usually the CT orbital study is performed in one of two ways. In the first, direct axial scanning is followed immediately by direct coronal scanning, with the patient's head hyperextended in the scanner. The axial scans are obtained at 0° to 10° from the orbitomeatal baseline to approximate the plane of the orbital muscle cone. The coronal views are obtained at approximately 65° in order to avoid artifacts from either the molar teeth or the cervical spine. Usually a total of 15 to 20 slices are taken at 3- to 5-mm slice widths, covering the entire orbital region during a 25- to 30-min examination.

In the second method, the orbit is scanned in the axial plane only, 25 to 30 high-resolution continuous slices being made at 1- to 1.5-mm slice width. Displays of the orbit in different projections may be created with computer software techniques known as multiplane reformatting. The reformatted images use the original scanning data to produce coronal and lateral views. The second method achieves higher limits of resolution with less volume-averaging of small structures, and it can be used for patients who are unable to tolerate extensive head extension. However, it also requires good patient cooperation to hold the head absolutely still for longer scanning times. Only the second method serves to obtain the volume measurements of the orbital muscle and fat compartments as described below.

Although intravenous contrast material is employed in many orbital CT examinations, its usefulness is less critical in Graves' ophthalmopathy than in other types of orbital pathology. Iodine, 20 to 42 g, in contrast solution infused over several minutes before scanning enhances the clarity of the vessels and many vascular lesions, e.g., hemangiomas, varices, gliomas, and meningiomas. However, the high level of natural contrast provided by the orbital fat, globe, and muscles is sufficient in many cases to define pathology, particularly the muscle enlargement associated with endocrine disease.

Volume Measurements

Data from the original CT scans, processed by special computer software techniques, can yield volume measurements of the orbital structures. These techniques—still under study—are being employed for more specific categorization of different subclasses of ophthalmopathy according to their proportions of muscle and fat. The off-line processing defines specific structures through preassigned density ranges and boundary margins. Individual scanning volumes ("pixels") are then summated and calibrated to provide measurements in cubic millimeters or cubic centimeters (Fig. 1). The method is accurate within a few percent and may be used for any structures with density sufficiently different from the rest, which in the orbit includes muscle, fat, globe, and overall bony orbit volume (9).

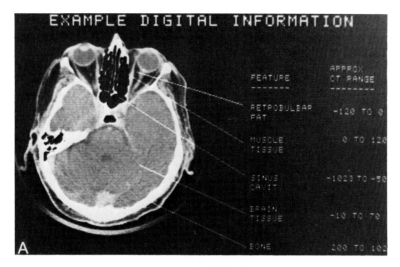

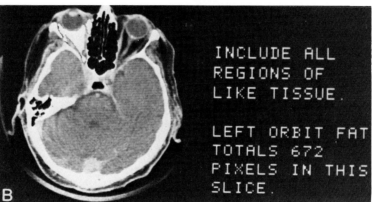

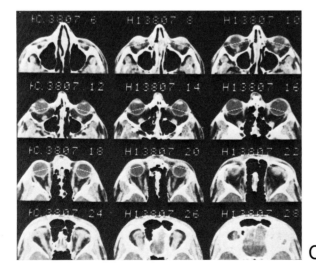

FIG. 1. Volume measurement technique. **A:** Density ranges are assigned to specific tissues within the orbit, including fat, muscle, bone, air, and fluid. **B:** Special programs then assign computer pixel counts from original scan data to assigned tissue ranges. **C:** Summated counts throughout orbits are calibrated to determine volumes of specific structures in cubic centimeters.

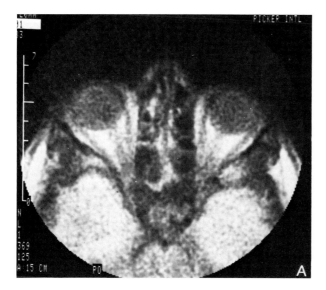 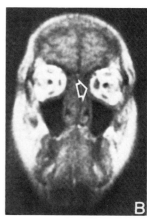

FIG. 2. Nuclear magnetic resonance. **A:** An intense signal is generated from orbital fat (which is represented as white in these views). **B:** Coronal views are easily obtained by rotating the magnetic field without moving the patient's head. These views are ideal for demonstrating cross-sectional muscle changes *(arrow)*. Note the marked contrast between muscles and orbital fat with this scanning technique.

Nuclear Magnetic Resonance

Nuclear magnetic resonance (NMR) scanning is currently being introduced to the study of head and neck problems. Experience with orbital imaging is limited, although preliminary indications are that NMR will lend itself very well to this use (Fig. 2). It offers a high degree of sensitivity for fat tissue and changes of hydration within soft tissue, and it involves no ionizing radiation. An added advantage is its ability to provide different projections in transverse, coronal, and sagittal planes without moving the patient or performing off-line analysis. Although spatial resolution does not yet match high-quality CT scanning of orbit, no ionizing radiation is used and the signal generated represents different physicochemical information of orbital structures. As spatial resolution and availability of the method increase, NMR may equal or surpass CT in orbital imaging (5). This will continue to be an area of active investigation in the future.

In NMR the information needed for an image is produced by stimulating tissue within a strong magnetic field by radio wave pulses at specific frequencies. The applied energy is absorbed by the hydrogen protons, which precess in the magnetic field because of their nuclear magnetic moments. As the excess energy is emitted, it creates a signal that is detected and analyzed by computer techniques similar to that used in a CT system. By changing the pulse sequences of the radio transmission, different types of images are formed, providing information based on different characteristics of the tissue. The marked differences of proton density and macromolecular environment of orbital fat and muscle result in excellent contrast between these types of structures in NMR images. Orbital fat and muscle also seem sensitive to small changes in NMR imaging, and its use in endocrine disease is likely to expand in the future.

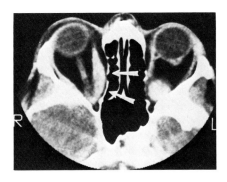

FIG. 3. Bone changes. Chronic pressure erosion from an enlarged medial rectus muscle has caused expansion of the orbital wall *(arrows)*. Bone expansion indicates long-standing pressure, whereas bone destruction may result from a more aggressive lesion.

IMAGING IN GRAVES' DISEASE

Late-generation scanning techniques can reveal characteristic CT changes in more than 90% of Graves' patients with clinical ophthalmopathy (7,24). This is not surprising in itself, as CT imaging is quite sensitive for discerning small anatomic changes in the orbits. However, many Graves' patients without eye changes and euthyroid patients with clinical proptosis also exhibit the characteristic changes on CT. This has been reported in up to 40% of asymptomatic Graves' patients with standard CT (7), and with more advanced techniques the proportion will likely be shown to be higher. Also, subtle abnormal changes may be discerned in the contralateral orbit in Graves' patients who have unilateral clinical proptosis. Altogether, this experience leads to several conclusions: (a) most, if not all, Graves' patients eventually have some orbital involvement; (b) in many of them the involvement is detectable with computerized scanning techniques recently brought to clinical use; (c) the abnormalities usually are quite characteristic for endocrine ophthalmopathy; and (d) as more refined scanning techniques are used, subtler abnormalities are detected in clinically asymptomatic orbits.

Bony Changes

Plain films of the skull or orbit occasionally show some bony changes associated with orbital tumor or infection but do not demonstrate the soft tissues: Generally they contribute little regarding endocrine ophthalmopathy. However, Graves' ophthalmopathy, though it principally involves the muscles and retrobulbar fat, can be of such long standing as to have caused bony changes of the orbital wall; and these are best seen on high-resolution CT (13). The lateral or the medial wall, or both, may show expansion, which is always associated with prominent enlargement of the adjacent ocular muscles (Fig. 3). It is the slow, indolent nature of the pressure from enlarging retrobulbar structures that causes the expansion and thinning of the bone, whereas aggressive neoplasia causes bone destruction.

Although orbital wall expansion is not often seen in Graves' disease, its occasional occurrence raises the question of the effect of bony orbit volume in decompressing or accentuating the retrobulbar pressure related to muscle enlargement. Orbital foraminal anatomy, as well as total orbital volume, warrants consideration as a precipitating cause of optic nerve compressive effects that may occur with the endocrine muscle enlargement. The relationships of these anatomic factors with the development of eye changes in Graves' disease remain areas for future investigation (14).

Soft Tissue Changes

The classic imaging of Graves' ophthalmopathy is CT demonstration of muscle enlargement in one or both orbits (Figs. 4 and 5). There may also be an apparent increase in the

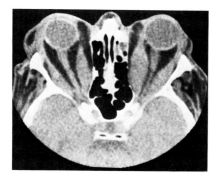

FIG. 4. Muscle enlargement. Classic changes in endocrine ophthalmopathy include a uniform increase in size that is most prominent at the belly of the muscle and tapers to a narrow line at the point of tendon insertion; mild expansion of medial orbital walls from long-standing pressure effects; and bilateral proptosis—although distribution in the two orbits is not symmetrical.

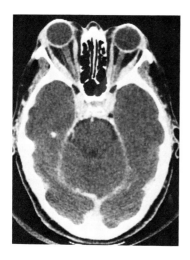

FIG. 5. Diffuse muscle enlargement only. Note the generalized enlargement of all muscles, causing bilateral proptosis. The fat compartment seems to be within normal limits. Compare with Fig. 6. (From ref. 9.)

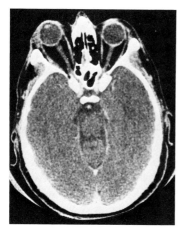

FIG. 6. Diffuse fat compartment enlargement only. Note the generalized enlargement of the fat compartment only in both orbits, causing bilateral proptosis. Muscles are of normal size. Sometimes enlargement of the fat compartment is thought to represent vascular congestion with mechanical compression from large muscles. Occasionally, however, such increased fat compartment volume occurs in the absence of muscle enlargement, raising the question of another type of infiltrative mechanism. Such changes were not recognized until late-generation CT scanning became available, and observations are being refined with more sensitive computer volume studies. Compare with Fig. 5. (From ref. 9.)

orbital fat compartment, with or without muscle enlargement (Fig. 6). Lacrimal gland enlargement has been mentioned as an occasional finding (19,24). Trokel and Hilal (22) also reported enlarged optic nerves on CT of some severely affected patients.

The overall increased volume of the retrobulbar structures produces a noticeable forward displacement of the globe in most cases. However, both ultrasound and recent quantitative

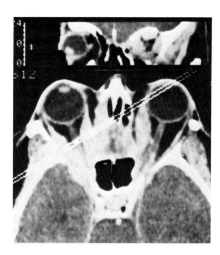

FIG. 7. Optic nerve encroachment. Marked swelling of all muscle bundles surrounds the optic nerve. In an extreme case, it may begin to compress the nerve at the orbital apex. Because the distribution of involvement frequently is asymmetrical, this compression may occur either unilaterally or bilaterally.

CT volume studies have revealed abnormalities in the retrobulbar muscles of Graves' patients without clinical proptosis (8,27,30); and the quantitative volume studies may detect small changes in the muscles of patients without proptosis observable either clinically or on the scan. Extreme enlargement may compress the optic nerve at the orbital apex (Fig. 7). All of the abnormal changes are invariably confined to orbits, and the sinuses and intracranial contents are otherwise normal.

Muscle

Muscle enlargement within the orbit of many Graves' patients was recognized easily with early-generation CT scanners (4). The principal findings were globe protrusion and thickening of the retrobulbar muscles, which might occur in asymmetrical patterns within one or both orbits. The limited resolution of the early scanners emphasized changes in the lateral and medial muscles, and the clumping of several enlarged muscles often gave the appearance of an orbital mass (21). The adjacent floor and roof of the orbit made visualization of the inferior and superior groups difficult because of volume averaging. As scanning improved, more subtle distinctions were made regarding the patterns in any of the muscle groups, the fat and bony changes, and the differentiation of true orbital masses from pure muscle enlargement (22,23).

The pattern of muscle involvement is often asymmetrical, involving single or multiple muscles, frequently in a different distribution in each orbit (Fig. 4). Overall, the medial and inferior rectus muscles have been reported to be more commonly involved—though as mentioned previously, scanning technique may influence the observation of these distributions (7,16,29) (Fig. 8). Among any series of patients, all possible patterns of distribution may be found in individual cases.

The muscle enlargement generally is seen as a symmetrical swelling of the entire muscle bundle, more pronounced in the middle portion (which is the thickest to begin with). The ends of the muscle bundle taper to a small point, although the crowding of several ends at the orbital apex may produce a picture of uniform density within the region. This sparing of the muscle tendon insertion helps distinguish Graves' disease from other infiltrative or inflammatory muscle conditions. The muscles often appear denser than normal muscles, but this may be due only to the increased size and lack of partial volume-averaging of the

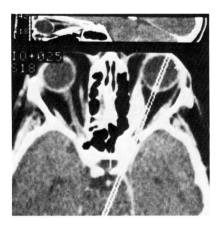

FIG. 8. Reformatted scan imaging: a common pattern of medial and inferior muscle bundle enlargement, seen with the aid of reformatted sagittal images. Such images are reconstructed from original computer scanning data and are particularly useful for displaying inferior and superior structures, adjacent to the floor or roof, that may be difficult to visualize on standard axial or transverse views. (From ref. 8.)

relatively small muscles related to the CT pixels. With intravenous contrast studies there is some generalized enhancement indicative of the vascular nature of the neuromuscular bundles. Attempts to characterize the density changes more specifically are restricted by poor reliability in comparisons of CT attenuation values under different scanning conditions (17).

Fat

An increase in the orbital fat compartment has now been recognized as a common occurrence in Graves' patients. Usually this is associated with muscle enlargement, though occasionally it may be an isolated finding with normal-sized muscles (Fig. 6). Whether it represents a true increase of fat material, an infiltrative process within the fat structure, or edema due to vascular congestion is unknown (24). Sometimes this appearance of increased fat is noted on CT, although histologic studies of orbital tissue removed after surgical decompression have shown that fatty material is partly replaced by increased connective tissue. Increased mucopolysaccharides, edema, and vascular congestion may also contribute to this appearance on CT (19). Our preliminary studies indicate that the phenomenon of increased volume of the fat compartment may be more common in men than in women.

Differential Diagnosis

Aside from their anatomic distribution, the muscle changes of Graves' disease can usually be differentiated from other causes of muscle enlargement by close observation of detail (22). Inflammatory pseudotumor often results in more asymmetrical enlargement of the muscle bundle and is associated with a soft tissue infiltrate or mass separate from the muscle bundle (Fig. 9). Graves' disease, which produces uniform symmetrical enlargement, is seldom if ever associated with infiltrative masses outside the confines of the muscle. Occasionally a tumor infiltrates a muscle, producing enlargement; but usually the tumor is identified along with the muscle change. Orbital myositis often is characterized by the more pronounced changes in the periorbital tissues anterior to the cone (Fig. 10). Rarely, what appears to be the uniform muscle enlargement of Graves' disease is an effect of a small dural arteriovenous malformation that causes engorgement of vessels along the course of the muscle bundles. The process is almost always unilateral, sometimes is suggested by identification of tortuous vessels and an enlarged superior ophthalmic vein on CT, and is confirmed by arteriography.

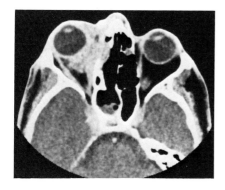

FIG. 9. Pseudotumor: infiltrative mass extends outside the muscle bundle and in this case even invades the adjacent sinus. The process is amorphous and unilateral, with characteristic thickening of the sclera.

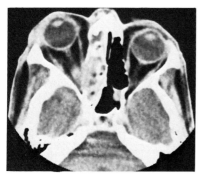

FIG. 10. Inflammatory changes. Infection in the adjacent ethmoid sinus may penetrate the orbital wall to produce myositis in the muscle bundle. This characteristic pattern is unilateral, with the epicenter outside the orbit.

Angiographic Findings

Orbital venography and (carotid) arteriography have had little part in the evolution of imaging of endocrine ophthalmopathy. In endocrine disorders, venography may provide only nonspecific findings of venous occlusion or stasis, which are also seen in pseudotumor, myositis, and orbital malignancy (28). In a single case of biopsy-proved Graves' ophthalmopathy, carotid arteriography has revealed multiple irregular small vessels branching from the ophthalmic artery, with diffuse staining and postcapillary puddling (13). It should be recognized that arteriography is not widely used in intraorbital diagnosis, except for evaluation of arteriovenous fistula and malformations.

Determinations of Muscle and Fat Volume

The next step in the development of computer-image studies of Graves' ophthalmopathy is to begin correlating the wide spectrum of changes with the different clinical variants. This should advance understanding of the underlying mechanisms as well as guide prognostic and therapeutic considerations in patients afflicted with early changes (6,15). This step has awaited the advent of refined techniques for measuring the extent of pathologic enlargement of the orbital muscle and fat detected in Graves' patients by *in vivo* tests (20,25,26). B-mode ultrasound has been used to determine increases of muscle and fat volume in Graves' patients as a group. Although no means has been shown for substantiating the quantitative data obtained by this technique, it does provide significant relative observations in Graves' disease: volume increases proportional to proptosis, increased fat volume in severe cases, and abnormalities of muscle in patients without clinically apparent proptosis. By this method, single-orbit muscle volumes were found to average 6.57 cm³ ± 2.70 in Graves' patients and 3.32 cm³ ± 1.31 in normal controls (30).

In CT studies, quantitative work can be carried further by off-line analyses of clinical CT data; additionally, the accuracy and reliability of the CT technique may be confirmed by reproducible phantom studies. Late-generation CT scanners are able to discriminate differences of density even in structures as small as 1 to 2 mm. Summation of computer pixel counts based on density ranges in successive cross-sectional areas can provide volume measurements of three-dimensional structures. The reliability of the volume measurement is dependent on technique, but accuracy within 5% has been achieved with very thin scanning slices and refined computer programs (3,18). Our own team has applied these special techniques to off-line analysis of normal controls and several clinical subdivisions of Graves' patients (9) (Fig. 1).

Normal adult retrobulbar soft tissue volumes, as measured by special CT analysis, range from 12 to 20 cm^3 and average 14 to 15 cm. Orbital muscle volumes average 4 to 5 cm^3 and orbital fat volumes 10 to 11 cm^3. Similar total volumes in Graves' patients with clinical ophthalmopathy may range up to 25 and 28 cm^3 and average 8 to 10 cm^3 and 12–14 cm^3 for muscle and fat, respectively. Most Graves' patients with even minimal clinical eye signs have some measurement abnormalities, although standard CT images seem normal; and many Graves' patients without clinical eye signs show some measurement abnormality, suggesting early subclinical involvement.

Several interesting concepts have developed from early quantitative studies of orbital structures in Graves' disease. First, it is clear that there is a spectrum of change in the degree of muscle enlargement. Second, there are definite changes in the fat compartment in some patients. Our early studies indicate that females tend to have muscle enlargement only, whereas males often have abnormally increased volume in the fat compartment in addition to muscle enlargement. Proptosis in some patients results from increased fat volume without any measurable enlargement of muscles. Most patients with unilateral proptosis have some small but measurable increase in either muscle or fat volume in the clinically normal orbit. Finally, some patients may have normal total volumes of the retrobulbar soft tissues and still have measurable increased muscle or fat volumes suggesting subclinical ophthalmopathy.

Future Considerations

The correlation of different patterns of retrobulbar muscle enlargement and fat infiltration with clinical subgroupings remains an area for investigation. Better understanding of the relationship to bony orbit structure and endocrine ophthalmopathy is also needed. It is possible that total bony orbit volume, as well as bony orbit morphology, is significant in determining whether proptosis, muscle movement limitations, or optic nerve compression occurs. The potential for further differentiating muscle and fat by their NMR properties will continue to be an area of active investigation (Fig. 2). More sophisticated imaging and analyses of muscle and fat volume should have both prognostic and therapeutic value in the future.

REFERENCES

1. Bernardino, M. E., Zimmerman, R. D., Citrin, C. M., and Davis, D. O. (1977): Scleral thickening: a CT sign of orbital pseudotumor. *AJR*, 129:703–706.
2. Bilaniuk, L. T., and Zimmerman, R. A. (1980): Computer-assisted tomography: sinus lesions with orbital involvement. *Head Neck Surg.*, 2:293–301.
3. Brenner, D. E Whitley, N. O., Houk, T. L., Aisner, J., Wiernik, P., and Whitley, J. (1982): Volume determinations in computed tomography. *JAMA*, 247:1299–1302.
4. Brismar, J., Davis, K. R., Dallow, R. C., and Brismar, G. (1976): Unilateral endocrine exophthalmos: diagnostic problems in association with computed tomography. *Neuroradiology*, 12:21–24.

5. Bydder, G. M., Steiner, R. E., Young, I. R., Hall, A. S., Thomas, D. J., Marshall, J., Pallis, C. A., and Legg, N. J. (1982): Clinical NMR imaging of the brain: 140 cases. *AJNR*, 3:459–480.
6. Daicker, B. (1979): Das gewebliche Substrat der verdickten äuberen Augenmuskeln bei der endokrinen Orbitopathie. *Klin. Monatsbl. Augenheilkd.*, 174:843–847.
7. Enzmann, D. R., Donaldson, S. S., and Kriss, J. P. (1979): Appearance of Graves' disease on orbital computed tomography. *J. Comput. Assist. Tomogr.*, 3:815–819.
8. Forbes, G. (1982): Computed tomography of the orbit. *Radiol. Clin. North Am.*, 20:37–49.
9. Forbes, G., Gorman, C. A., Gehring, D., and Baker, H. L., Jr. (1983): Computer analysis of orbital fat and muscle volumes in Graves' ophthalmopathy. *AJNR*, 4:737–740.
10. Forbes, G. S., Earnest, F., IV, and Waller, R. R. (1982): Computed tomography of orbital tumors, including late-generation scanning techniques. *Radiology*, 142:387–394.
11. Forbes, G. S., Sheedy, P. F., II, and Waller, R. R. (1980): Orbital tumors evaluated by computed tomography. *Radiology*, 136:101–111.
12. Harr, D. L., Quencer, R. M., and Abrams, G. W. (1982): Computed tomography and ultrasound in the evaluation of orbital infection and pseudotumor. *Radiology*, 142:395–401.
13. Healy, J. F., Metcalf, J. H., and Brahme, F. J. (1981): Thyroid ophthalmopathy: bony erosion on CT and increased vascularity on angiography. *AJNR*, 2:472–474.
14. Jensen, S. F. (1971): Endocrine ophthalmoplegia: is it due to myopathy or mechanical immobilization? *Acta Ophthalmol. (Copenh.)*, 49:679–684.
15. Kroll, A. J., and Kuwabara, T. (1966): Dysthyroid ocular myopathy: anatomy, histology, and electron microscopy. *Arch. Ophthalmol.*, 76:244–257.
16. Leonardi, M., Barbina, V., Fabris, G., and Penco, T. (1977): Sagittal computed tomography of the orbit. *J. Comput. Assist. Tomogr.*, 1:511–512.
17. Levi, C., Gray, J. E., McCullough, E. C., and Hattery, R. R. (1982): The unreliability of CT numbers as absolute values. *AJR*, 139:443–447.
18. Rhodes, M. L. (1979): Towards fast edge detection for clinical 3-D applications of computer tomography. *Proc. Conf. Comp. Appl. Rad. Anat. Radiol. Images, 6th, Newport Beach, June 18–21, 1979*, pp. 321–327. IEEE Society, New York.
19. Riley, F. C. (1972): Orbital pathology in Graves' disease. *Mayo Clin. Proc.*, 47:975–979.
20. Solomon, D. H., Chopra, I. J., Chopra, U., and Smith, F. J. (1977): Identification of subgroups of euthyroid Graves's ophthalmopathy. *N. Engl. J. Med.*, 296:181–186.
21. Susac, J. O., Martins, A. N., Robinson, B., and Corrigan, D. F. (1977): False diagnosis of orbital apex tumor by CAT scan in thyroid eye disease. *Ann. Neurol.*, 1:397–398.
22. Trokel, S. L., and Hilal, S. K. (1979): Recognition and differential diagnosis of enlarged extraocular muscles in computed tomography. *Am. J. Ophthalmol.*, 87:503–512.
23. Trokel, S. L., and Hilal, S. K. (1980): Submillimeter resolution of CT scanning of orbital diseases. *Ophthalmology*, 87:412–417.
24. Trokel, S. L., and Jakobiec, F. A. (1981): Correlation of CT scanning and pathologic features of ophthalmic Graves' disease. *Ophthalmology*, 88:553–564.
25. Werner, S. C. (1969): Classification of the eye changes of Graves' disease. *J. Clin. Endocrinol. Metab.*, 29:982–984 (letter to the editor).
26. Werner, S. C. (1977): Modification of the classification of the eye changes of Graves' disease: recommendations of the Ad Hoc Committee of the American Thyroid Association. *J. Clin. Endocrinol. Metab.*, 44:203–204 (letter to the editor).
27. Werner, S. C., Coleman, D. J., and Franzen, L. A. (1974): Ultrasonographic evidence of a consistent orbital involvement in Graves's disease. *N. Engl. J. Med.*, 290:1447–1450.
28. Wilner, H. I., Gupta, K. L., and Kelly, J. K. (1980): Orbital pseudotumor: association of orbital vein deformities and myositis. *AJNR*, 1:305–309.
29. Wing, S. D., Hunsaker, J. N., Anderson, R. E., VanDyk, J. L., and Osborn, A. G. (1979): Direct sagittal computed tomography in Graves' ophthalmopathy. *J. Comput. Assist. Tomogr.*, 3:820–824.
30. Yamamoto, K., Itoh, K., Yoshida, S., Saito, K., Sakamoto, Y., Matsuda, A., Saito, T., and Kuzuya, T. (1979): A quantitative analysis of orbital soft tissue in Graves' disease based on B-mode ultrasonography. *Endocrinol. Jpn.*, 26:255–261.

The Eye and Orbit in Thyroid Disease, edited by
C. A. Gorman et al. Raven Press, New York 1984.

Ultrasonic Diagnosis of Graves' Ophthalmopathy

Karl C. Ossoinig

Department of Ophthalmology, University of Iowa Hospitals and Clinics, Iowa City, Iowa 52242

Three types of noninvasive ultrasound have evolved in ophthalmology during the past two decades (1): (a) Ultrasonic biometry primarily serves the measurement of axial eye length for the computation of intraocular lens power prior to lens implantation. The biometric instruments are designed exclusively for those measurements and cannot be used for proper diagnosis. (b) B-scan echography and (c) standardized echography are the two major methods presently applied for diagnosis. B-scan echography utilizes mostly contact, real-time B-scan units with or without simultaneous (nonstandardized) A-mode displays. Standardized echography is based on the standardized A-scan that was specifically designed for tissue differentiation; it is complemented by contact, real-time B-scan and, in the orbit, by Doppler techniques. Standardized echography and B-scan echography differ clearly and profoundly in the design and use of instrumentation and examination techniques; consequently, they differ in their spectrum of clinical applications and, most importantly, in their results (1,2).

It is *standardized echography* (2) that has become increasingly effective in the diagnosis of Graves' disease over the past two decades. By the mid-1960s, orbital mass lesions could be detected or ruled out reliably and accurately by standardized A-scans. With this method, the diagnosis of Graves' disease was also aided more directly by demonstrating diffusely widened and more coarsely structured orbital soft tissues (3). Since the early 1970s accurate measurement of the straight extraocular muscles, and since the mid-1970s such measurement of oblique extraocular muscles, greatly improved the diagnosis of Graves' ophthalmopathy (1,4–8). Any thickening of extraocular muscles in both orbits of a patient as the primary or only cause of exophthalmos strongly indicated Graves' disease. However, there remained those few cases of early, truly unilateral Graves' ophthalmopathy as well as some conditions with bilateral thickening of extraocular muscles of a different etiology, e.g., acute myositis or tumors, which occasionally caused confusion. It was therefore a decisive improvement of the diagnosis of Graves' ophthalmopathy when a specific acoustic property of the diseased muscles, i.e., an increased heterogeneity and reflectivity of the thickened muscles, was discovered to be typical of, and indeed specific for, Graves' ophthalmopathy (1,9–11). During the past 6 years this acoustic hallmark has been used effectively and has made standardized echography today's most sensitive and specific diagnostic test for Graves' ophthalmopathy, regardless of whether the patient is hyperthyroid, hypothyroid, or, as is most frequently the case, euthyroid (1). Standardized A-scan is the method of choice for confirming or ruling out a diagnosis of Graves' disease when it is suspected or indicated by the clinical examination. Often enough standardized echography secures the correct diagnosis of Graves' ophthalmopathy when the clinical picture or computed tomographic (CT) scan findings suggest an orbital tumor or inflammation.

In addition to the exact measurement and evaluation of the acoustic properties of extraocular muscles, the standardized A-scan reveals several other findings that are typical of

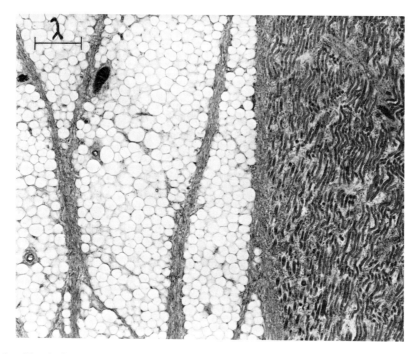

FIG. 1. Histological section of normal extraocular muscle and adjacent orbital fat tissues. Note the pronounced difference in surface size between the muscle fibers and the connective tissue septa, which explains the lower reflectivity of the muscle versus the higher reflectivity of the surrounding tissues. Wavelength of diagnostic ultrasound (λ), 0.19 nm.

Graves' ophthalmopathy (1,2): a solid thickening of the optic nerve sheaths and the periorbit, and occasionally swelling of the lacrimal glands. With standardized A-scans, compressive optic neuropathy (2,10,12–14) can be confirmed or predicted to be imminent by detecting increased subarachnoidal fluid around the more anterior portion of the optic nerve.

ACOUSTIC IDENTIFICATION OF EXTRAOCULAR MUSCLES

Normal and diseased extraocular muscles differ clearly in their acoustic properties from the surrounding orbital tissues by displaying a more homogeneous internal structure, a lower internal reflectivity, and a particularly high reflectivity of the surfaces of the muscle sheaths. Figure 1 explains this acoustic difference by demonstrating the different sizes of anatomical and acoustic interfaces in a histological section. The small surfaces of individual muscle fibers weakly scatter the ultrasound unlike the large surfaces of the connective tissue septa, which strongly reflect the ultrasound. The much larger and dense muscle sheaths produce even stronger echo signals than the orbital septa. The fat lobules, vessels, and nerves within the soft tissue surrounding an extraocular muscle contribute to a greater heterogeneity of that tissue compared to the more homogeneous muscle tissues. When using the standardized A-scan with the high, defined "tissue sensitivity," those acoustic differences between the extraocular muscles and the surrounding tissues are optimally displayed and allow the examiner to clearly identify the muscles in the echograms.

The typical shape and course of extraocular muscles can be traced by dynamic A-scans (Figs. 2 and 3) and B-scans (Fig. 5). A straight extraocular muscle can easily be seen to insert into the globe at the typical location. More posteriorly, the muscle body becomes

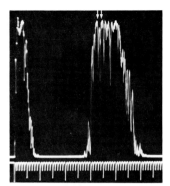

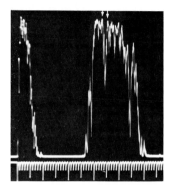

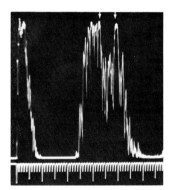

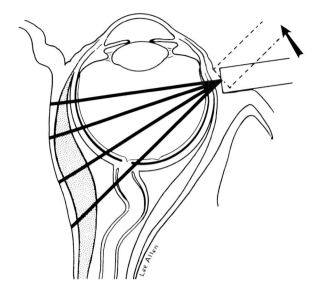

FIG. 2. Standardized A-scan examination of a right medial rectus muscle. The probe is placed on the temporal bulbar conjunctiva and is angled so that the ultrasonic beam scans the muscle in a transocular approach, from its insertion into the globe back to the orbital apex. The four A-scan echograms show cross sections of the normal medial rectus muscle, which correspond to the beam paths drawn into the picture on the right. *Arrows* mark the left and right surface spikes which correspond to the temporal and nasal sheaths of the muscle. N = cross section of the optic nerve.

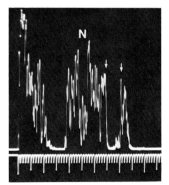

wider and shifts away from the globe into the immediate neighborhood of the bony orbital wall. It can further be followed back to the orbital apex, where it narrows and ends, remaining at the side of the bony orbital wall. Similarly, oblique extraocular muscles can be identified acoustically by their location and course. The superior oblique muscle can be followed from the trochlea back to the orbital apex, staying next to the bony orbital wall throughout its course. Its inserting tendon can be recognized overlying the sclera superiorly and posteriorly. The inserting tendon of the inferior oblique muscle likewise can be displayed next to and behind the insertion of the lateral rectus muscle.

Most extraocular muscles are examined with a transocular ultrasonic beam (Fig. 2). The ultrasonic probe is placed opposite the muscle, and the beam is aimed through the globe at the muscle. The belly of the inferior muscle, however, is best demonstrated with a paraocular approach: The probe is placed directly over the lower lid, and the beam is aimed in a sagittal direction through the muscle immediately below the globe. Figure 3 illustrates A-scan cross sections of thickened straight and oblique extraocular muscles at the various stations discussed above. It must be emphasized that the echographic identification and display of an extraocular muscle is a very dynamic procedure, where the probe is shifted and angled so that the beam scans the muscle in an anteroposterior direction as well as across the muscle in order to: (a) identify the muscle; (b) evaluate its internal structures throughout its course; and (c) measure its various portions, particularly its maximum thickness at both the inserting tendon and the muscle belly. In addition to this active scanning, another dynamic evaluation helps to identify and evaluate extraocular muscles: While probe and sound beam are kept stationary, the patient's eye is rotated by appropriate changes in the direction of gaze so that the muscle or portions of it shift in and out of the beam in a typical fashion, which helps the echographer to clearly distinguish a normal or abnormal muscle (Fig. 4) from other abnormal orbital structures, e.g., a lymphoma or a sclerosing pseudotumor located between a muscle and the bony orbital wall. It is such dynamic examinations that make standardized echography superior in the evaluation of extraocular muscles in regard to both measuring muscle size and differentiating muscle disorders.

ACOUSTIC MEASUREMENT OF EXTRAOCULAR MUSCLES

Major thickening of straight extraocular muscles (particularly the horizontal ones) can be demonstrated well with B-scan echography or other imaging procedures such as CT or nuclear magnetic resonance (NMR). B-scans are particularly impressive when a muscle is markedly thickened and low-reflective (see later), as shown in Figs. 5 through 7. The standardized A-scan is required to accurately measure all extraocular muscles, both straight

FIG. 3. Series of A-scan cross sections of thickened extraocular muscles beginning at the muscle insertion *(top echograms)* through increasingly more posterior segments of the muscles *(echograms from top to bottom)* and from the orbital apex *(bottom echograms)*. The left sequence of echograms was recorded from a medial rectus muscle thickened because of Graves' disease. The central sequence was obtained from another thickened medial rectus muscle in a case of acute myositis. The right sequence shows cross sections from a markedly thickened superior oblique muscle in the case of a carcinoma metastatic to this muscle. *Arrows* indicate the left and right surface spikes representing the inner and outer sheaths of the muscles. The echo spikes between the arrows represent the muscle body. Note the shift of the muscle pattern from a place immediately next to the sclera *(S)* (insertions of the medial rectus muscles) to a place next to the orbital bone *(B)* away from the globe echogram (bellies of the rectus muscles). The patterns of the superior oblique muscle stays next to the bone spike *(B)*. Also note the differences in spike heights recorded from the muscles in the various disease processes.

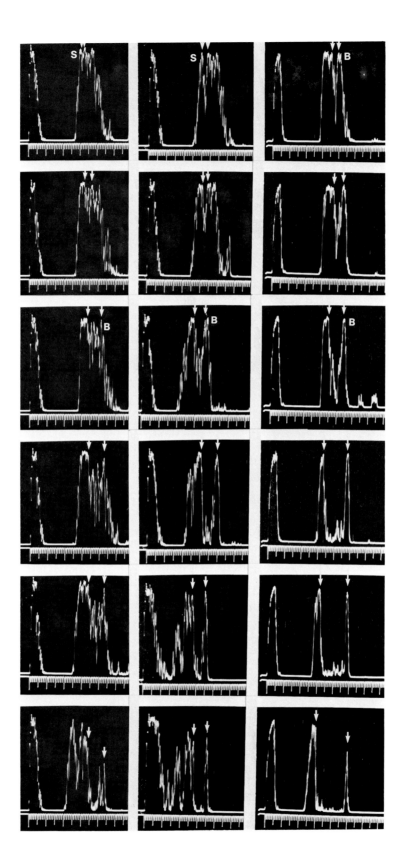

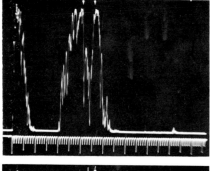

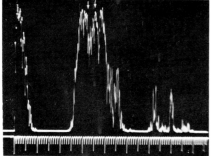

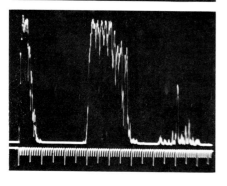

FIG. 4. Dynamic A-scan examination is one of the echographic means of identifying an extraocular muscle. The top echogram represents a cross section through the belly of a medial rectus muscle; it was recorded in straight gaze direction of the examined eye. The muscle sheaths are indicated by *arrows*. The center echogram was obtained by having the patient look away from the probe; the probe position and direction were kept stationary. Because of the gaze shift, the muscle belly slipped out of the beam (more posteriorly into the orbit), and a more anterior (narrower) cross section of the muscle is now displayed. Note that this cross section is located halfway between the scleral and bone spikes, unlike the cross section in the top echogram, which is located next to the bone. The bottom echogram was recorded when the patient looked even further away from the probe. This time even the inserting tendon of the muscle slipped out of the path of the ultrasonic beam. The orbital pattern was recorded from the paraocular space, anterior to the muscle.

and oblique ones, and thus detect minor thickening of a muscle. The measuring sensitivity of the standardized A-scan ranges from 0.1 to 0.2 mm at the muscle insertion, from 0.2 to 0.5 mm at the muscle belly, and from 0.5 to 0.8 mm near the orbital apex. The optimum measuring sensitivity can be achieved for the horizontal straight and the superior oblique muscles, provided they are normal or thickened by diseases other than Graves' ophthalmopathy. In Graves' disease the muscle sheaths tend to be thicker and less regularly delineated, which slightly decreases the measuring accuracy to the larger values given above. These larger figures also apply to the measurement of the superior and inferior straight muscles and the inferior oblique muscle, which all are more difficult to expose to a perfectly perpendicular sound beam.

For muscle measurement, one or two drops of Ophthaine are instilled to anesthetize the conjunctiva; the small pen-like A-scan probe is then placed on the bulbar conjunctiva opposite the muscle to be measured (Fig. 2). By angling the probe and scanning the muscle in an anteroposterior direction, the muscle is displayed and can be measured throughout its course in a dynamic fashion. Naturally, the measuring techniques for the inferior oblique

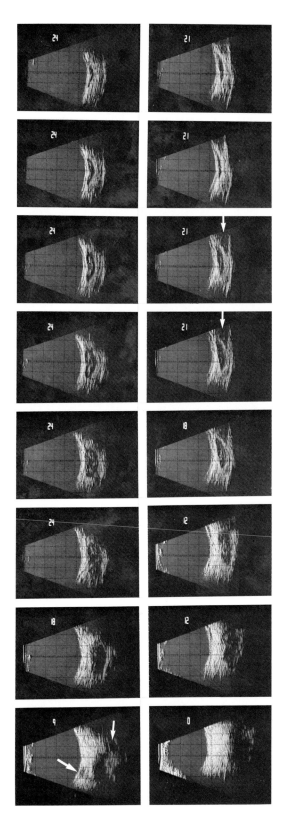

FIG. 5. Sequences of B-scan cross sections of a medial rectus muscle *(left)* and a lateral rectus muscle *(right)* in a patient with acute orbital myositis. The top echograms display cross sections of the thickened and infiltrated inserting tendons, whereas the lower echograms display cross sections of increasingly more posterior segments of the muscles. Note the shift of the muscle patterns from the sclera to the bony orbital wall as they get thicker in the more posterior orbit. *Arrows* mark the partial cross sections of the superior rectus muscle, the superior oblique muscle, and the anterior portion of the optic nerve.

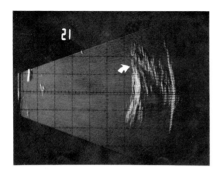

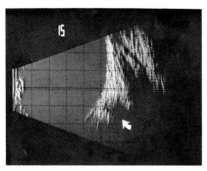

FIG. 6. Acoustic long sections of a thickened and infiltrated medial rectus muscle in a patient with orbital myositis. The top echogram shows the most anterior segment of that muscle including the inserting tendon. The bottom echogram shows a more posterior segment of the muscle and an oblique section of the most anterior portion of the optic nerve. *Arrows* point out the inserting tendon of the medial rectus muscle *(top echogram)* and the optic nerve *(bottom echogram).*

muscle must be modified according to its different course. By slightly angling the probe in a direction across the muscle, its maximum thicknesses are promptly recognized (Fig. 8).

Two echographic criteria guide the examiner during this dynamic procedure and ensure the accurate measurement of true cross sections of a muscle: (a) the width of the muscle pattern in the echogram; and (b) the height and steepness of both surface signals received from the sheaths of the muscle. The examiner angles and shifts the beam in order to maximize the width of the pattern. At the same time the examiner has to ensure that the beam hits both muscle surfaces perpendicularly in order to avoid an oblique cross section of the muscle, which naturally is wider than the true cross section. Perpendicularity is ensured when maximally high and steeply rising or falling surface spikes are displayed. The standardized A-scan utilizes a parallel though narrow ultrasonic beam. It is inherent in such beam characteristics and in the design and signal processing of the standardized A-scan instrument that a steeply rising, maximally high surface spike is displayed only when the beam reaches a large surface perpendicularly. The more the beam deviates from such perpendicularity, the lower and wider the surface spike becomes, and the less steeply it rises and falls (Fig. 9). Focused ultrasonic beams, as utilized for the B-scan, are far less sensitive to the direction of the beam and are much less suited to indicate perpendicularity of the sound beam. The unique features of the standardized A-scan make the accurate measurement of true cross sections of the muscle possible. Together with the dynamics of the procedure, they allow the examiner to quickly find and measure the maximum thickness of an extra-ocular muscle. In the posterior orbit, the application of a perpendicular sound beam becomes more difficult. However, refraction of the beam toward the muscle surface aids in this task (14).

SPECIFIC ACOUSTIC SIGN

Thickened muscles in Graves' disease clearly differ in their acoustic properties from muscles thickened by other diseases, e.g., acute myositis (15), chronic myositis (pseudotu-

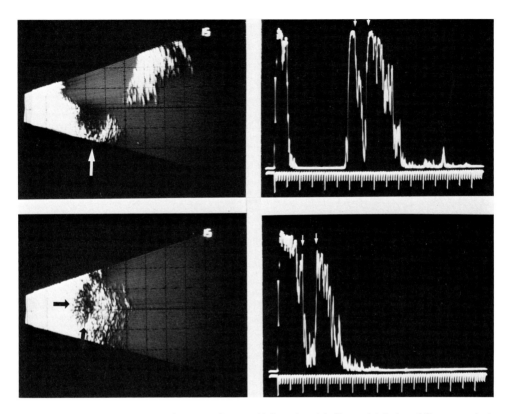

FIG. 7. B-scan and A-scan echograms from a thickened and infiltrated inferior oblique muscle in a patient with acute orbital myositis. The top B-scan echogram represents a vertical section through the inferior half of the globe and a cross section through the inferior oblique muscle at 6 o'clock. The bottom B-scan echogram is a horizontal sagittal section through the thickened oblique muscle just below the eyeball. The transocular A-scan echogram *(top)* shows a cross section of the markedly thickened inserting tendon of the inferior oblique muscle. The bottom A-scan echogram shows a sagittal cross section through the belly of the inferior oblique muscle at 6 o'clock (the probe was placed on the lower lid, and the beam was aimed in a sagittal direction just below the eyeball). The *arrows* indicate the inferior oblique muscle in the B-scan echograms, and the muscle's sheaths in the A-scan echograms.

mor), lymphoma, pseudolymphoma, sarcoidosis, metastatic carcinoma, hematoma, hypertrophy, and congestion (hyperemia) (2). Whereas all these other conditions display an often marked decrease in reflectivity and a much more homogeneous pattern than normal muscles, thickened muscles in Graves' disease are characterized by an increase in reflectivity and heterogeneity. This *increased heterogeneity and reflectivity* is specific for thickened muscles in Graves' disease, with the one exception of "pseudo-Graves' disease" (see below). The histological sections in Fig. 10 explain this acoustic behavior of extraocular muscles in Graves' disease versus the quite different acoustic properties in the other conditions. The increased fluid content of tissues in Graves' disease effectively separates and thus enhances and accentuates the acoustic interfaces normally present in the muscles, e.g., the surfaces of muscle fibers and bundles, and those of vessels and fat tissues within the muscle. In the other conditions, those interfaces are diminished or destroyed, resulting in a more homogeneous and much less reflective pattern than is characteristic of normal muscles (Fig. 1) and Graves' disease muscles. Figures 11 and 12 highlight the heterogeneity (irregular spike

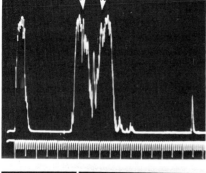

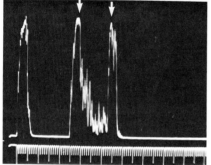

FIG. 8. A-scan echograms representing cross sections of a thickened lateral rectus muscle in a case of a carcinoma metastatic to this muscle. The center echogram shows a true cross section through the most thickened part of the muscle belly. Note the steeply falling and rising surface spikes *(arrows)* on either side of the low-reflective muscle pattern. The top and the bottom echograms were obtained from the same segment of the muscle but with sound beams aimed slightly above *(top echogram)* and below *(bottom echogram)* the muscle center. Note the V-shape of the top and bottom echographic muscle patterns and their slowly and irregularly falling and rising surface spikes indicating nonperpendicularity of the sound beam at their sheaths *(arrows)*.

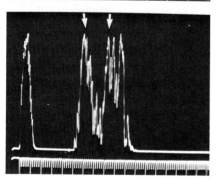

height) and high reflectivity (higher spikes) of muscles thickened in Graves' ophthalmopathy and contrast both with the homogeneity (regular spike height) and decreased reflectivity (lower spikes) encountered in muscles thickened from inflammation (acute myositis).

Like the measurement of extraocular muscles, their acoustic evaluation in regard to internal structure and reflectivity is a dynamic procedure. The reflectivity should be evaluated in the most anterior third of a muscle, where the sound beam passes through the ocular wall in a perpendicular direction and is not attenuated by the ocular wall (Figs. 2, 3, and 12). When displaying cross sections of more posterior segments of a muscle, the ultrasonic beam passes through the ocular wall in an increasingly oblique direction and is attenuated because of this. A thickened muscle's reflectivity then tends to seem low, regardless of whether Graves' disease or other conditions are present (Fig. 3). Unlike the reflectivity, the heterogeneity can be evaluated throughout the course of a muscle, but again it is more pronounced anteriorly. When recognizing and considering these particularities, the examiner can safely rely on the acoustic sign of increased heterogeneity and reflectivity in Graves' disease.

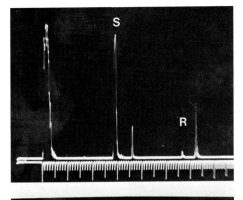

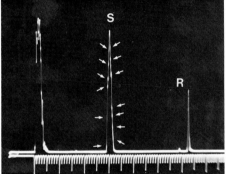

FIG. 9. Demonstration of the outstanding directional sensitivity of the parallel ultrasonic beam in standardized A-scan. The ultrasonic beam was aimed in a perfectly perpendicular direction at a large, coarse surface *(top echogram)*. Note the maximum height of the surface spike *(S)* with its steeply rising *(left)* and falling *(right)* limbs indicating perpendicularity. The second echogram (from the top) was obtained with slightly less perpendicularity. Both the ascending and descending limbs of the surface spike are less steep and show several high-frequency nodules *(arrows)*. The third and fourth echograms (from the top) were recorded with increasingly oblique sound beams and show a deteriorating height and an irregular widening of the surface spike. By angling and shifting the A-scan beam in order to produce maximum height and steeply rising and falling limbs of a surface spike (as shown in the top echogram), the examiner can ensure perpendicularity of the ultrasonic beam at that surface and, in measurements of extraocular muscles and optic nerves, the display of true cross sections through these structures. *R* = reverberation signals (artifacts).

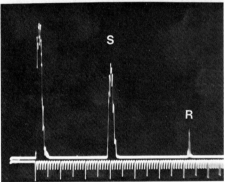

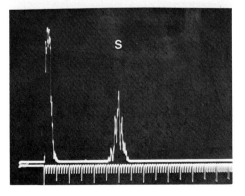

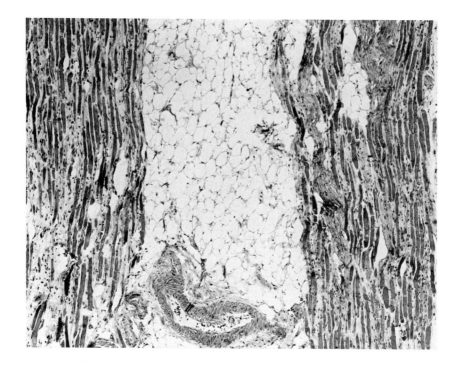

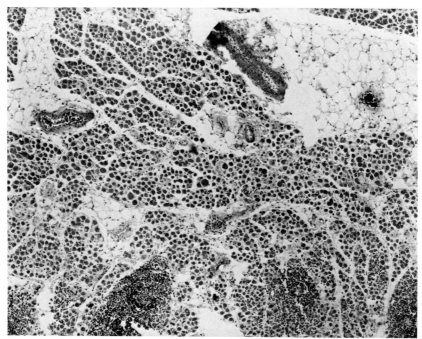

FIG. 10. Histological sections through thickened extraocular muscles: in a patient with Graves' disease *(left sections)*; in a patient with carcinoma metastatic to an extraocular muscle *(top right)*; and in a patient with orbital pseudotumor *(bottom right)*. Note how the acoustic surfaces in the Graves' disease muscles are enhanced. This explains their higher reflectivity and greater heterogeneity. In the

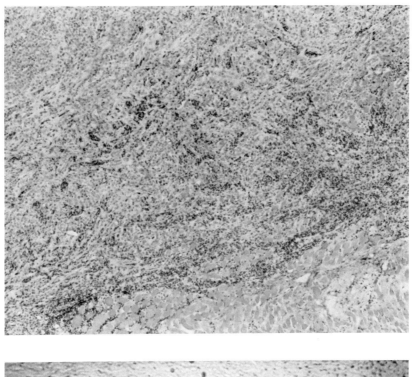

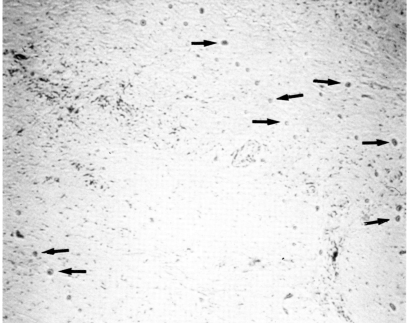

other conditions the muscle fibers are pushed to the side, and much more homogeneous and less reflective tumor tissue fills the widened space between the muscle sheaths (e.g., metastatic carcinoma) or the muscle fibers are wiped out and replaced by homogeneous connective tissue with a few atrophic fibers remaining *(arrows)*, as is the case in the pseudotumor.

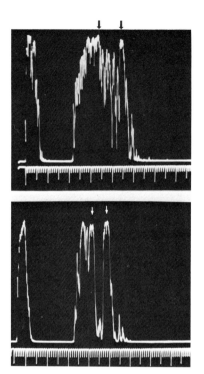

FIG. 11. A-scan cross sections through thickened medial rectus muscles in a case of Graves' disease *(top echogram)* and in a patient with acute myositis *(bottom echogram)* highlighting the pronounced acoustic difference between thickened muscles in these two conditions. Both echograms were obtained from muscle segments just anterior to the muscle belly, and both were recorded at the "standardized tissue sensitivity" setting of the A-scan instrument. The *arrows* point at the temporal and nasal muscle sheaths that outline the muscle body. The muscle patterns between the arrows contrast conspicuously by displaying high reflectivity (high spikes) in Graves' ophthalmopathy versus extremely low reflectivity (very low spikes) in acute myositis. Also, the internal muscle structure is heterogeneous (long spikes) in the Graves' muscle, whereas it is homogeneous (short spikes) in the acutely inflamed muscle.

There is only one other condition, "pseudo-Graves' disease," in which muscles, although only mildly thickened, display a relatively high heterogeneity and reflectivity. Patients who have been treated with lithium over a long period of time and those with longstanding, disseminated cancer who have undergone chemotherapy or extensive radiation therapy tend to show thicker extraocular muscles than the normal population. The same phenomenon was observed in patients with kidney transplants. However, muscles in these patients are equally thickened in both orbits—and not to a different and varying degree as seen in Graves' ophthalmopathy (see below). If those patients who suffer from widespread cancer or who are being treated with lithium are excluded from the echographic differentiation, the acoustic sign of increased heterogeneity and reflectivity is specific for Graves' ophthalmopathy.

OTHER ECHOGRAPHIC FINDINGS TYPICAL OF GRAVES' DISEASE

It is well known that muscles in Graves' disease typically are thickened more in their posterior segments. Accordingly, the inserting tendons often seem to be not or only slightly thickened in the A-scans (Figs. 3 and 12) and actually may not even be identifiable because of their higher reflectivity and heterogeneity. This is in sharp contrast to other frequent causes of muscle thickening, e.g., acute myositis and tumors, where the inserting tendons are markedly thickened, show decreased reflectivity, and are thus very prominent in the echogram (Figs. 3 and 12). In acute myositis the inserting tendon may at first be the only thickened and infiltrated portion of the affected muscle.

When observing a case of Graves' disease over a longer period of time (whether the patient is treated or not), the echographer will find quite a variation in the number and types of muscles most involved as well as in the thickness of the individual muscles. Whereas in one examination an inferior rectus muscle may be markedly thickened, it may barely be

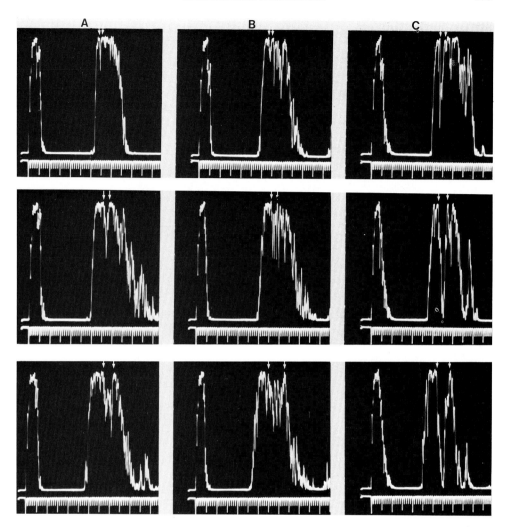

FIG. 12. Sequences of A-scan cross sections through the inserting tendons *(top line)*, the most anterior segments *(center line)*, and more posterior segments (still anterior to the muscle bellies) of **(A)** a normal medial rectus muscle *(left echograms)*, **(B)** a medial rectus muscle in a patient with Graves' disease *(middle echograms)* and, **(C)** a medial rectus muscle in a case of acute myositis *(right echograms)*. Note how prominent (lower-reflective and wider) the tendon and anterior portions of the myositic muscles are compared to the normal muscle on the left and, in particular, to the muscle structures in Graves' disease *(center)*. The *arrows* indicate the left and right surface spikes that correspond with inner and outer sheaths of the tendons and muscles.

detectable (fibrotic and thin) the next time. In the same patient, a muscle that was normal or mildly thickened during the first examination may become markedly swollen the next time. This is characteristic of the natural course of Graves' ophthalmopathy and was not observed in any of the other diseases that cause muscle thickening (e.g., myositis, tumors, or even pseudo-Graves' disease).

In addition to the thickening and internal acoustic changes of extraocular muscles, Graves' disease is characterized by a number of other related findings (Fig. 13). The optic nerve sheaths are thickened throughout the course of the nerve. This thickening may become quite

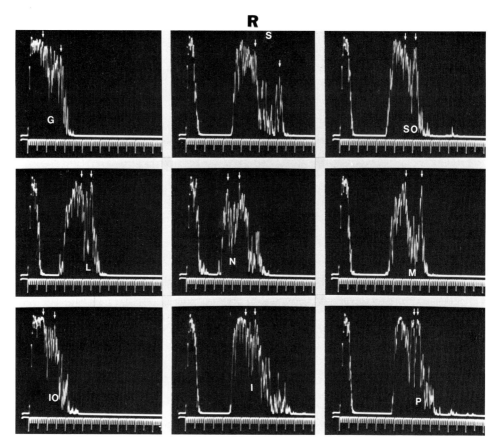

FIG. 13. Standardized A-scan echograms representing affected structures in the two orbits of a patient with Graves' ophthalmopathy. The various A-scan echograms are placed within the figure according to the location of the represented structures in the two orbits of the patient as the examiner would see facing the patient. *R* displays the structures of the right orbit, whereas *L* displays the structures of the left orbit of the patient. In the center, for instance, the echograms which represent the cross sections of the optic nerves are shown. *N* = optic nerve cross section. *M* = cross section of medial rectus muscle. *L* = lateral rectus muscle. *S* = superior rectus muscle. *I* = inferior rectus muscle. *SO* = superior oblique muscle. *IO* = inferior oblique muscle. *G* = lacrimal gland. *P* = thickened periorbit. The *arrows* outline the borders of the various structures displayed. Note the heterogeneity of all extraocular muscle patterns; the reflectivity of some of the muscle cross sections seems to be low only because of posterior acoustic beams (sound attenuation at obliquely crossed ocular wall).

marked but rarely amounts to an overall thickening of the nerve beyond 5.0 mm (see next paragraph). Likewise, the periorbit, hardly identifiable in normal patients, becomes prominent and clearly thickened in Graves' disease. Occasionally, both lacrimal glands in a patient with Graves' disease appear swollen, although the reflectivity of these glands generally remains high. This is in contrast to other causes of lacrimal gland swelling, e.g., dacryoadenitis or (pseudo)tumors of the lacrimal gland, where the reflectivity is always decreased in comparison to normal glands. As mentioned in the beginning, the orbital fat tissues also appear coarsened and thickened in patients with Graves' ophthalmopathy. Although these additional acoustic findings support the diagnosis of Graves' disease, they are not as specific and not always as obvious as the increased heterogeneity and reflectivity of thickened muscles, which remain the centerpiece of the echographic diagnosis of Graves' disease.

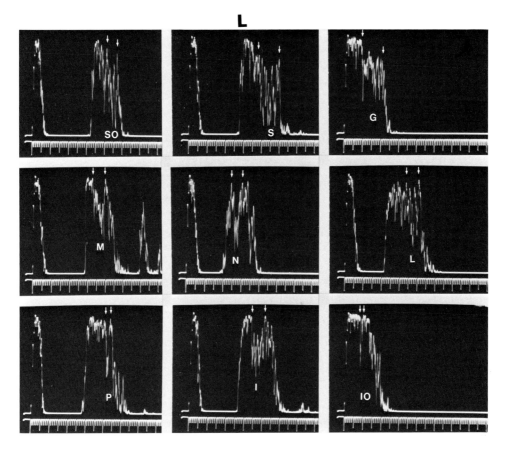

FIG. 13 *(Continued).*

ACOUSTIC SIGNS OF OPTIC NEUROPATHY

Two types of optic nerve involvement can be identified in patients with Graves' ophthalmopathy: (a) A widening of the optic nerve sheaths and consequently a moderate increase in optic nerve thickness is regularly detected in these patients. This "simple Graves' optic neuropathy" is usually asymmetrical in the two orbits of a patient. If marked enough, this sheath thickening strongly supports the diagnosis of Graves' disease. (b) Compressive optic neuropathy produces a very different echographic picture and is characterized by increased subarachnoidal fluid surrounding the anterior portion of the nerve; it also may lead to larger values of optic nerve thickening than are seen with sheath swelling.

For an optic nerve evaluation and measurement, the A-scan probe is usually placed on the bulbar conjunctiva near the temporal equator of the globe (Fig. 14). The beam is first aimed at the anterior portion of the medial rectus muscle, which serves as a landmark. By angling the beam posteriorly along this muscle and then tilting it slightly superiorly, the optic nerve pattern is quickly detected and then identified and evaluated. Occasionally the optic nerve inserts into the globe in an inverse fashion and is then easier displayed with the probe placed near the nasal equator of the globe.

Like the extraocular muscles, the thickness of the optic nerves can be measured accurately with standardized A-scans. The measuring sensitivity ranges from 0.2 to 0.4 mm along the

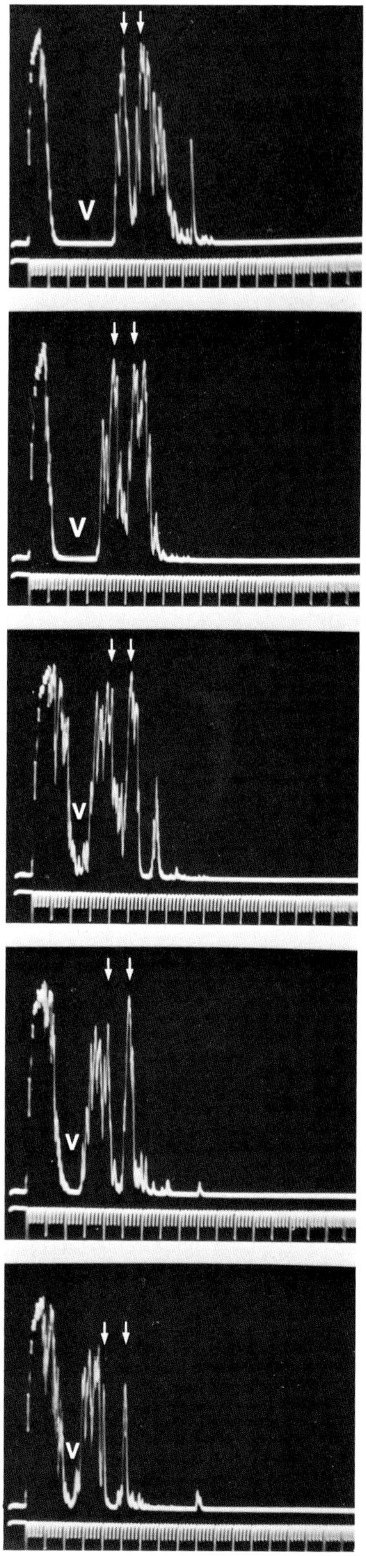

FIG. 14. A-scan cross sections of a normal optic nerve and a drawing of the examination technique. *Arrows* mark the distinct surface spikes that represent the temporal *(left)* and nasal *(right)* inner arachnoidal surfaces of the optic nerve. The five A-scan cross sections *(from top to bottom)* correspond to the five beam paths drawn in the picture (from retrobulbar space to posterior orbit). Perpendicularity of the ultrasonic beam at the arachnoidal surfaces is achieved only because the beams are refracted toward the optic nerve at the outer layers of the dura, as indicated in the drawings. Note that the ultrasonic beams cut through increasingly peripheral portions of the globe when aimed at more posterior segments of the optic nerve. Accordingly, the baseline representing the vitreous cavity *(V)* in the A-scan echograms becomes shorter.

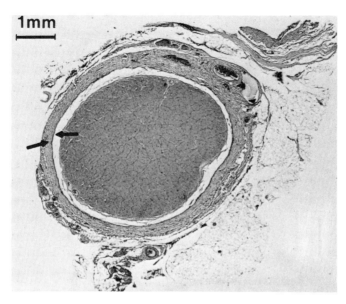

FIG. 15. Histological cross section of a normal nerve. Note that the inner arachnoidal surface *(arrows)* is separated by fluid from the pia that is attached to the nerve. This inner arachnoidal surface is the strongest and most regular reflector in normal optic nerve structures. The outer dural surface, by comparison, is much less distinct and less reflective.

anterior path of the orbital portion of the nerve, and from 0.3 to 0.6 mm along the nerves' posterior orbital section; the measuring sensitivity lies between 0.5 and 0.8 mm in the orbital apex. In normal and moderately swollen optic nerves, as well as those with any degree of distention of the optic nerve sheaths caused by increased (normal or abnormal) subarachnoidal fluid, the optimal measuring accuracy can be achieved (see above). The inner arachnoidal surface is then the most prominent of the nerve structures and is both a regular and a smooth surface (Fig. 15). It produces distinct and high (steeply rising and falling) surface spikes on either side of the optic nerve pattern (Fig. 14). It is the distance between the two opposite (inner) arachnoidal surfaces that is measured most easily and accurately with ultrasound and represents the echographically measured optic nerve thickness in the cases mentioned above.

Optic nerve measurements are a dynamic procedure during which the sound beam is shifted along the curved optic nerve structures from the retrobulbar space toward the apex and vice versa. As in muscle measurements, the beam is also angled slightly across the nerve to quickly recognize its maximum diameter. The relatively lower reflectivity of the optic nerve fibers and the particularly high reflectivity of the smooth arachnoidal surfaces (Fig. 15) make identification and measurement of the optic nerve easy. The measurements are significantly aided by the fact that the ultrasonic beam is refracted toward the optic nerve at the outer layers of the nerve's dural sheaths (Fig. 14). As in the muscle measurements, the examiner is guided by the width of the echographic optic nerve pattern and the display of maximally high and steeply rising or falling surface spikes from the arachnoidal surfaces.

As is true of muscle measurements, the measuring sensitivity of the standardized A-scan is decreased in Graves' disease, and the larger sensitivity values given above apply. In Graves' ophthalmopathy the optic nerve sheaths are thickened to some degree. Therefore

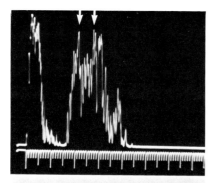

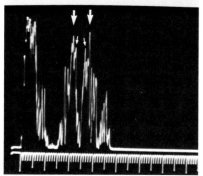

FIG. 16. A-scan cross sections of an optic nerve with moderately thickened sheaths in Graves' ophthalmopathy. The top echogram was recorded with the eye in straight gaze position. The bottom echogram was obtained when the gaze was directed toward the ultrasonic probe with a deviation of at least 30° from the straight direction (see drawings in Fig. 18). Note that the overall thickness of the nerve (dura/dura diameter) does not decrease in the 30° direction; this is typical for "simple" optic neuropathy in Graves' disease. The *large arrows* mark the temporal *(left)* and nasal *(right)* outer dural surfaces of the nerve. The less-high but also quite distinct pair of spikes *(small arrows)* within the optic nerve structures in the lower echogram corresponds to the interfaces between pia and arachnoid; these inner arachnoidal surfaces are much less prominent in this condition than in normal nerves or nerves with increased subarachnoidal fluid (see Figs. 17 and 18).

the separation of the inner arachnoidal surface from the pia is incomplete or absent, and the inner arachnoidal surface is no longer prominent in the echogram. In Graves' ophthalmopathy, then, optic nerve thickness measurements are taken from the outer dural, instead of the inner arachnoidal, surfaces. The outer dural surface, however, is less regular and smooth as well as less reflective (Fig. 15). Its maximal surface signals are not as easy to display as the surface signals from the arachnoid in the other conditions mentioned above. Therefore simple Graves' optic neuropathy (consisting of the thickening of the optic nerve sheaths) has two echographic consequences: The maximum nerve thickness is clearly increased compared to normal optic nerves, and the nerve patterns are more difficult to display. When measuring such nerves first in straight and then in 30° gaze direction, no significant decrease in the measurements is noted (Fig. 16). As a matter of fact, many times the 30° measurement may come out slightly (0.1 to 0.3 mm) larger than the measurement in a straight gaze direction. Rarely, the optic nerve thickness as measured echographically then reaches or surpasses a value of 5.0 mm.

In *compressive optic neuropathy* the echographic picture changes dramatically. The increased subarachnoidal fluid distends the thickened outer optic nerve sheaths (arachnoid and dura) from the pia, again making the inner arachnoidal surface the most prominent reflector and allowing for easier and more accurate optic nerve thickness measurements (Fig. 17). In this condition, the 30° measurements (Fig. 18) come out clearly decreased compared to measurements in straight gaze direction (fluid sign). The more severe the compression, the more subarachnoidal fluid there is surrounding the optic nerve anteriorly. Thus the amount of measured optic nerve thickness parallels the presence and severity of dysfunction of the optic nerve (afferent pupillary defects, decreased visual acuities, visual field deficits). Experience has shown that most nerves with functional compressive optic neuropathy have a measured optic nerve thickness of greater than 4.7 mm; many of these

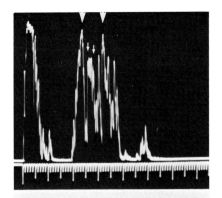

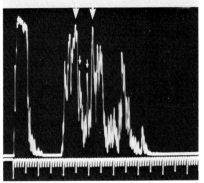

FIG. 17. A-scan cross sections of an optic nerve in a case of compressive optic neuropathy caused by Graves' disease. The upper echogram was obtained in straight-gaze position of the eye, whereas the bottom echogram was recorded when the gaze was shifted at least 30° toward the ultrasonic probe (see Fig. 18). The *large arrows* mark the inner arachnoidal surfaces; because of the increased subarachnoidal fluid these surfaces have regained their prominence in the echogram. Note the low reflectivity of the subarachnoidal space (homogeneous fluid) between the inner arachnoidal surfaces and the also enhanced pial surfaces *(small arrows)* of the nerve. In compressive optic neuropathy the overall thickness of the optic nerve (arachnoid/arachnoid diameter) clearly decreases (by at least 10%) in the 30° gaze direction (for explanation see Fig. 18).

optic nerves are wider than 5.2 mm and all show the fluid sign. On the other hand, optic nerves which have a diameter greater than 4.7 mm many times, but not always, display loss of function, whereas those beyond 5.2 mm are always accompanied by severe functional deficits, provided the fluid sign is present.

Measurements of the optic nerve thickness and, in particular, detection of increased subarachnoidal fluid surrounding the anterior portion of the optic nerve, and thus the objective proof of compressive optic neuropathy with the help of standardized A-scans, are invaluable for the management of patients with Graves' disease. The A-scan measurements in Graves' ophthalmopathy are comparable with, and fulfill the same function as, tonometry in patients with glaucoma: The echographic detection of increased subarachnoidal fluid together with a measurement of optic nerve thickness surpassing 4.7 mm helps to confirm functional compressive optic neuropathy (particularly in eyes where cataracts, other intra-ocular opacities, or other lesions make it difficult to pinpoint the cause of functional loss). Most importantly, it is an alarming sign and indicates that functional loss, if not yet present, may occur at any time. We repeatedly observed that patients who had the echographic but not the clinical signs of compressive optic neuropathy developed such clinical signs soon thereafter. Patients who have an optic nerve thickness increased beyond 4.7 mm and the fluid sign should therefore be observed much more closely and actually should be taught to screen their optic nerve function regularly themselves. By contrast, patients who lack the acoustic signs of compressive optic neuropathy may be followed on a much longer time scale.

RESULTS AND CONCLUSIONS

Among more than 500 consecutive cases of exophthalmos examined in the Echography Service of the Department of Ophthalmology at the University of Iowa over a 2-year period

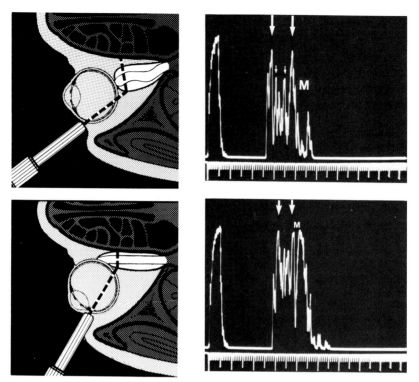

FIG. 18. Explanation of the 30° measurements. In this case of papilledema the thickness of the optic nerve (arachnoid/arachnoid diameter) was markedly increased, as shown in the top echogram. When the gaze direction was shifted by at least 30° toward the ultrasonic probe, the optic nerve was stretched and the subarachnoidal fluid was distributed over a longer distance, thus clearly decreasing the overall width of the nerve *(bottom echogram)*. The *large arrows* indicate the temporal *(left)* and nasal *(right)* arachnoidal surfaces. The *small arrows* mark the pial surfaces of the optic nerve. Note the lower reflectivity of the subarachnoidal space (between the large and the small arrows). Also, note the width of the medial rectus muscle *(M)* which in 30° examinations is also thinner (muscle is being stretched).

(1981–1982), 20% were diagnosed as Graves' ophthalmopathy. This is consistent with the well-known statements in ophthalmic literature that Graves' ophthalmopathy is the single most frequent cause of exophthalmos and stresses the importance of the correct diagnosis of this condition. Among these more than 500 cases of exophthalmos were 154 patients in whom the exophthalmos was primarily or solely caused by thickening of extraocular muscles in one or both orbits. Only 105 (68%) of these patients were found to suffer from Graves' ophthalmopathy (Table 1). This points out the importance of correctly identifying Graves' disease and differentiating it from other causes of muscle thickening.

   The second most frequent cause of muscle thickening was acute myositis. In this condition the thickened muscles were extremely low-reflective, and their inserting tendons were conspicuous (both thickened and low-reflective). There were three cases which seemed to represent a combination of myositis and Graves' ophthalmopathy (or atypical courses of Graves' disease with unusually dense cellular infiltration). In these three patients, the signs of acute myositis were overwhelming at first but disappeared during high-dose steroid therapy, and all three turned into typical Graves' ophthalmopathy patients thereafter (with high reflectivity and heterogeneity of the continuously thickened muscles and lack of prominence of the inserting muscle tendons). All six patients with "pseudo-Graves' disease"

TABLE 1. *Summary of 157 consecutive
cases with thickened extraocular muscles as
the primary or only cause of exophthalmos,
observed during a 2-year period[a]*

Cases	No.	%
All cases	154	100
Two-thirds:		
Graves' disease	105	68.2
One-third:		
Myositis	27	17.5
Mixed myositis–Graves' disease	3	1.9
Pseudo-Graves' disease[b]	6	3.9
Metastatic carcinoma	5	3.3
Slow-flow intracranial A–V fistula	3	1.9
Pseudotumors	2	1.3
Hematomas within muscle sheaths	2	1.3
"Thick muscle"	1	0.7

[a]From the Echography Service, Department of Ophthalmology, The University of Iowa (1981–1982).
[b]Chemotherapy for: carcinomatosis, 3; psychosis (lithium), 2; kidney transplant, 1.

had long-term chemotherapy. Three suffered from carcinomatosis, two from psychosis (lithium therapy), and one had undergone a kidney transplant. The metastatic carcinoma in the five patients listed was confined to the space within the muscle sheaths (Fig. 3); these patients had no other orbital metastases or bony metastases next to the orbit. In the three cases with slow-flow intracranial arteriovenous fistula, the muscle thickening was caused by severe hyperemia in the congested orbits. There was no specific diagnosis in only one of the 154 patients with thickened muscles; the one thickened extraocular muscle in this patient was labeled as "thick muscle." Apart from the 105 cases diagnosed as Graves' disease, only the three "mixed cases" and the six cases with "pseudo-Graves' disease" showed high reflectivity and pronounced heterogeneity of the thickened muscles. In all other causes of muscle thickening, the muscles appeared homogeneous and low-reflective.

Table 2 summarizes the acoustic signs of Graves' disease as utilized for the echographic diagnosis. Most prominent among these signs are the special distribution and mode of muscle thickening and the high reflectivity and pronounced heterogeneity of the muscle tissues. In the absence of these two key criteria, the diagnosis of Graves' ophthalmopathy should not be made in a patient with thickened muscles. These key criteria are also found in patients with pseudo-Graves' disease. In addition to the obvious medical history in these patients, the muscles are thickened more equally and mildly and do not vary in thickness during follow-up examinations, as they do in Graves' ophthalmopathy. Therefore this group of patients does not represent a problem for an accurate diagnosis of Graves' ophthalmopathy.

When evaluating the Graves' disease patients listed in Table 1, three cases were eliminated because other lesions (i.e., metastatic carcinomas in two patients and an optic nerve meningioma in the third patient) additionally affected one of their orbits. In all three of these cases, several muscles were thickened in both orbits, and the high heterogeneity and reflectivity was clearly present in the thickened muscles; in two of the cases Graves' disease was confirmed by positive thyroid studies. Although there was no question that Graves' disease was involved, these three cases were nevertheless excluded from the following comparisons.

TABLE 2. *Acoustic signs of Graves' ophthalmopathy as evaluated with standardized A-scan*

1. Absence of tumors
2. Diffuse swelling of orbital fat tissues (mostly in anterior orbit; coarser structure than in normal tissues)
3. *Thickened extraocular muscles*
   a. Most often in both orbits
   b. Inserting tendons poorly visible in echograms
   c. Thickening more pronounced in posterior orbit
   d. Muscle thicknesses vary greatly over time
   e. Different muscles affected over time
4. *New sign:* High reflectivity (must be evaluated in anterior one-third of muscle) and pronounced heterogeneity of thickened muscles
5. Thickened optic nerve sheaths (markedly distended by increased subarachnoidal fluid in compressive optic neuropathy)
6. Thickened periorbit
7. Enlarged lacrimal glands

Table 3 compares the echographically measured thickening of extraocular muscles with the clinical appearance, i.e., the presence or absence of noticeable exophthalmos, the presence or absence of lid signs, e.g., lid retraction (Dalrymple's sign) and lid lag (Graefe's sign), and the clinical course of the disease in the 102 patients with diagnosed Graves' disease. It is notable that only two-thirds of the patients with Graves' ophthalmopathy displayed typical clinical signs, and only about two-thirds of the cases (not always the ones with a typical clinical appearance) had a clinically evident bilateral exophthalmos. Nevertheless, the echographic measurements showed bilaterality of the disease in almost 90% of the cases. Two-thirds of the cases were confirmed by positive thyroid tests at some point along the course of the disease, either before, at the time of, or after the clinical and echographic evaluations. It is, however, quite remarkable that about one-third of all patients remained euthyroid. Sixty-five (63.7%) of the 102 cases of Graves' disease (and even 31 of the 68 cases confirmed by positive thyroid tests at one time during their observation) were euthyroid at the time of the echographic diagnosis. A large number of the confirmed cases had positive thyroid tests only long before the onset of Graves' orbitopathy and had negative tests at the time of onset of ocular problems. In six of the confirmed cases, the thyroid status became abnormal for the first time several weeks to months after the echographic diagnosis. In four of these six cases, the clinical appearance had been atypical; in two of them the exophthalmos had been unilateral; but in all six the thickening of the extraocular muscles, as measured with standardized A-scans, was found to be bilateral, and the acoustic sign of high reflectivity and heterogeneity was clearly positive.

Table 4 specifies the degree of the acoustic sign of high reflectivity and pronounced heterogeneity of the thickened muscles in the 102 cases of Graves' disease studied. This acoustic sign was present in all cases diagnosed as Graves' disease. In six (5.9%) of the patients, the heterogeneity and reflectivity were only borderline. Four of these patients, who displayed typical lid signs, obviously represented very mild, early stages of Graves' disease, as the thickening of extraocular muscles was also slight. In the other two borderline cases, most of the muscles in both orbits were markedly thickened posteriorly. However, in none of the borderline patients was the internal structure homogeneous enough or the reflectivity low enough to be consistent with any of the other causes of muscle thickening listed in Table 1 (except for the group of mixed myositis and Graves' disease). So far, no attempt has been made to correlate the degree of the acoustic sign of high reflectivity and pronounced heterogeneity of the thickened muscles with different types of Graves' disease.

TABLE 3. *Case material studied (and diagnosed as Graves' ophthalmopathy) with standardized echography[a]*

Cases	Total No. (examined 1981–1982)	Clinical appearance		Exophthalmos			Thickened muscles detected with echography	
		Typical	Atypical	Unilateral	None	Bilateral	Bilateral	Unilateral
Confirmed[b] (66.7%)	68 (100%)	49 (72.1%)	19 (27.9%)	16 (23.5%)	2 (3%)	50 (73.5%)	61 (89.7%)	7 (10.3%)
Unconfirmed[b] (33.3%)	34 (100%)	19 (55.9%)	15 (44.1%)	14 (41.2%)	2 (5.9%)	18 (52.9%)	29 (85.3%)	5 (14.7%)
All (100%)	102 (100%)	68 (66.7%)	34 (33.3%)	30 (29.4%)	4 (3.9%)	68 (66.7%)	90 (88.2%)	12 (11.8%)
		2/3	1/3	1/3		2/3	9/10	1/10

[a]Using, among others, the high reflectivity and pronounced heterogeneity of thickened extraocular muscles as objective criteria. Study by K. C. Ossoinig and V. M. Hermsen, 1982.
[b]By thyroid studies.

TABLE 4. *High acoustic reflectivity and pronounced acoustic heterogeneity of thickened extraocular muscles is a typical, newly described sign of Graves' ophthalmopathy[a]*

Cases	Total No.	No. by degree of new acoustic sign			
		+ + +	+ +	+	±
Confirmed[b] (66.7%)	68 (100%) (7)[c]	34 (50.0%) (3)[c]	15 (22.0%) (1)[c]	18 (26.5%) (3)[c]	1 (1.5%) (0)[c]
		[Clear-cut: 67 (98.5%)]			[Borderline: 1 (1.5%)]
Unconfirmed[b] (33.3%)	34 (100%)	12 (35.3%)	10 (29.4%)	7 (20.6%)	5 (14.7%)
All (100%)	102 (100%)	46 (45.1%)	25 (24.5%)	25 (24.5%)	6 (5.9%)
		[Clear-cut: 96 (94%)]			[Borderline: 6 (6%)]

[a]Grading of this sign in cases studied with standardized echography.
[b]By thyroid tests.
[c]Cases of unilateral thickening of muscles as indicated by echography.

Standardized echography has become a highly reliable and specific method for diagnosing Graves' disease ever since the new objective acoustic sign of high reflectivity and pronounced heterogeneity of the thickened muscles was introduced. As can be seen from Table 3, 15 patients were diagnosed as having Graves' disease in spite of euthyroid status and atypical clinical appearance. All 15 cases clearly displayed the new acoustic sign. It is certainly difficult to confirm the echographic diagnosis in these patients. However, follow-up periods of 1 to 2 years have not turned up any other cause for the exophthalmos in these patients. Likewise, none of the other patients who were echographically diagnosed to have Graves' disease and were confirmed by thyroid tests or clinical appearance developed signs or symptoms that would have changed the diagnosis. The same thing holds true for the cases of acute myositis or other conditions (listed in Table 1) that were echographically differentiated from Graves' disease.

During the 15 months that have passed since the 2-year study, 128 more patients were diagnosed with standardized echography to have Graves' disease. The acoustic sign of increased reflectivity and heterogeneity was clearly present in 120 (93.7%) and borderline in only eight (6.3%) of these patients. These 128 additional Graves' disease patients represent 41% (a clear increase from the 20% of the previous study) of 375 new patients with orbital problems who have been examined echographically during the last 15 months. This figure too is higher than the number of orbital cases seen in corresponding time periods of previous years. This growing popularity of standardized echography as a reliable and specific diagnostic test in patients with orbital disorders, and in particular when Graves' disease is suspected or is to be ruled out, expresses not only an increasing awareness of the availability of such a test but also a growing appreciation of its achievements.

REFERENCES

1. Ossoinig, K. C. (1983): Advances in diagnostic ultrasound. In: *Acta: XXIV International Congress of Ophthalmology*, edited by P. Henkind, pp. 89–114. Lippincott, Philadelphia.
2. Ossoinig, K. C. (1979): Standardized echography: basic principles, clinical applications and results. *Int. Ophthalmol. Clin.*, 19:127–210.
3. Ossoinig, K. C. (1971): Echo-orbitography—a reliable method for the differential diagnosis of endocrine exophthalmos. In: *Further Advances in Thyroid Research*, edited by K. Fellinger and R. Hoefer, pp. 871–877. Verlag Wiener Med. Akademie, Vienna.

4. McNutt, L. C., Kaefring, S. L., and Ossoinig, K. C. (1977): Echographic measurement of extraocular muscles. In: *Ultrasound in Medicine*, Vol. 3A, edited by D. White and R. E. Brown, pp. 927–932. Plenum Press, New York.
5. Ossoinig, K. C. (1979): The technique of measuring extraocular muscles. In: *Diagnostica Ultrasonica in Ophthalmologia*, edited by H. Gernet, pp. 166–172. Remy, Muenster.
6. Skalka, H. W. (1979): Clinical presentation, extraocular muscle and perineural optic nerve changes in endocrine orbitopathy. In: *Diagnostica Ultrasonica in Ophthalmologia*, edited by H. Gernet, pp. 155–158. Remy, Muenster.
7. Shammas, H. J. F., Minckler, D. S., and Ogden, C. (1980): Ultrasound in early thyroid orbitopathy. *Arch. Ophthalmol.*, 98:277–279.
8. Byrne, S. F., and Glaser, J. S. (1983): Orbital tissue differentiation with standardized echography. *Ophthalmology*, 90:1071–1090.
9. Ossoinig, K. C. (1982): A new echographic sign for the reliable differential diagnosis of endocrine exophthalmos. *Klin. Monatsbl. Augenheilkd.*, 180:189–197.
10. Ossoinig, K. C. (1982): Diagnostic ultrasound. In: *Neuro-Ophthalmology 1982*, Vol. 2, edited by S. Lessel and J. T. W. van Dalen, pp. 373–388. Excerpta Medica, Amsterdam.
11. Ossoinig, K. C. (1982): A new echographic sign for reliable differential diagnosis of Graves' disease. In: *Proc. AIUM/SDMS Annual Convention*, Denver.
12. Ossoinig, K. C., Kaefring, S. L., McNutt, L., and Weinstock, S. J. (1977): Echographic measurement of the optic nerve. In: *Ultrasound in Medicine*, Vol. 3A, edited by D. White and R. E. Brown, pp. 1065–1066. Plenum, New York.
13. Skalka, H. W. (1978): Perineural optic nerve changes in endocrine orbitopathy. *Arch. Ophthalmol.*, 96:468–473.
14. Ossoinig, K. C., Cennamo, G., and Frazier-Byrne, S. (1981): Echographic differential diagnosis of optic-nerve lesions. *Doc. Ophthalmol.*, 29:327–332.
15. Ossoinig, K. C., and Hermsen, V. M. (1983): Myositis of extraocular muscles diagnosed with standardized echography. In: *Ophthalmic Ultrasonography*, edited by J. S. Hillman and M. M. LeMay, pp. 381–392. Dr. W. Junk Publishers, The Hague.

The Eye and Orbit in Thyroid Disease, edited by
C. A. Gorman et al. Raven Press, New York 1984.

Endocrine Ophthalmopathy:
Differential Diagnosis

*Robert R. Waller and †David H. Jacobson

*Department of Ophthalmology and †Division of Endocrinology and Department of Internal
Medicine, Mayo Clinic, Rochester, Minnesota 55905*

Endocrine ophthalmopathy commonly presents as bilateral eye disease characterized by signs of inflammation and vascular congestion associated with eyelid retraction, proptosis, and extraocular muscle dysfunction. These eye findings, when coupled with an abnormality of thyroid function or regulation, leave little question about the diagnosis. Unfortunately, not all patients present with the full constellation of symptoms and signs. Eye findings may be subtle or unilateral and may be present without a readily demonstratable thyroid abnormality. Furthermore, a number of vascular, inflammatory, and neoplastic disorders may closely mimic endocrine ophthalmopathy. This chapter describes those eye disorders that are most commonly confused with Graves' disease as well as the clinical, anatomic, and laboratory features that play an important role in the differential diagnosis of orbital inflammation. Table 1 lists the signs of orbital inflammation. Table 2 includes the major disease categories for consideration in the differential diagnosis of orbital inflammation. While reviewing these various disorders it should be remembered that a pathologic diagnosis of orbital inflammation may often be associated with no clinical signs of inflammation.

TABLE 1. *Signs of orbital
inflammation*

Chemosis
Lid swelling
Erythema
Proptosis
Displacement
Strabismus
Visual disturbance

TABLE 2. *Differential diagnosis of inflammatory ophthalmopathy*

Endocrine ophthalmopathy
Idiopathic inflammatory orbital pseudotumor
Chronic orbital myositis
Systemic manifestations of lymphoma, sarcoidosis, amyloidosis, and vasculitis
Inflammation secondary to contiguous sinus disease
Other organism-related inflammations
Cysts
Neoplasms
Vascular malformations
Foreign bodies

The clinical features of endocrine ophthalmopathy are described in great detail elsewhere in this text. It is important to remember, however, that these features are present in varying combinations and that they can be expected to change during the course of the disease. Indeed, subtle remissions and exacerbations are characteristic of endocrine ophthalmopathy. Retrospective review of the eye findings in an individual patient often demonstrates this clearly. The degree of eyelid retraction, for example, may vary not only from week to week but even from minute to minute. Furthermore, individual findings in endocrine ophthalmopathy differ in their diagnostic specificity. Eyelid retraction and lid lag are quite characteristic of Graves' disease, especially when they are present bilaterally. Other causes of lid retraction are the following (9):

Upper lid retraction
   Graves' disease
   Neurologic disorders—Marcus Gunn phenomenon; midbrain disease;
      hydrocephalus; Parinaud's syndrome; trauma to cranial nerve III;
      aneurysm involving cranial nerve III
   Sympathomimetic drugs
   Cirrhosis
   Congenital abnormality
   Postsurgical lesion—operation for ptosis; lid reconstruction

Lower lid retraction
   Graves' disease
   Postsurgical lesion—recession of the inferior rectus muscle;
                        repair of a blowout fracture
   Posttraumatic impairment
   Postinflammatory lesion
   Congenital abnormality

Periorbital edema, chemosis, conjunctival injection, and ophthalmoplegia are rather nonspecific. Bilateral proptosis can be associated with a variety of neoplastic, vascular, and inflammatory processes, some of which are the following:

Endocrine disorders—Graves' disease; Hashimoto's thyroiditis
Orbital neoplasms—neoplasms arising in the orbit; metastatic malignancy
Orbital cysts
Granulomatous diseases—sarcoidosis; Wegener's granulomatosis
Inflammatory disorders—orbital pseudotumor; chronic orbital myositis
Infectious diseases—orbital cellulitis; syphilis; mucormycosis;
   parasitic diseases
Neuromuscular disorders—myotonia congenita; myasthenia gravis
Miscellaneous problems—eosinophilic granuloma; lithium treatment;
   mediastinal irradiation

Unilateral proptosis is even less specific, although endocrine ophthalmopathy constitutes its single most common cause.

Although no single eye finding is pathognomonic, certain patterns can be considered diagnostic of Graves' disease and exclude the other disorders in the differential diagnosis. Figure 1 displays the major clinical and laboratory findings associated with Graves' eye disease. When all of the features are present, the diagnosis is assured. When all of the

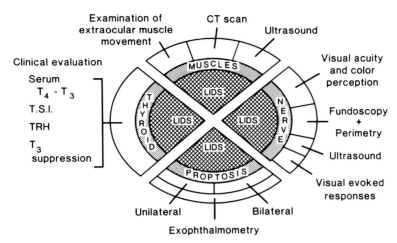

FIG. 1. Clinical and laboratory findings associated with endocrine ophthalmopathy. When all features are present the diagnosis is ensured. When all features displayed in one quadrant are present, the diagnosis is likely. Isolated involvement of the eyelids, muscles, or nerves leaves the diagnosis open to question. (From ref. 4.)

features in one quadrant are present, the diagnosis is considered likely. Isolated involvement of the eyelids, muscles, or nerves leaves the diagnosis open to question. Finding choroidal folds, papilledema, or an orbital apical density on computed tomography does not exclude the diagnosis because crowding of the apex by diffuse enlargement of the extraocular muscles may mimic an orbital tumor. Newer generation imaging machines can often clarify the nature of the apical density.

The majority of patients with endocrine ophthalmopathy have a readily identifiable abnormality of thyroid function. This may precede or follow the diagnosis of ophthalmopathy but usually appears within 18 months of the onset of eye symptoms. Some investigators have suggested that a small percentage of patients with Graves' ophthalmopathy develop no thyroid abnormality. The number of patients fitting this description has dwindled steadily as more sensitive tests of thyroid regulation, including thyrotropin stimulation and triiodothyronine suppression tests, have been applied. Abnormal blood levels of thyroid stimulating or binding immunoglobulins may also be identified in many patients with endocrine ophthalmopathy who are clinically euthyroid. These have been implicated as important elements in the pathogenesis of Graves' disease.

ORBITAL PSEUDOTUMOR AND CHRONIC ORBITAL MYOSITIS

The diagnostic categories of orbital pseudotumor and chronic orbital myositis are surrounded by a considerable amount of confusion primarily because of the varying definitions of each disorder which have appeared in the medical literature. The term "orbital pseudotumor" was coined by Birch-Herschfeld in 1930 and was used to describe three clinical situations: (a) orbital tumors which subsided spontaneously; (b) exophthalmos which was shown to be unrelated to distinct tumefaction at the time of surgery but displayed chronic inflammation microscopically; and (c) exophthalmos which was surgically proved to be associated with a nonspecific inflammatory mass. Currently, orbital pseudotumor is defined as an idiopathic, localized inflammatory infiltration of orbital tissues associated with a fibrovascular tissue reaction. This probably represents a common response to a variety of etiologic factors. It

TABLE 3. *Comparison of orbital pseudotumor and orbital myositis[a]*

Parameter	Orbital myositis	Pseudotumor
Age (years)	20–30	50–60
Muscle inflammation	Yes	Sometimes
Systemic disease	No	Sometimes
Painful ophthalmoplegia	Yes	Sometimes (30%)
Orbital mass	No	Yes
Response to prednisone	Yes	Sometimes
Visual loss	No	Sometimes
Recurrence, relapse	Often	Sometimes

[a]From ref. 1.

may simulate neoplasm and has a variable but self-limited course. Eye findings are usually unilateral at the onset but can become bilateral. Bilateral eye involvement, however, requires exclusion of systemic disease. Signs of vascular congestion, inflammation, and proptosis are commonly present. Systemic symptoms, including lethargy, anorexia, fever, headache, and abdominal pain, are not uncommon. The erythrocyte sedimentation rate is frequently elevated. Vision may be threatened when the inflammatory process is severe.

When inflammation primarily involves the eye muscles, ophthalmoplegia may be the most prominent finding. This is referred to as chronic orbital myositis and is characterized by ocular pain, ophthalmoplegia, histologic and radiographic evidence of inflammation of the extraocular muscles, a remitting and recurring course, and a dramatic clinical response to corticosteroids. Patients with chronic orbital myositis tend to be younger than those with pseudotumor. They develop no systemic symptoms and are usually not at risk for visual loss even after multiple recurrences. A comparison of the clinical features of orbital pseudotumor and orbital myositis is found in Table 3.

Orbital pseudotumor and orbital myositis can often be distinguished from endocrine ophthalmopathy when eyelid retraction and typical ophthalmoplegia patterns are present to support the latter diagnosis. Subtle differences in appearance by computed tomography (CT), e.g., thickening of Tenon's capsule and the presence of feathery orbital densities, favor the diagnosis of pseudotumor as does the presence of a palpable orbital mass.

SYSTEMIC DISEASES WITH ORBITAL INVOLVEMENT

A variety of systemic diseases, including lymphoma, sarcoidosis, amyloidosis, and vasculitis, may involve the orbit and present with symptoms and signs similar to those of endocrine ophthalmopathy. Certain clinical clues are helpful in distinguishing these diseases from Graves' ophthalmopathy. Lymphoma has a predilection for the trochlear area and should be suspected when palpation of the superonasal aspect of the orbit reveals nodular areas. The presence of paraorbital disease involving the lacrimal excretory system, upper eyelid, and forehead should also raise the specter of lymphoma. Bilateral involvement with lymphoma does occur. When lymphoma is suspected, a biopsy is indicated for confirmation and histologic classification.

Sarcoidosis and amyloidosis may involve the orbit and may resemble endocrine ophthalmopathy because of their protean manifestations. Sarcoid nodules and amyloid deposits can produce proptosis and may result in extraocular muscle enlargement which becomes apparent by CT scanning. Involvement of the eyelids may also occur. Sarcoidosis and amyloidosis are suspected when typical involvement of other organ systems is present. A biopsy allows definitive diagnosis.

Wegener's granulomatosis should be strongly suspected in any patient with bilateral eye disease, nasolacrimal duct obstruction, or a saddle nose deformity in the presence of systemic findings including epistaxis, hemoptysis, hematuria, or arthralgias. The diagnosis may be confirmed by a biopsy of the nasal mucosa.

CONTIGUOUS SINUS DISEASE

Orbital cellulitis resulting from contiguous sinus infection can produce signs of orbital vascular congestion and inflammation along with proptosis and painful ophthalmoplegia. This may closely mimic endocrine ophthalmopathy or orbital pseudotumor. Furthermore, in the case of ethmoidal sinusitis, computed tomography may demonstrate enlargement of the medial rectus muscle if the orbital soft tissues are inflamed secondarily. Biopsy findings may resemble those of pseudotumor. A high index of suspicion must be maintained in any patient with a history of sinusitis, as prompt diagnosis of orbital cellulitis is essential to minimize risk of visual impairment. Careful palpation of the orbit looking for bone tenderness or evidence of fistulous tracts is important. Fever, leukocytosis, or other evidence of an acute infectious process should alert the clinician to the possibility of orbital cellulitis. Treatment must be aggressive, as vision may be lost quickly with this disorder.

OTHER ORGANISM RELATED ORBITAL INFLAMMATORY PROCESSES

A wide variety of viral, bacterial, fungal, and parasitic infections can involve the orbit and may, especially early in their course, be difficult to distinguish from endocrine ophthalmopathy. The most lethal of these is mucormycosis, which most commonly occurs in diabetics with ketoacidosis or patients who are immunosuppressed from a variety of causes. Survival of the patient depends on early diagnosis and aggressive treatment. Infectious mononucleosis, syphilis, trypanosomiasis, schistosomiasis, cystocercosis, and echinococcal disease have all been associated with orbital inflammation producing lid edema, conjunctivitis, proptosis, and eye muscle dysfunction.

ORBITAL CYSTS AND NEOPLASMS

Cysts can develop in a number of orbital structures and can produce proptosis by mass effect. The degree of proptosis may vary because of fluid shifts across their boundaries. Moreover, rupture of a cyst may produce inflammatory changes, bringing cysts within the framework of the differential diagnosis of endocrine ophthalmopathy. Epidermoid and dermoid cysts are the most common. Their unilateral nature and characteristic appearance on orbital CT scans are important diagnostic features.

Neoplasms arising within the orbit or metastatic to the orbit can present with proptosis and/or signs of inflammation. Meningiomas, gliomas of the optic nerve, benign and malignant tumors of the lacrimal gland, choroidal melanomas, metastatic breast carcinomas, neuroblastomas, and rhabdomyosarcomas have each been described as presenting with eye pain, chemosis, proptosis, and eyelid erythema resembling endocrine ophthalmopathy. Careful palpation of the orbit along with computed tomography or ultrasonography usually allows orbital neoplasms to be distinguished from endocrine eye disease. When uncertainty exists and an abnormality of thyroid function or regulation cannot be demonstrated, a biopsy is indicated.

ORBITAL VASCULAR LESIONS

High-flow and low vascular shunts can involve the orbit, producing conjunctival injection, chemosis, proptosis, and ophthalmoplegia. These eye signs are frequently bilateral, and orbital CT scanning may reveal extraocular muscle enlargement. A careful history may be helpful in distinguishing vascular lesions from endocrine ophthalmopathy, as high-flow shunts, e.g., carotid-cavernous fistulas, usually follow significant orbital trauma. Orbital ultrasound and CT studies may show dilatation of the intraorbital vessels. Angiography is the most definitive diagnostic procedure.

INTRAORBITAL FOREIGN BODIES

Occult intraorbital foreign bodies can result in signs of inflammation which may be confused with endocrine ophthalmopathy. The history of trauma may be somewhat obscure and the pattern of inflammatory signs atypical; however, orbital computed tomography or conventional x-ray techniques usually allow identification of foreign bodies.

DIAGNOSTIC APPROACH TO INFLAMMATORY OPHTHALMOPATHIES

A careful and detailed history is an essential part of the evaluation of all patients with inflammatory eye disease. Information dealing with the onset and progression of symptoms is important. A relatively abrupt onset and rapid progression of symptoms are common in orbital pseudotumor, chronic orbital myositis, and various infectious diseases, whereas patients with endocrine ophthalmopathy tend to have a more gradually progressive course punctuated by exacerbations and partial remissions. A history of constitutional symptoms, including fever, malaise, and weight loss, may point to systemic disease, e.g., lymphoma, metastatic malignancy, or sarcoidosis, whereas skin and nail abnormalities, palpitations, and heat intolerance suggest hyperthyroidism associated with Graves' disease. A history of chronic or recurrent sinus infections or orbital trauma is of obvious importance. Finally, a family history of goiter, hyperthyroidism, or proptosis points in the direction of endocrine ophthalmopathy.

The physical examination should include a thorough examination of the eyes with quantitation of congestive signs, proptosis, and extraocular muscle function. The orbit and paraorbital areas should be carefully palpated looking for masses or bone tenderness. Ophthalmoscopy and biomicroscopy are essential. The thyroid should be examined, preferably by someone experienced in thyroid palpation. Any evidence of pretibial myxedema or acropachy should be noted.

The basic laboratory evaluation should include a complete blood count and an erythrocyte sedimentation rate. Because a large majority of patients with endocrine ophthalmopathy have a readily demonstrable abnormality of thyroid function, total thyroxine and triiodothyronine blood levels and a radioiodine uptake should be determined in all patients with orbital inflammatory disease. If these are normal, a more subtle abnormality of thyroid regulation should be excluded, using thyrotropin stimulation or triiodothyronine suppression testing. Serum levels of thyroid-stimulating or thyroid-binding immunoglobulins can be measured. These are present in 50 to 90% of patients with Graves' disease depending on the assay used. Antimicrosomal and antithyroglobulin antibodies are present in a smaller percentage of patients.

Orbital imaging using ultrasonography or computed tomography is occasionally necessary to establish the etiology of inflammatory eye disease. The diagnostic accuracy of ultrasonography has been reported to be in the range of 80 to 95%. The diagnostic accuracy of computed tomography is reported to be 70 to 90%. When combined their accuracy is 97%. New techniques for imaging the orbit, including the use of nuclear magnetic resonance, are currently under study.

CONCLUSIONS

The differential diagnosis of endocrine ophthalmopathy includes a variety of local and systemic diseases which involve the orbit. Graves' disease can usually be distinguished from other inflammatory eye disorders by a careful search for: (a) specific patterns of eye findings characteristic of ophthalmopathy; and (b) abnormalities of thyroid function or regulation. Careful attention should be paid to any evidence of local or systemic infection, as orbital cellulitis can result in loss of vision and mucormycosis can be lethal if not treated promptly and aggressively. Orbital cysts, neoplasms, and vascular anomalies can all produce inflammatory changes which clinically mimic endocrine ophthalmopathy. These are usually readily distinguished by their characteristic findings on ultrasound or CT scans and because of the absence of a thyroid abnormality. Orbital pseudotumor and orbital myositis may be difficult to differentiate from endocrine ophthalmopathy. A relatively abrupt onset of symptoms and response to treatment with corticosteroids in the absence of any abnormality of thyroid function or regulation points toward orbital pseudotumor or orbital myositis. They remain, however, diagnoses of exclusion. Biopsy of intraorbital tissues is sometimes necessary to exclude systemic diseases or neoplasia.

REFERENCES

1. Bullen, C. L., and Younge, B. R. (1982): Orbital myositis. *Arch. Ophthalmol.*, 100:1751.
2. Dallow, R. L. (1975): Evaluation of unilateral exophthalmos with ultrasonography, analysis of 258 consecutive cases. *Laryngoscope*, 85:1905.
3. Gorman, C. A. (1978): The presentation and management of endocrine ophthalmopathy. *Clin. Endo. Metab.*, 7:67.
4. Gorman, C. A. (1984): Extrathyroidal manifestations of Graves' disease. In: *The Thyroid*, edited by S. H. Ingbar and L. E. Braverman. Lippincott, Philadelphia (submitted for publication).
5. Henderson, J. W. (1980): *Orbital Tumors*, edited by B. C. Decker, New York.
6. Jakobiec, F. A. (1978): *Ocular and Adnexal Tumors*. Aesculapius, Birmingham.
7. Jellinek, E. H. (1969): The orbital pseudotumor syndrome and its differentiation from endocrine exophthalmos. *Brain*, 92:35.
8. Mottow-Lippa, L., Jakobiec, F. A., and Smith, M. (1981): Idiopathic inflammatory orbital pseudotumor in childhood. II. Results of diagnostic tests and biopsies. *Ophthalmology*, 88:565.
9. Waller, R. R. (1982): Eyelid malpositions in Graves' ophthalmopathy. *Trans. Am. Ophthalmol. Soc.*, 80:854–930.

The Eye and Orbit in Thyroid Disease, edited by
C. A. Gorman et al. Raven Press, New York 1984.

Orbital Decompression Techniques

Stephen G. Harner

Mayo Clinic, Rochester, Minnesota 55905

The first three sections of this book dealt with the anatomy and physiology of the eye in Graves' ophthalmopathy and the work-up of a patient with this problem. The final section explores treatment options. Whenever the pathophysiology of a disease is incompletely understood, treatment tends to be multifaceted and directed toward alleviation of symptoms rather than resolution of the disease. This is true of Graves' ophthalmopathy. The basic problem is too much tissue in a limited space. The only naturally available relief is anterior protrusion of the globe, which leads to the cosmetic and functional problems that are associated with this disease.

Graves' ophthalmopathy ranges from a very mild prominence of the eye to the severe malignant exophthalmos first described by von Basedow in 1840 (1). In addition to being variable in degree, the disease tends to have a natural history of exacerbation followed by remissions and occasionally even regression.

The ideal treatment would be to identify the process which causes massive enlargement of the extraocular muscles and periorbital fat, stop the process, and then reverse it. Unfortunately, this is not possible at this time. Systemic steroids and radiation therapy do have effects on the process (discussed in the chapters by Pinchera et al. and by McConahey, *this volume*). Surgical decompression of the orbit is usually recommended when control of thyroid disease, local ophthalmic therapy, systemic steroids, and tincture of time fail.

Early attempts at surgical control of this process included enucleation of the eye, tarsorrhaphy, and complete closure of the eyelids. At one time the cervical sympathetics were believed to control the disease, and there were reports of cervical sympathectomy being used for treatment (2). This was referred to as the Jaboulay operation after the French surgeon who popularized it. In 1920 Moore reported a case which he managed by opening the inferior fornix and removing periorbital fat (3). He did not remove any of the bony orbit.

Orbital decompression is not an ideal treatment. It does nothing to alter the basic process. In fact, the orbital contents are merely displaced rather than reduced. There is consistent alleviation of certain problems, but other problems are created, i.e., extraocular muscle imbalance.

The concept of orbital decompression is relatively simple. There is too much tissue in a limited space, and either the tissue must be removed or the space enlarged. Removal of tissue is not practical; therefore the space must be enlarged. The bony orbit can be thought of as a pyramid (see Figs. 1C, 2C, and 3C, below), in which the vertex represents the optic canal and the base the orbital rim. This leaves four walls designated as superior, inferior, medial, and lateral. The superior wall is primarily the orbital process of the frontal bone. The lesser and greater wings of the sphenoid and zygomatic bones form the lateral wall. Inferiorly is the maxilla. The medial wall is comprised of ethmoid and lacrimal bones (see

Figs. 1A,B, 2A,B, and 3A,B, below). Orbital decompression procedures involve the removal of one or more of these walls, which alleviates pressure and creates space to accommodate excess orbital tissue.

Indications for orbital decompression fall into three categories: decreasing visual acuity, impaired function of the orbital contents, and appearance of the eye. The most significant complication of Graves' ophthalmopathy is loss of vision. Decreasing visual acuity, papilledema, and increasing visual field defect are the unquestioned indications for orbital decompression. In fact, these are emergency situations. The more usual surgical indications relate to function of the eye. Inability to close the lids leads to drying of the cornea with pain, corneal ulceration, and possible perforation. The extraocular muscles become massively enlarged, are stretched to their limit, and ultimately are unable to move the globe. Keratitis, chemosis, diplopia, and lid edema are also relative indications for surgery. Early reports dealing with Graves' ophthalmopathy were not concerned with cosmetic appearance as an indication for surgery. This is an important fact to remember when evaluating results. A series that includes patients operated for cosmetic reasons should have better results and fewer complications.

There have been many reports of surgical decompression of the orbit. They are found in ophthalmologic, neurosurgical, otolaryngologic, plastic surgical, endocrine, and general medical literature. Generally, the results are good. The time period covered is approximately 100 years; most series are relatively small; indications for surgery and criteria for success varies; and information included is incomplete. The operative procedures can be placed into one of three groups: the lateral approach, the superior approach, and the inferior approach. The following discussion deals with these three groups, the people who have popularized them, the general concepts of the procedures, their modifications, their advantages and disadvantages, and general comments regarding the results.

LATERAL APPROACH

The lateral approach was used in the first reported orbital decompression. Dollinger in 1910 operated on a patient, removing the lateral orbital wall but leaving the lateral orbital rim intact. This was reported in the German literature in 1911 with photographs of the patient and several drawings outlining the procedure (4). It is the same surgical approach which Krönlein had described in 1888 to remove tumors in the infratemporal fossa and retro-orbital area (5). Review shows that Krönlein did remove a segment of the lateral orbital rim as part of this procedure. Except for Dollinger and Guyton (6), authors who use the lateral approach remove a segment of the orbital rim. It is therefore appropriate to designate this as the Krönlein procedure even though it was not initially described for Graves' ophthalmopathy.

The lateral approach has been used primarily by ophthalmologists. Very little literature is available on this method, apparently reflecting the infrequent performance of the procedure and the fact that other surgical specialists have done most of the decompressions using different techniques. There is one series by Swift (7), and Berke published another in 1954 (8). He was presenting the lateral orbitotomy technique, and most of the patients presented had orbital tumors rather than Graves' ophthalmopathy. The photography in his article is excellent. Knauer (9) and Kroll and Casten (10) each published a small series of patients. In 1966 Long et al. reviewed 67 cases they had collected over 16 years (11). The most recent experience is by Kennerdell and Maroon (12,13), who used the lateral approach to gain access to all four orbital walls.

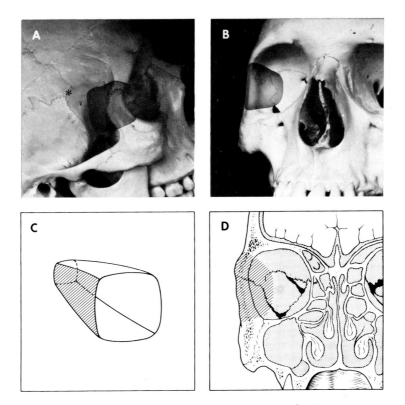

FIG. 1. Lateral approach in orbital decompression. **A:** Straight lateral view of the right bony orbit. The area of resection is shaded. This includes the orbital rim, portion of the zygomatic bone, and greater wing of the sphenoid; (*) pterion. **B:** View of the lateral wall of the orbit from anterior and medially. The area of bone resection is shaded. **C:** Outline of the right bony orbit. The area of bone removal is shown by hatch marks. **D:** Vertical section through the facial bones. The areas of bone removal for the lateral approach are indicated by hatch marks.

The lateral approach requires a skin incision somewhere in the region of the lateral canthus or over the zygomatic arch. The lateral rim of the orbit is exposed (Fig. 1), and usually a significant portion of the temporalis muscle is removed. The lateral rim and wall of the orbit are removed from anterior to posterior, which is shown very nicely in the article by Long and Ellis (11). Finally, the periorbita is incised to allow further expansion of the orbital contents. The work of Kennerdell and Maroon (12,13) shows how the bony walls can be removed superiorly across the midline nearly to the ethmoid complex. The inferior wall and approximately one-half of the medial wall can also be removed by this approach. With a lateral orbitotomy the degree of recession is difficult to assess because of loss of the lateral orbital rim. Baylis et al. reported 2 to 3 mm as the usual amount (14). Generally the recession is considered to be less than that achieved with the inferior approach and roughly even with that of the superior approach. The four-wall dissection of Kennerdell is reported to yield 10 to 17 mm of recession (12,13).

It seems that preservation or improvement in vision, relief of lid edema, protection of the cornea, etc., are quite satisfactory with the lateral approach. Although results are satisfactory, there are some negative aspects to this approach. Generally, only one side is operated at a time; therefore bilateral disease requires two operations. In order to expose the lateral orbital rim, some type of external incision is necessary. This, combined with the removal of a segment of the lateral orbital rim and temporalis muscle, creates a noticeable change in facial appearance. The space available with the lateral approach is limited. Removal of the temporalis muscle helps, but there are no air cells or sinuses in the lateral bone. This lack of space can be partially alleviated by extending the decompression superiorly and/or inferiorly. There is also increased bleeding. Still other problems include paralysis of the frontalis muscle and weakness of the lateral rectus muscle. The frontalis muscle is paralyzed when the frontal branch of the facial nerve is transected in the skin incision. The lateral rectus muscle may become involved in fibrosis following incision of the periorbita. It seems as though the lateral approach is used only occasionally, primarily for cases of proptosis of 30 mm or greater as described by Kennerdell and Maroon (12,13).

SUPERIOR APPROACH

The second broad classification of procedures is the superior approach. This group includes those procedures in which removal of the superior orbital wall is a major goal. The first example was the frontal craniotomy approach described and popularized by Naffziger (15). The second was the pterion approach described by Welti and Offret (16) and used by a number of other surgeons (17–20).

Naffziger was a neurosurgeon who in 1931 first described decompressing an orbit into the anterior cranial fossa (15). At that time it was recognized that severe, progressive Graves' ophthalmopathy (malignant exophthalmos) could progress to blindness, meningitis, and ultimately death. When one appreciates the natural history of the disease and the limited treatment options, a frontal craniotomy does not seem unreasonable. Initially, Naffziger described removing only the superior roof on one side (15). Later he recognized that the lateral orbital wall should also be removed and that both sides could be done as one procedure (12). There are three transfrontal series published with reasonably large numbers of patients. Naffziger reviewed his overall experience in 1954 (21). He had a total of 40 patients he had collected over a 20-year span. Poppen, a neurosurgeon in Boston, used the same procedure and presented 66 patients from his experience in 1950 (22). The most recent series, in 1970, was by MacCarty et al., in which the Mayo Clinic neurosurgeon and his colleagues presented 46 patients (23).

The procedure begins with a scalp incision (Soultan) (15). Three burr holes are placed and a bone flap lifted. The frontal lobes are gently lifted, and the floor of the anterior cranial fossa is exposed. The bone is then removed from the roof of the orbit (Fig. 2). Medially, this extends to the ethmoid air cells. Laterally the dissection is carried downward and includes the entire lateral wall of the orbit; the lateral orbital rim is left intact. In the early years Naffziger unroofed the optic canal, but later this was not considered necessary. The periorbita is incised, and the bone flap is returned to its usual position and wired in place. The burr holes are filled and the scalp incision closed. It is important to recognize that this procedure is intracranial but extradural. There are drawings in the articles by these neurosurgeons which are excellent (21,23,24).

The results of this approach are good. Vision is stabilized or improved, ocular motility is improved, and the appearance is satisfactory in most cases. The degree of recession varies, but the average (from series in the literature) seems to be around 3 mm. There are a number of comments in the literature about the morbidity and possible mortality of this procedure, but there were no deaths in the reports by Naffziger, Poppen, and MacCarty et al. When one considers the type of patients and circumstances at the time of these operative

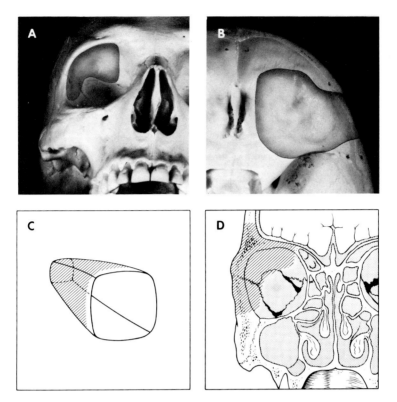

FIG. 2. Superior approach in orbital decompression. **A:** Superior wall of the right orbit as viewed from anterior and inferiorly. The area of resection of the superior and lateral walls is shaded. The bones involved are the frontal, the greater wing of the sphenoid, and the zygomatic ones. Note that the orbital rim is intact. **B:** Right superior orbital wall as seen superiorly, i.e., from the anterior cranial fossa. The cribriform plate is on the left. The anterior cranial wall is at the top of the photograph. The area of resection extends from the ethmoid medially and includes the frontal bone and greater wing of the sphenoid, extending laterally to the cranial wall. **C:** The right orbit. The area of bone removal of the superior approach (transcranial or pterional) is hatched. Note that the orbital rim remains intact. **D:** Vertical section through the facial bones. The areas of bone removal for the superior approach are indicated by hatch marks.

procedures, this is a remarkable statistic. Frontal lobe injury, intracranial hemorrhage, cerebrospinal fluid rhinorrhea, and meningitis, are potential problems but in fact are very uncommon. The limited space available for a decompression is a much more significant criticism of this procedure. The external incision and deformity secondary to the bone flap can also be distressing. Another criticism has been pulsation of the globe. There is no question that pulsation of the cerebrospinal fluid is transmitted to the globe, and the globe is observed to move. However, this did not seem to be a problem from the patient's point of view (23).

The pterion approach to orbital decompression has the same goals as the transcranial, i.e., removal of the superior and lateral orbital walls. The reports using this approach have come from neurosurgeons and plastic surgeons. During World War II Welti and Offret described this approach in the French surgical literature (16), and Hamby (18) and Backlund (19) have each reported on a small series of patients. Moran, a plastic surgeon, summarized his experience in 1972 with over 100 patients (20).

The pterion is the point where the sphenoid, frontal, and parietal bones and the squamous portion of the temporal bone meet in the infratemporal fossa (Figs. 1A and 3A). The pterion can be exposed through an incision anterior to the ear in a hair-bearing area. The fibers of the temporalis muscle are split, and some of the muscle may be removed. An opening is made into the anterior and medial cranial fossa, and the superior and lateral walls of the orbit are removed. As in the transfrontal procedure, the lateral rim of the orbit is preserved. Medial dissection of the superior wall is somewhat difficult, but the lateral portion of the inferior wall can be removed rather easily. The scar created by the procedure is inconspicuous and the bony defect well covered by temporalis muscle. The basic results and potential complications are otherwise the same as with the transfrontal procedure. It is possible to do this as a bilateral procedure, but generally the two sides are operated on at different sessions.

INFERIOR APPROACH

Currently the inferior approach is the most widely used and accepted decompressive technique. This procedure can be done either transantrally or transorbitally. The greatest number of decompressions have been done by otolaryngologists using a transantral approach. There are now a number of reports in which ophthalmologists remove the same bone using an orbital approach. Hirsch and Urbanek presented a case in the German literature in 1930 (25) in which they removed the roof of the maxillary antrum on one side to alleviate severe exophthalmos. There was 3 mm of recession, and it was considered a successful procedure. In 1936 Sewall described orbital decompression through an external ethmoidectomy (26). He commented that this was based on laboratory dissection, and apparently he never performed a decompression. It seems that Kistner was the first to perform an actual decompression using the method which Sewall described (27). There were two cases, and the results reported were satisfactory. Schall and Reagen (28) and Boyden (29) also used an ethmoidectomy approach.

Hirsch carefully reviewed the available decompressive procedures and suggested the transantral approach (30). It remained, however, for Walsh and Ogura to publish the first series of transantral decompressions in which the inferior and medial walls of the orbit were removed (31). The inferior approach has tremendous appeal because it provides the greatest space for the orbital contents (Fig. 3). There were a series of articles by Ogura et al. (31–35) outlining the Washington University experience from the years 1946 through 1980 which encompassed 252 patients. Other series using the transantral approach include: Stell, six cases (36); Golding-Wood, 10 cases (37); Sessions et al., nine patients (38); Calcaterra and Thompson, 104 patients (39); Baylis et al., 24 patients (14); and DeSanto, 200 patients (40). The concept of the transantral orbital decompression is to remove the bony wall between the orbit and the ethmoid and maxillary sinuses. The technique is thoroughly described in DeSanto (this volume). The ability to preserve or restore vision, improve ocular motility, and enhance appearance are excellent. Potential complications include blindness, cerebrospinal fluid leakage, orbital cellulitis, sinusitis, nasolacrimal duct obstruction, and persistent numbness of the face. The advantages are no external incision, no facial deformity, and minimal morbidity. The most consistent criticism of the transantral approach has been a relatively high incidence of extraocular muscle imbalance, ptosis of the globe, the need for secondary eye muscle surgery, and persistent diplopia.

In 1972 Schimek presented his experience with removal of the inferior orbital floor transorbitally (41). Leone and Banjandas used an orbital approach to remove the inferior

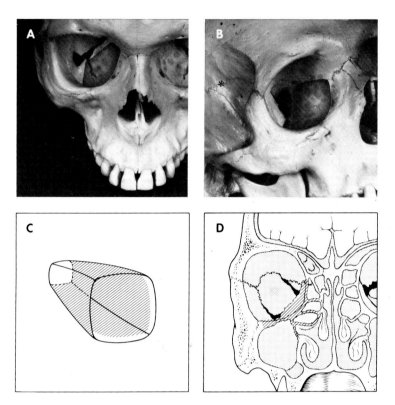

FIG. 3. Inferior approach in orbital decompression. **A:** The inferior wall of the orbit as seen from anterior and superiorly. The area of bone removed for the inferior approach is shaded. The bone involved is primarily the maxilla. The inferior orbital fissure is visible, as is the canal for the inferior orbital nerve. The resection should include bone lateral to the inferior orbital nerve. **B:** The medial wall of the right bony orbit as viewed from anterior and laterally. The area of resection for the inferior approach is shaded. The bone removed is primarily ethmoid and some lacrimal bone. (*) pterion. **C:** The right orbit. The area of bone removal for the inferior approach (transantral or transorbital) is hatched. The orbital rim remains intact. **D:** Vertical section through the facial bones. The area of bone removal for the inferior approach is indicated by hatch marks.

and a portion of the medial orbital walls (42,43), but this approach has been criticized because it utilized a transcutaneous lid incision with scarring and some degree of deformity (44). In 1979 McCord and Moses presented a technique of exposure through the inferior fornix combined with a lateral canthotomy (44). They published their results with 34 patients in 1981 (45), and the procedure is well demonstrated in that report. The incision is inconspicuous except for the lateral extension. They showed that the medial, inferior, and lateral walls can be approached. As with all of the various approaches, the results seem quite good. The authors believe that this approach avoids injury to the inferior rectus muscle and, as a result, there are fewer problems with diplopia. The average recession achieved approached 6 mm, which is slightly higher than most reports of the transantral procedure. The complications, morbidity, and mortality of this procedure should be the same as with the transantral procedure.

COMMENT

Preparation for this review of surgical decompression of the orbit has led to certain general observations. This study covers nearly 100 years and involves many specialties. It becomes apparent that line for line comparison of indications, operative techniques, and results is not possible. Comments by some authors on results of previous publications are frequently self-serving and taken out of context. Many patients develop Graves' ophthalmopathy, but very few go on to the malignant exophthalmos of von Basedow. Until 1970 nearly every patient who was surgically decompressed had malignant exophthalmos. By definition they had failing vision, corneal ulcers, ophthalmoplegia, and grotesque-appearing eyes. Multiple treatment options had been utilized and failed. The goal in these patients was the prevention of blindness or possible death. Over the past 10 to 15 years the success of orbital decompressions has led to significant changes in indications for surgery. This means greater numbers of patients with milder degrees of disease, better results, and few complications.

The lateral and superior approaches can achieve reasonable results in the preservation of vision, prevention of corneal ulcers, etc. However, in the milder cases seen today, the cosmetic defects of these procedures are unacceptable. The transantral inferior approach achieves excellent results with preservation of vision, prevention of corneal ulcers, etc. It has the logical appeal of greater space for orbital contents, no cosmetic defects, short hospitalization, and acceptable morbidity and mortality. Even the incidence of diplopia has decreased as milder cases are treated surgically. For these reasons it seems that the transantral inferior approach is the best of the surgical options.

It is obvious that consistently successful surgical decompression requires the removal of two walls or the orbit. Single wall removal has helped, but results always improved when a second wall was removed. It now seems that three or more walls can be removed when indicated. The number of patients who need surgical decompression is relatively small. The surgical techniques involved are difficult. If decompression is indicated it still represents only one stage in the overall rehabilitation of a patient with Graves' ophthalmopathy. Control of thyroid function, correction of extraocular muscle imbalance, and relief of residual lid retraction requires the coordinated effort of several medical and surgical disciplines. Until we understand the pathophysiology of Graves' disease and can control the disease process itself, we are limited to treatments which at least have the merit of effectively relieving symptoms, protecting vision, and restoring appearance.

REFERENCES

1. Von Basedow, C. (1840): Exophthalmos durch Hypertrophie des Zellgewebes in der Augenhöhle. *Wehnscher. Ges. Heilk.*, 6:197–204, 220–228.
2. Mayo, C. H. (1914): The surgical treatment of exophthalmos. *JAMA*, 63:1147–1149.
3. Moore, R. F. (1920): Exophthalmos and limitation of the eye movements of Graves' disease. *Lancet*, 2:701.
4. Dollinger, J. (1911): Die Druckentlastung der Augenhöhle durch Entfernung der äussen Orbitalwand bei Lochgradigern Exophthalmos (morbus Basedowii) und konsekutiver Hornhauterkrankeun. *Dtsch. Med. Wochenschr.*, 37:1888–1890.
5. Krönlein, R. U. (1888): Zur Pathologie und operativen Behandlung der Dermoidcysten der Orbita. *Beitr. Klin. Chir.*, 4:149–163.
6. Guyton, J. S. (1946): Decompression of the orbit. *Surgery*, 19:790–809.
7. Swift, G. W. (1935): Malignant exophthalmos and operative approach. *West. J. Surg. Obstet. Gynecol.*, 43:119–126.
8. Berke, R. N. (1954): A modified Krönlein operation. *Arch. Ophthalmol.*, 51:609–632.
9. Knauer, W. J. (1957): The surgical treatment of exophthalmic ophthalmoplegia. *Am. J. Ophthalmol.*, 43:58–66.
10. Kroll, A. J., and Casten, V. G. (1966): Dysthyroid exophthalmos palliation by lateral orbital decompression. *Arch. Ophthalmol.*, 76:205–210.
11. Long, J. C., and Ellis, G. D. (1966): Temporal decompression of the orbit for thyroid exophthalmos. *Am. J. Ophthalmol.*, 62:1089–1098.
12. Kennerdell, J. S., and Maroon, J. C. (1982): An orbital decompression for severe dysthyroid exophthalmos. *Ophthalmology*, 89:467–472.

13. Maroon, J. C., and Kennerdell, J. S. (1980): Radical orbital decompression for severe dysthyroid exophthalmos. *J. Neurosurg.*, 56:260–266.
14. Baylis, H. I., Call, N. B., and Shibata, C. S. (1980): The transantral orbital decompression (Ogura technique) as performed by the ophthalmologist. *Ophthalmology*, 87:1005–1012.
15. Naffziger, H. C. (1931): Progressive exophthalmos following thyroidectomy; its pathology and treatment. *Ann. Surg.*, 94:582–586.
16. Welti, H., and Offret, G. (1943): Indications et technique de la trépanation décompressive de l' orbite dans le traitement des exophtalmies malignes basedowiennes. *Lyon Chir.*, 38:542–554.
17. Rowbotham, G. F., and Clarke, P. R. R. (1956): Progressive exophthalmos treated by orbital decompression. *Lancet*, 1:403–405.
18. Hamby, W. B. (1964): Pterional approach to the orbits for decompression or tumor removal. *J. Neurosurg.*, 21:15–18.
19. Backlund, E-O. (1968): Pterional approach for orbital decompression. *Acta Ophthalmol. (Copenh.)*, 46:535–540.
20. Moran, R. E., Letterman, G. S., and Schuster, M. A. (1972): The surgical correction of exophthalmos: history, technique and long term follow-up. *Plast. Reconstr. Surg.*, 49:595–608.
21. Naffziger, H. C. (1954): Progressive exophthalmos. *Ann. R. Coll. Surg. Engl.*, 15:1–24.
22. Poppen, J. L. (1950): The surgical treatment of progressive exophthalmos. *J. Clin. Endocrinol.*, 10:1231–1236.
23. MacCarty, C. S., Kenefick, T. P., McConahey, W. M., and Kearns, T. P. (1970): Ophthalmopathy of Graves' disease treated by removal of roof, lateral walls and lateral sphenoid ridge: review of 46 cases. *Mayo Clin. Proc.*, 45:488–493.
24. Poppen, J. L. (1944): Exophthalmos, diagnosis and surgical treatment of intractable cases. *Am. J. Surg.*, 64:64–79.
25. Hirsch, V. O., and Urbanek, J. (1930): Behandlung eines exzessiven Exophthalmus (Basedow) durch Entfernung von Orbitalfelt von der Kieferhöhle aus. *Monatsschr. Ohrenheilkd. Laryngorhinol.*, 64:212–213.
26. Sewall, E. C. (1936): Operative control of progressive exophthalmos. *Arch. Otolaryngol.*, 24:621–624.
27. Kistner, F. B. (1939): Decompression for exophthalmos. *JAMA*, 112:37–38.
28. Schall, L. A., and Reagan, D. J. (1945): Malignant exophthalmos. *Ann. Otol. Rhinol. Laryngol.*, 54:37–42.
29. Boyden, G. L. (1956): An otolaryngologic approach to malignant exophthalmos. *Laryngoscope*, 66:623–627.
30. Hirsch, O. (1950): Surgical decompression of malignant exophthalmos. *Arch. Otolaryngol.*, 51:325–334.
31. Walsh, T. E., and Ogura, J. H. (1957): Transantral orbital decompression for malignant exophthalmos. *Laryngoscope*, 67:544–568.
32. Ogura, J. H. (1968): Transantral orbital decompression for progressive exophthalmos: a follow-up of 54 cases. *Med. Clin. North Am.*, 52:399–407.
33. Ogura, J. H. (1971): Surgical approach to the ophthalmopathy of Graves' disease. *JAMA*, 216:1627–1631.
34. Ogura, J. H., and Lucente, F. E. (1974): Surgical results of orbital decompression for malignant exophthalmos. *Laryngoscope*, 84:637–644.
35. Ogura, J. H., and Thawley, S. E. (1980): Orbital decompression for exophthalmos. *Otolaryngol. Clin. North Am.*, 13:29–38.
36. Stell, P. M. (1968): Transantral orbital decompression in malignant exophthalmos. *J. Laryngol. Otol.*, 82:613–621.
37. Golding-Wood, P. H. (1969): Trans-antral ethmoid decompression in malignant exophthalmos. *J. Laryngol. Otol.*, 83:683–694.
38. Sessions, R. B., Wilkins, R. B., and Weycer, J. S. (1972): Endocrine exophthalmos. *Arch. Otolaryngol.*, 95:46–52.
39. Calcaterra, T. C., and Thompson, J. W. (1980): Antral-ethmoidal decompression of the orbit in Graves' disease: ten-year experience. *Laryngoscope*, 90:1941–1949.
40. DeSanto, L. W. (1980): The total rehabilitation of Graves' ophthalmopathy. *Laryngoscope*, 90:1652–1678.
41. Schimek, R. A. (1972): Surgical management of ocular complications of Graves' disease. *Arch. Ophthalmol.*, 87:655–664.
42. Leone, C. R., and Bajandas, F. J. (1980): Inferior orbital decompression for thyroid ophthalmopathy. *Arch. Ophthalmol.*, 98:890–892.
43. Leone, C. R., and Bajandas, F. J. (1981): Inferior orbital decompression for dysthyroid optic neuropathy. *Ophthalmology*, 88:525–532.
44. McCord, C. D., and Moses, J. L. (1979): Exposure of the inferior orbit with fornix incision and lateral canthotomy. *Ophthalmic Surg.*, 10:53–63.
45. McCord, C. D. (1981): Orbital decompression for Graves' disease: exposure through lateral canthral and inferior fornix incision. *Ophthalmology*, 88:533–541.

The Eye and Orbit in Thyroid Disease, edited by
C. A. Gorman et al. Raven Press, New York 1984.

Transantral Orbital Decompression

Lawrence W. DeSanto

Mayo Clinic, Rochester, Minnesota 55905

Until the cause of the eye changes in Graves' disease is found and prevention becomes possible, some patients will require treatment for their eyes. There are many approaches to treatment, as noted by Harner and by McConahey in other chapters in this book. Because the disease is so variable, treatment that is useful for one patient may be excessive or ineffective for the next. Hence there is no standardized therapy that is universally useful or effective. Some patients require no treatment, whereas others have not been helped by any.

The concept of enlarging the orbital space for orbital decompression has been proposed, performed, criticized, and even condemned. For a detailed account of various types of surgery available, see chapter by Harner, *this volume*. The principle of enlarging the space for some patients is usually acceptable. Controversy remains, however, because of the several approaches for enlarging the orbital space and because of differing opinions in regard to selecting patients for whom this seemingly radical therapy should be offered.

No uniform opinion exists concerning: (a) whether the orbital space should be enlarged; (b) the indications for enlarging the space; (c) the sequence of therapy that is most successful in restoring the eyes to near-normal; (d) the value of mechanical enlargement of the orbital space; and (e) the nonsurgical alternatives that are useful in the seriously affected patient.

In October 1969 I was asked if I could remove the bone from the floor and the medial wall of the orbit through the sinuses in patients with severe ophthalmopathy of Graves' disease. This was part of a study to compare the contemporary forms of orbital decompression in the most severely afflicted patients: those with visual field defects and visual loss. Since that time this personal experience has involved the use of transantral orbital decompression in about 450 patients, or 900 eyes. From this experience some opinions have been formed and some data have been accumulated to substantiate those opinions.

OBSERVATIONS IN THE FIRST 200 PATIENTS

The first 200 patients were sequentially studied. Of these, 199 had surgery on both eyes at the same anesthetic session, and one patient had a unilateral decompression. Hence this experience cites 200 patients and 399 eyes.

Of the 200 patients, 142 were female and 58 (29%) were male. The youngest patient was a 16-year-old girl and the oldest a 72-year-old woman. The mean age was 49.7 years. In both sexes the decade from 50 to 60 was the most frequent age for decompression.

Forty-five (78%) of the 58 males and 123 of the 142 females (87%) had clinical or chemical hyperthyroidism or were treated for it at some time before decompression. Thirteen males and 19 females never experienced a hyperthyroid state.

The time interval from the treatment of hyperthyroidism to orbital decompression in patients who were hyperthyroid varied (Table 1). The interval from hyperthyroidism to

TABLE 1. *Interval from diagnosis of hyperthyroidism to decompression in 200 patients*

Interval (years)	Males		Females	
	No.	%	No.	%
<1	8	17	26	21
1–2	15	34	28	23
2–3	8	17	18	15
3–4	4	9	9	7
4–5	2	5	16	13
>5	8	17	26	21

TABLE 2. *Treatment for hyperthyroidism in a series of 200 transantrally decompressed patients*

Treatment	Males		Females	
	No.	%	No.	%
Thyroidectomy	7	16	12	10
^{131}I	26	58	74	60
Antithyroid drugs	9	20	36	29
Iodides	2	4	1	1
Propranolol	1	2	0	0
Total:	45	100	123	100

orbital decompression in patients who were hyperthyroid ranged from 7 months to 30 years in the females and 2 months to 30 years in the males. The mean interval in both sexes was 28 months.

Treatment of Hyperthyroidism

No single method was used in the treatment of hyperthyroidism (Table 2). Only 19 of the 200 patients had thyroidectomy, and each had some residual thyroid gland present. No patient who had a proved total thyroidectomy was seen for decompression.

A frequently encountered sequence was the diagnosis and treatment of clinical hyperthyroidism followed by slowly progressive ophthalmopathy. Multiple and commonly ineffective treatments for the ophthalmopathy were tried until orbital decompression was finally recommended.

The exceptions to this common sequence were found in the 32 patients who were never diagnosed to be hyperthyroid and in the occasional patient whose hyperthyroidism spontaneously remitted to a euthyroid state without antithyroid therapy. At the time of decompression, only seven of the 200 patients had persisting hyperthyroidism preoperatively. Each of these were treated as an emergency because their eyes were so threatened that time would not allow treatment of their hyperthyroidism.

Other Treatment Before Orbital Decompression

Oral corticosteroids were taken by 103 patients (41 males and 62 females) before orbital decompression. Duration of therapy and drug dosage varied considerably. Prednisone equiv-

TABLE 3. *Prior therapy in 44 patients with ophthalmopathy*

Procedure	Males	Females
Tarsorrhaphy	1	2
Orbital irradiation	2	7
Lateral decompression	0	3
Neurosurgical decompression	2	7
Extraocular muscle surgery	6	14
Total:	11	33

alent dosage of 40 to 120 mg/day was usual. The mean interval of this drug therapy was 3 months, but it ranged from less than 1 month to as long as 25 months.

Of the 103 patients, 26 improved on steroids, as estimated by the patient and the endocrinologist. A meaningful response was recorded if congestive symptoms regressed and pain was reduced or eliminated. A positive effect was also recorded if vision improved in a measurable way or proptosis recessed by more than 3 mm. With these broad and mixed criteria, a positive therapeutic effect was noted in one of four patients treated with corticosteroids. The 26 patients who improved while receiving corticosteroids were nevertheless advised to have orbital decompression because of steroid side effects (facial swelling, emotional changes, diabetes, and osteoporosis) or the clinical judgment that the dosage required to maintain remission of eye symptoms could not be safely sustained. Some of the patients requested that steroid therapy be discontinued.

The criteria we employed to assess the effectiveness of steroid therapy are stringent. Our results should not be considered representative of steroid effectiveness in the larger population of patients with Graves' ophthalmopathy. The 200 patients were studied only because they underwent orbital decompression, and the number of others who were not seen because steroids were helpful is not known. Nevertheless, steroid intolerance or failure was a major secondary indication for orbital decompression.

Table 3 cites the other forms of therapy used in patients along with, before, or after corticosteroids. Each of the 44 patients had received corticosteroids, as well as undergoing surgical procedures or irradiation before orbital decompression.

Indications for Orbital Decompression

Data concerning indications for decompression were derived from the first 7 years of using orbital decompression. In the beginning only patients with vision-threatening problems were considered for the operation and then only after all other therapeutic efforts had failed. We used the traditional indications, which excluded patients in whom vision was not in danger. Over the years the indications for surgery have expanded as the value of orbital decompression was appreciated, the risks better understood, and the concept better accepted. Currently, a larger proportion of our patients have orbital decompression for reasons other than threatened loss of vision than was true for the first 200 patients, whose indications for surgery are shown in Fig. 1.

Bilaterality

Ophthalmopathy of Graves' disease may not affect both eyes equally or in the same way at the same time. The orbital process may seem unilateral yet be bilateral but asymmetrical.

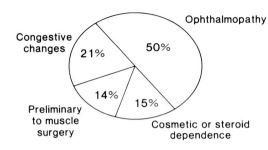

FIG. 1. Indications for orbital decompression in 200 patients.

In this situation, the lesser affected eye can seem to be normal. It is, however, not usually normal, or if it is it is unlikely to stay that way if its mate is so involved as to be a candidate for orbital decompression. Because of this fact, it makes little practical sense to operate on only the most involved eye in asymmetrical ophthalmopathy. In this series, with one exception, both eyes were decompressed, even if only one orbit was obviously diseased. Thus unilateral indications led to bilateral operations. Fourteen years later there is no reason to alter this approach.

Orbital decompression was not offered to explore the orbit when the diagnosis was in doubt in unilateral situations. Even with this attitude several patients with a bilateral process were operated on who did not, on orbital examination, have Graves' disease. (See conditions that mimic Graves' disease in Hay, *this volume*.)

The availability of high-resolution computed tomography (CT) scanning in questionable situations has greatly reduced the possibility of diagnostic error.

The vision-threatening indications for orbital decompression are well recognized. Visual loss with a field defect characteristic of Graves' disease, chronic papilledema, choroidal folding, and corneal ulcerations that resist simple treatment are some of these. It is of interest that there were so few patients who have corneal ulcers as the sole indication for surgery in this group. The few patients who had a corneal ulcer also had some other more pressing indication for surgery. The nonvision-threatening indications are: (a) a preliminary operation to expedite muscle surgery for diplopia: (b) the congestive changes of ophthalmopathy of Graves' disease with painful eyes, photophobia, tearing without visual loss; (c) the need to stop corticosteroids because of a steroid-related complication after steroids have or have not stabilized the orbital process; and (d) cosmetic adjustment. A young woman, for example, who requires 80 to 120 mg of prednisone each day for many months to maintain vision has very little difficulty deciding on a more direct treatment with surgery. In this case the treatment with steroids can be as distressing as the orbital disorder. To the ocular muscle surgeon, a 4- to 6-mm (or more) relief of proptosis might make a difference in the ease of extraocular muscle surgery and the final appearance of the eyes.

RESULTS

Vision

Eighty-seven patients (143 eyes) had decompression that was performed for vision-threatening problems. In each, the vision was jeopardized either by optic neuropathy and its associated visual field defect or by serious corneal ulceration that did not respond to conservative treatment. There were far more patients with optic neuropathy than ulcers. A few patients had chronic papilledema. Follow-up visual acuity measurements and field plots

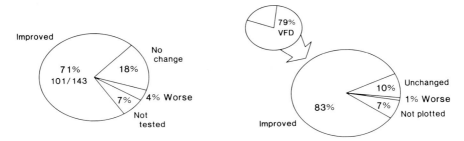

FIG. 2. Results of transantral orbital decompression in 143 eyes with preoperatively impaired visual acuity and in 113 eyes with preoperative visual field defects.

were obtained in 84 of the 87 patients. The follow-up interval ranged from 6 months to 3 years, with a mean follow-up of 9 months. Of the 84 patients available for study, 79 had improved visual acuity and the field defect was eliminated in both eyes. One of these patients had a deep corneal ulcer that healed, with an opaque scar being left. One patient in the group with chronic papilledema and finger-counting vision in both eyes experienced improvement in vision in one eye. Three patients with dense field defects had no improvement (Fig. 2).

Four of the five patients who were considered decompression failures had some initial improvement of their visual acuity and lessening of the density of their field defect, but later had regression of their vision and a return of a denser field defect. Corticosteroid therapy was resumed for three patients, and although the visual loss stabilized they were considered surgical failures. All patients but the five cited had improvement of their vision at some time between the operation and the first follow-up.

There is usually some improvement noted during the first week, but in those patients with measurable field defects improvement can continue slowly for months. Of the 79 patients who had improvement of vision, 20 had objective improvement between the first and second follow-up visit (3 to 12 months). Six patients had continued objective improvement up to 1 year.

The fact that usually improvement rapidly followed orbital decompression is not of itself proof that decompression caused the improvement. It is well known that untreated ophthalmopathy of Graves' disease often stabilizes and improves spontaneously. Nevertheless, the dramatic return of vision was impressive in 79 of the 87 patients with serious loss of vision and dense field defects in whom prior treatment with steroids, radiation, or other forms of decompression failed.

Patients usually comment on perceptible vision improvement within 3 days of surgery, but this seldom exceeds one or two lines on the eye charts. Then at the first follow-up visit (about 3 months), there is clearing of the field defect by measurement. After that, vision stabilizes or improves slightly. Patients with dense field defects that were present for many months and those with longstanding papilledema or disc pallor may not improve, or if they do they tend to do so at a slower rate.

All patients who were receiving corticosteroids before decompression also received steroids before surgery and in tapering doses after the operation. The steroid bolus before surgery may also have had a role in visual improvement.

Ocular Protrusion

The changes in ocular protrusion as measured by Krahn or Hertel exophthalmometers were determined by subtracting the last measurement from the immediate preoperative

TABLE 4. *Changes in ocular protrusion after orbital decompression in 334 eyes*

Change (mm)	No.	Change (mm)	No.
<1	3	6	55
1	11	7	31
2	32	8	30
3	31	9	21
4	45	10	22
5	52	13	1

TABLE 5. *Effect of orbital decompression on extraocular muscle function*

Muscle motion	Before decompression		After decompression	
	No.	%	No.	%
Females				
Normal	26	18	10	7
Myopathy, no diplopia	45	32	21	15
Myopathy, diplopia	71	50	111	78
Total:	142		142	
Males				
Normal	5	8	2	3
Myopathy, no diplopia	18	32	9	16
Myopathy, diplopia	35	60	47	81
Total:	58		58	

measurement. At least two measurements were available in 334 eyes. A mean recession of 5.5 mm was observed (Table 4). The range of change was 0 to 13 mm. A test retest error of 2 mm is usually cited as the limits of exophthalmometer accuracy.

There were 28 patients who had an increase in protrusion in one eye between the first and second follow-up visits, the increase being 1 to 4 mm. In other words, eyes that recede sometimes do not stay back. Slight recession was noted in 273 other eyes in which measurements were taken at a second follow-up, but the recession was seldom more than the range of error of the measuring instrument.

As a rule, most of the changes of eye position occurred during the first month after decompression. The exophthalmometer reading at 4 to 6 months was usually maintained.

Extraocular Muscle Function

The effect of the ophthalmopathy of Graves' disease on extraocular muscles varies. Orbital decompression does nothing to improve the muscles directly but may have an indirect beneficial effect by decreasing the pressure and tension on the muscles and enhancing the blood supply within the orbit. On the other hand, recession of the eye leaves lax muscles. Some of these muscles have been damaged by the orbital process and have only slight potential for spontaneous recovery of contractility. The change in eye position after decompression also influences extraocular muscle function but in an unpredictable way. Table 5 demonstrates the best estimate of muscle status before and after decompression in 200 patients.

Some patients had normal muscles and no diplopia, but these were a minority (18% of the females and 8% of the males). Others had clinical evidence of muscle disease but no diplopia. The majority in both sexes had both myopathy and diplopia before decompression. Decompression did not improve muscle function as a rule. Rather, muscle function and diplopia were more apparent after the operation in the majority. Preoperatively, 92 male and 82 female patients had clinical evidence of myopathy, and diplopia was present in 60 males and 50 females. Following decompression 81 males and 78 females had some diplopia.

Even if normal extraocular muscle function exists before decompression (an infrequent event, seen in 31 of the 200 patients), muscle dysfunction is still possible after surgery (Table 5). When myopathy exists before decompression, it will exist after. Some of the diplopia that was manifest after orbital decompression occurred in patients with severe Graves' ophthalmopathy. Before decompression they were unable to see well enough in one or both eyes to have diplopia. Diplopia was experienced after decompression with return of vision. In this situation diplopia is a positive event compared to blindness. Nearly 70% of our total group of patients required extraocular muscle surgery as discussed in Chapter 19. Some of these patients had been advised to have decompression as a planned preliminary to muscle surgery.

Eyelids

The elevator and depressor muscles of the upper and lower eyelids have the same myopathic changes as the oculorotatory muscles in Graves' ophthalmopathy. These inflammatory changes ultimately result in upper lid retraction. Orbital decompression with axial recession and inferior displacement of the globe can depress the lower lid. Either lid retraction or lower lid depression allows scleral baring and the appearance of a stare. Lid retraction is more likely than the other ophthalmic expressions of Graves' disease to improve with time. Nevertheless, lid surgery is helpful in the ultimate rehabilitation of some of these patients. Lid surgery, both upper and lower, was done in 50 of the 200 patients in the series (see Waller, *this volume*).

Complications

It is difficult to establish consistent criteria for evaluating complications of an operation such as orbital decompression because of the different indications and goals of the operation. For example, a sensory disturbance of the upper lip from a sublabial incision might be considered a complication if the operation was done for cosmetic improvement. The same residual in a patient who has a severe visual loss, painful proptosis, congested orbits, and a field defect or chronic papilledema may be looked on differently. Likewise, diplopia that evolves in a legally blind individual might be a positive benefit rather than a complication in that diplopia is preferable to no vision at all.

Another "complication," an oral-antral fistula after a Caldwell-Luc antrostomy, might be looked on as a complication or an inevitable sequela of the operation depending on the patient. For example, an oral-antral fistula is highly probable in the patient with steroid-induced diabetes who presents for surgery with failing vision in spite of 120 mg of prednisone daily for months or years, whereas in the nonmedicated, nondiabetic patient it is a complication.

It is clear that differing value judgments may be applied to analysis of complications encountered during transantral decompression. Our judgments are cited in Table 6. All

TABLE 6. *Complications in 200 patients
undergoing orbital decompression*

Complication	No. of patients
Cerebrospinal fluid rhinorrhea	4
Nasolacrimal duct obstruction	9
Nasolacrimal duct obstruction requiring surgery	5
Oroantral fistula requiring surgery	7
Blindness (one eye)	2
Steroid used postoperatively	3
Diplopia	159
Numb lip (temporary)	200
Numb lip (permanent)	8

TABLE 7. *Length of
hospitalization in 200 patients*

Days	No. of patients	%
2	16	8
3	52	26
4	82	41
5	30	15
6	18	9
>6	2	1

patients with cerebrospinal fluid (CSF) leak had closure during the transantral decompression procedure and did not require further therapy.

Since these data were analyzed, there have been 250 more patients operated on. One patient died of meningitis within 6 weeks of surgery—an elderly woman who had been taking 160 mg of prednisone for 9 months and who had diabetes and osteoporosis. Her surgical wounds did not heal.

Surgical Morbidity

The surgical morbidity as measured by hospital time is documented in Table 7. The mean hospital stay was 3.5 days with a range of 1 to 13 days. The day of admission was counted as day 1, and the day of dismissal was the final day in the hospital.

DISCUSSION

Planning Prior to Decompression

The technical aspect of the transantral ethmoidal orbital decompression are straightforward and well within the capabilities of the otolaryngologist who is comfortable with antral and ethmoid surgery. There are a few technical details that seem to make a difference between a successful operation and a disappointing one, but these can be learned. If the surgery was all that was required of the otolaryngologist, his role would be simple. He operates, supervises the convalescent period, and steps aside. Patient satisfaction and personal involvement require much more (see chapter by Gorman, *this volume*, p. 325).

The patient with ophthalmopathy of Graves' disease who is a candidate for orbital decompression requires considerable counseling. First, he or she should be provided with detailed insight into the rationale, risks, limitations, and pitfalls of the procedure in order to attain a realistic estimate of the likelihood of benefit from decompression for the specific problem. If the patient's expectations for improvement exceed the potential of the operation, that fact should be established preoperatively; assuming that his or her goals are realistic, the patient must be made aware of the further efforts which may be required to attain the stated goals.

The surgeon's objectives and those of the patient must be compatible. For example, a young woman with significant and deforming proptosis, as well as vision-threatening effects of ophthalmopathy, must be aware that vision preservation is the primary goal and that her appearance may be unsatisfactory after what is in usual terms a successful operation. When the two parties to this operation have different ideas of what constitutes success, both will be disappointed.

When an otolaryngologist operates on eyes, the patient should be aware that he is not an eye doctor but only serving in a technical role for which he is well qualified. He should also know that the otolaryngologist is functioning in a technical role as a consultant of the endocrinologist and ophthalmologist. Likewise, he should be aware that the otolaryngologist will not be involved in whatever other rehabilitative procedures that may be needed. The patient should also be informed of the other options for his problem, and that decompression is not always successful. The more that has been done to the patient surgically or with radiation before decompression, the less predictable the procedure becomes. The patient should also know that the operation does not treat the cause of the ophthalmopathy but is a palliative step to provide more space in a crowded orbit.

The team concept needs to be reinforced in the preliminary discussion. Total rehabilitation may require the services of the ocular muscle surgeon, oculoplastic surgeon, and facial plastic surgeon after a successful orbital decompression.

Preoperative Evaluation

The preoperative evaluation involves endocrine studies. If time permits, patients with hyper- or hypothyroidism are rendered euthyroid before transantral decompression. If urgent decompression is required, hyperthyroidism can be controlled with propranolol.

Eye studies should include measurements of uncorrected and corrected visual acuity, exophthalmometer readings, assessment of extraocular and levator muscle function, palpebral fissure measurements, and a complete funduscopic examination.

Patients with visual loss that is not correctible with lenses require visual field assessment. The field measurements document the seriousness of the eye problem and provide an objective baseline for determining the effectiveness of the operation.

Roentgenograms of the sinuses were routinely obtained in the early years but are no longer used as they are not helpful. In patients with a history suggestive of sinus disease, the actual status of the sinuses is determined at surgery. Usually modest sinus membrane changes or polypoid disease are not contraindications to orbital decompression as these are treated with decompression. Computerized scans are interesting but usually not helpful either. The exception is the patient with asymmetrical exophthalmos who does not have a history of hyperthyroidism. In patients in whom the least-involved eye falls into the normal range of exophthalmometer measurement, the computerized scan can secure the diagnosis by showing the characteristic eye muscle thickening, the absence of an orbital mass, and proptosis. (See Forbes, *this volume*).

Patients who are receiving corticosteroids systemically or who have taken these drugs during the previous 9 months require special precautions during and after operation. It has been our policy to prepare these patients with an intramuscular injection of 200 mg of cortisone acetate the evening before surgery and again on the morning of the operation; 40 mg of prednisolone is given intravenously during the operation.

Complete decompression is possible only if a complete ethmoidectomy is performed and all the bony projections at the periphery are removed. In secondary decompressions that have been done after a previous operation failed, it is the failure to accomplish a complete ethmoidectomy that seems to be responsible for the inadequate result. I have performed a second operation on 10 patients who have had previous decompression through the lower lid. It is failure to complete the ethmoidectomy that limits that approach. When teaching the transantral approach, it has been repeatedly observed that residents are reluctant to complete the ethmoidectomy. However, with repetition the proper ethmoid operation is learned. The importance of the ethmoidectomy cannot be overemphasized.

The operation is usually done under general anesthesia and can be accomplished in less than an hour or so. If the patient's condition is so precarious as to preclude general anesthesia, the operation could be done with a second-division trigeminal nerve block.

SURGICAL TECHNIQUE

The patient is placed supine on the table with a tilt of about 15° of reverse Trendelenburg (i.e., sitting slightly upright). This position allows more comfort for the surgeon and assistant in relationship to the operating microscope.

The microscope provides two benefits: (a) it permits the assistant to observe directly through the side piece or television monitor and makes resident supervision practical; and (b) the brilliant light and magnification provided by the microscope helps limit trauma to the eyes and infraorbital nerves. A 300-mm lens provides adequate working distance for use with conventional paranasal sinus instruments.

The eyes are left uncovered but are protected with boric acid ointment. If the lids do not close, a single suture can be passed between them to close them during the operation.

A standard sublabial incision for anterior antrostomy exposes the face of the maxillary antrum. A generous anterior bone removal is done. Bone is removed up to the infraorbital rim but without trauma to the infraorbital nerve bundle. The microscope is then positioned and the ethmoid capsule entered with a Wilhelminski punch. The ethmoid is best entered at a point along the superior border of the nasoantral wall one-half the distance from front to back. The ethmoid cells are then crushed gently with an ethmoid exenteration instrument. One can estimate the angle between the cribriform area and the roof of the ethmoid capsule from front to back, remembering that with the head slightly up the posterior cribriform is lower than the anterior. A complete ethmoidectomy is accomplished with the exenteration instruments or curettes. The most anterior ethmoid dissection should be completed. This area is the least visible and the easiest part to neglect. The superior limits of the dissection are easily identified by the smooth bone of the cribriform area. If exenteration is carried out parallel to the plane of the cribriform, rather than angling into the bone, trauma to the cribriform plate and CSF leaks can be avoided. Usually a completed ethmoidectomy accommodates three 0.75×2 inch cottonoid strips soaked in epinephrine solution. If the three strips do not fit easily into the ethmoid capsule, the ethmoidectomy is not complete. This is an important point of the technique.

The bone of the orbital floor is then fractured with a small chisel. This bone is usually very thin medial to the course of the infraorbital nerve and comes away easily with a curette

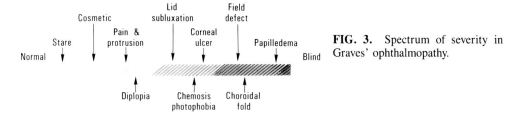

FIG. 3. Spectrum of severity in Graves' ophthalmopathy.

or periosteal elevator. The bone around the infraorbital nerve and lateral to it should also be removed. Lateral to the nerve the bone is much thicker, and a sphenoid punch type of instrument is needed. Likewise, the bone just behind the infraorbital rim is removed with the same instrument. After the bony orbital floor is removed, the paper plate of the ethmoid can be fractured into the previously dissected ethmoid capsule and removed. After rinsing out the pieces of bone, the orbital fascia is slit. This is done by placing linear slits from front to back. The first slit is placed high in the ethmoid, and the succeeding ones are made working from medial to lateral. Usually the fascia is excised in two places medial to the infraorbital nerve and in one place lateral to the nerve. At times the neurovascular bundle is quite lateral, and all the slits can be made medial to it. If proptosis is a major concern, orbital fat can be teased down and out of the orbit into the sinuses. If lesser amounts of proptosis are present, that is not necessary. In other words, the operation can be tailored somewhat to the patient's problem and needs.

One of the major technical difficulties is retraction of the sublabial incision to gain proper exposure of the orbital floor and ethmoid. We have tried a number of the available self-restraining retractors and designed a few of our own. None work very well, and the best we can recommend is a hand-held retractor and an assistant who is patient and steady.

Decompression is usually immediate. In most instances the ethmoid capsule is filled completely with fat, and the antrum is filled in its upper one-half. Only rarely are the muscles of the eye seen.

ILLUSTRATIVE CLINICAL VIGNETTES

Ophthalmopathy of Graves' disease is associated with a range of severity (Fig. 3). Enlarging the orbital space by orbital decompression is useful to a degree in some but not all the variations within the spectrum. Enlarging the orbital space obviously is not needed in the normal-appearing and functioning eye. Likewise, the patient with a minimal stare from lid retraction and mild proptosis has little to gain from that operation. In these patients time and aging will minimize the stare. If that is not acceptable, the ophthalmologic plastic surgeon has predictable techniques to lower the upper eyelids and raise, when required, the lower eyelids. A simple tarsorrhaphy can camouflage a stare if more sophisticated correction is not needed.

Decompression for cosmetic reasons alone is an attractive but unrealistic concept. Mere recession of the globe alone is unlikely to satisfy the patient who requires cosmetic decompression. When the globe recedes—and most do recede far enough—the lids widen, the horizontal axis of the globe goes down, or both. The upper sclera is visible, and the eyes still appear prominent. This is not to say that cosmetic decompression should not be done. Among the first 200 patients, six were operated for primarily cosmetic reasons. All six were ultimately satisfied, and all required secondary procedures (four had muscle and lid surgery and two had lid surgery only).

Cosmetic Decompression

Case 1

In July 1974, when the patient was 14 years old, her eyes became prominent; and in November 1974 the diagnosis of hyperthyroidism was made. She was treated with propylthiouracil and eventually subtotal thyroidectomy. There was some improvement in the eyes. In early 1976 the eyes rapidly protruded from 23 to 28 mm at base 93 over a period of 3 months. The upper eyelids subluxed on two occasions. There was no diplopia or visual loss. Decompression was carried out in June 1976, with a 6-mm recession of both globes (Plates I and II, color plates, p. 136). In December 1976 the inferior and medial rectus muscles were recessed, and in September 1977 upper lid retraction was treated by a Müller's muscle myotomy and recession with bilateral transection of the levator aponeurosis to the anterior tarsal plate.

In this case, with the return of the eyes to a more normal position in the orbit, the upper lid retraction became more obvious. With this retraction, the cosmetic appearance was unsatisfactory and lid surgery was needed to complete rehabilitation. In general, decompression alone in the presence of lid retraction does not totally solve the cosmetic problem.

Decompression for Steroid Dependence

Case 2

In early 1976 the patient experienced blurring, diplopia, lacrimation, and decreased vision. Prednisone at 120 mg/day relieved the symptoms, but when the dose was gradually reduced to 50 mg/day the symptoms returned. Because of limb muscle wasting and emotional lability, decompression was done in June 1977. The eyes receded 4 and 5 mm, and steroids were discontinued. This patient had muscle surgery on the inferior and medial rectus muscles.

Comment

Decompression to end steroid dependence is of predictable value. It is reasonable to use a short burst of high-dosage corticosteroids to relieve symptoms. Unfortunately, however, a short-term expedient can too easily become long-term dependence. In the presence of the secondary effects of corticosteroids (e.g., facial changes, osteoporosis, steroid diabetes, emotional lability, or psychosis), decompression is a conservative alternative. Of the 33 patients treated to eliminate steroid dependence, withdrawal was successful for all. That this could be accomplished without decompression in some is possibly true. Nevertheless, each patient was in deep distress because of the secondary effects of the steroids. Gradual withdrawal programs had failed in all because the eye symptoms returned as the drug dosage was reduced.

Decompression seems preferable to long-term high-dose steroids. The issue of how long is "long term" and how high is "high dose" is best left to the judgment of the endocrinologist, as should the question of what is a "serious" side effect.

Therapeutic decisions are most difficult for patients who have only moderate proptosis and diplopia. The question in these patients is whether muscle surgery alone will suffice or the surgery should be combined with decompression. The issue is simple. To produce single vision, muscle surgery is more predictable if the eye is back in a near-normal position, and the eyes look better if they are recessed and straight. Decompression after muscle surgery undoes the benefit of muscle surgery. (This is a lesson that has been relearned more than once.) Muscle surgery with proptosis may aggravate the orbital process. Decompression may actually facilitate the muscle surgery by lessening the tautness of the extraocular muscles. If muscle surgery is required and the eyes display marked proptosis, decompression should precede the muscle surgery. If vision is double before decompression, it will be double after. Some patients never attain single vision and thus must settle for prisms.

Decompression for Congestive Changes

The congestive changes of ophthalmopathy are often dramatic (Plates III and IV, color plates, p. 136). The pain, pressure, tearing, and unattractive appearance are most distressing. Seldom are these changes the only problem; features of diplopia or impaired visual acuity may coexist. Visual fields are often normal in the acute inflammatory phase of Graves' ophthalmopathy. The congestive changes are predictably reversed by transantral orbital decompression. Because changes in the congested eyes are dramatic—the reversal can occur within hours—these patients are easy to satisfy.

Decompression for Corneal Ulcer

The combination of corneal exposure, drying, and ulceration is an acceptable but infrequent indication for decompression. Recession of the globe is predictable, and the ulcer usually heals rapidly. One patient had an ulcer that did not heal, and the eye was lost after the anterior chamber ruptured.

Decompression for Visual Loss

Case 3

This patient was first seen in December 1976. Thyrotoxicosis had been diagnosed in 1968 and propylthiouracil was given. The eyes were prominent for 10 years, and visual loss began in January 1976. By October 1976 acuity was down to fingercount in the right eye and 20/80 in the left eye. (Fig. 4A) Disc pallor was noted. Decompression was done on October 7, 1976, and a residual field defect was noted 2 months later (Fig. 4B); some remained at the last check in February 1977 (Fig. 4C), and each eye recessed 6 mm. Subsequently muscle surgery was done to correct diplopia.

Case 4

A 48-year-old woman was first seen in July 1976. She had originally noted visual decrease in January 1972, and in July 1973 her vision was markedly decreased; visual field examination showed defects in both eyes at that time. Angiography and pneumoencephalography were normal. By September 1973, proptosis in both eyes was established. Diplopia on distant vision began in July 1975, and color obscuration was beginning. Hyperfunction of the thyroid was first diagnosed at this time. Treatment with cortisone and antithyroid drugs was followed by a dramatic improvement of the eyes but no change in vision.

When the patient was first seen by our group, the serum thyroxine level was elevated, and a diffuse goiter was palpated. Visual field examination on August 2, 1976 showed a bitemporal hemianopia; this finding was not typical of Graves' ophthalmopathy (Fig. 5A) and suggested a sellar or suprasellar lesion. Tomograms of the sellar region were not diagnostic of an intra- or suprasellar lesion. A computerized scan showed thickening of the

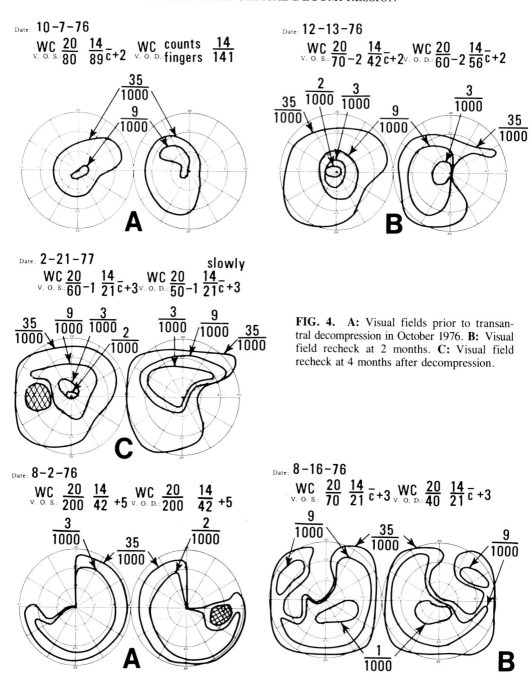

FIG. 4. **A:** Visual fields prior to transantral decompression in October 1976. **B:** Visual field recheck at 2 months. **C:** Visual field recheck at 4 months after decompression.

FIG. 5. Unusual bitemporal field defect due to Graves' ophthalmopathy. Fields were plotted before transantral orbital decompression (**A**) and were markedly improved 14 days later (**B**).

medial and lateral rectus muscles only. With this scan finding as the only clue to Graves' ophthalmopathy, a transantral orbital decompression was performed. Visual acuity improved from 20/200 right and left to 20/70 left and 20/40 right within 14 days (Fig. 5B). This acuity was sustained and muscle surgery followed.

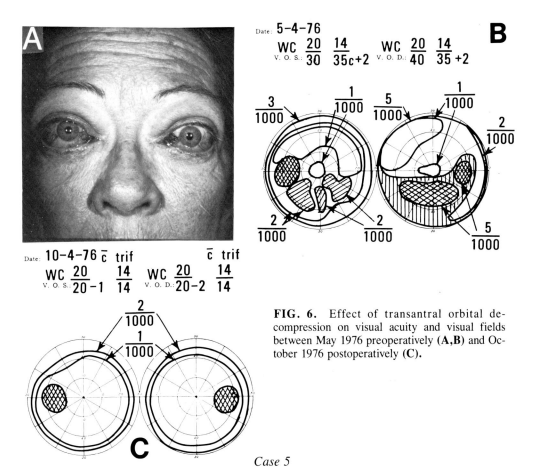

FIG. 6. Effect of transantral orbital decompression on visual acuity and visual fields between May 1976 preoperatively (**A,B**) and October 1976 postoperatively (**C**).

Case 5

This patient had classic hyperthyroidism manifested by weight loss, tremor, elevated serum thyroxine, and an enlarged thyroid in April 1974. Proptosis and intermittent diplopia were observed in July 1975. Hyperthyroidism was controlled with 400 mg of propylthiouracil daily. In May 1976 visual blurring, steady diplopia, and congestive changes were noted (Fig. 6A,B). Decompression and later extraocular muscle surgery were performed. Visual improvement followed decompression and was maintained (Fig. 6C).

Case 6

A 54-year-old woman was first seen in December 1975. Hyperthyroidism was diagnosed in 1970 and treated with [131]I. Proptosis occurred intermittently during the next 5 years. When the patient was first seen, her eye measured 22 mm right and 21 mm left at base 96. The fields were normal, and diplopia was absent. By September 1976 her eyes protruded to 26 mm right and 27 mm left at base 96, and there was a field defect on the left. Decompression was done on September 16, 1976. The field defect cleared, and later upper lid surgery was done.

Comment

The visual field defect is considered the most urgent indication for orbital decompression. The field defect, as illustrated by the case cited above, can occur before, after, or during thyroid hyperfunction and even in the absence of altered thyroid hormone levels. In the absence of current or past thyroid hyperfunction, the diagnosis is more difficult. The computerized scan is probably the most helpful tool to make this diagnosis in this situation.

In the series of 200 patients, most patients with field defects had a trial of corticosteroids, nine had orbital irradiation, and 12 had decompression by another route—all still had lost vision and retained field defects. Orbital irradiation for field defects in these patients did not seem to be effective.

Not every patient with field defects had changes in visual acuity. Early and less-dense defects can occur with normal acuity. Usually these patients complain of impaired vision and are distressed if they are told they have normal visual acuity. Visual field studies generally verify the correctness of the patient's observation. As a generalization, defects that are present for weeks to a few months clear with decompression. The field defects that do not improve or get worse are those longstanding ones associated with the ominous prognostic sign of disc pallor.

Decompression for Papilledema

Case 7

A 59-year-old male was first seen in June 1970 with diplopia, decreasing vision, and progressive proptosis. He was never hyperthyroid. Eye examination documented normal visual acuity for near and far vision, muscle imbalance, and one diopter of papilledema in both eyes. By August there were three diopters of papilledema, an enlarged blind spot on field examination, and exophthalmometer readings of 28 mm right and 27 mm left. Decompression was done. By January 1971 both fields were improved, the papilledema was gone, and the left eye receded 2 mm and the right eye 3 mm.

Comment

Chronic papilledema can be a serious and advanced complication of ophthalmopathy, short of blindness. This is a rare problem, but it occurred in 6% of all eyes in the series of 200 patients.

Papilledema rarely occurs alone, usually coexisting with a field defect and being considered an ischemic phenomenon. Papilledema, even of months' duration, is reversible. When associated with disc pallor, it is a more ominous sign. Some visual return is possible even with disc pallor, and decompression is worthwhile at times as a last desperate effort if the patient understands the seriousness of the problem. If eyes are blind from optic neuropathy with no measurable vision, in our experience they are not restorable by decompression. If there is not at least finger count vision, operation is not worthwhile.

Ophthalmopathy Without Clinically Detected Hyperthyroidism

Case 8

In September 1967 a 51-year-old woman was seen with unilateral proptosis that progressed. Thyroid function was normal. Corticosteroids in doses up to 80 mg of prednisone daily did not help. Intermittent diplopia followed. In July 1974 vision began to blur, with "gray-outs" lasting seconds. Bilateral papilledema was observed, and a hemorrhage into a 3-mm choked disc was seen on the left. Decompression was performed in December 1974.

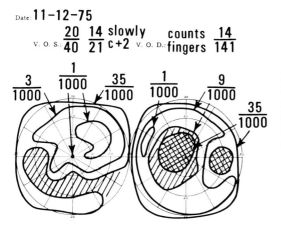

Date: 11-12-75

V. O. S.: $\frac{20}{40}$ $\frac{14 \text{ slowly}}{21}$ c+2   V. O. D.: counts $\frac{14}{\text{fingers } 141}$

$\frac{3}{1000}$ $\frac{\frac{1}{1000}}{}$ $\frac{35}{1000}$ $\frac{1}{1000}$ $\frac{9}{1000}$

$\frac{35}{1000}$

FIG. 7. Visual fields from a patient who had received three courses of irradiation to his orbits for Graves' ophthalmopathy. Visual acuity was not improved by radiation therapy or by surgical decompression via the transantral and transfrontal routes.

Papilledema cleared in 7 days. In 1976 when muscle surgery was performed, the discs were normal.

Conditions That Mimic Graves' Disease

Four other patients were treated (beyond the 200) who had conditions that turned out to be something other than Graves' ophthalmopathy. These patients were not included in the statistical analysis.

Case 9: Radiation Retinopathy

The first of these four patients was a man who may well have had ophthalmopathy at the onset, but by the time the patient got to decompression he had radiation retinopathy and was not helped by decompression.

A 55-year-old man was first seen in July 1975. He was treated with ^{131}I after classic clinical hyperthyroidism was diagnosed. In 1971 his eyes became prominent and vision decreased. Steroid therapy of unknown dosage failed to alter progressive visual deterioration. Cobalt irradiation was administered in 16 fractions to a dose of 2,857 rads, and vision returned. Steroid therapy was restarted 1 month after the radiation because the proptosis progressed. Diplopia began in January 1973. By March 1974 visual blurring was present. Fundus examination showed atropic choroidal retinal areas and papilledema. A second course of cobalt therapy in a dose of 1,052 rads was given with some improvement of the vision. In February 1975 a third course of cobalt radiotherapy was delivered. When first seen at the Mayo Clinic, visual acuity was 20/200 right and 20/30 left. A field defect was plotted (Fig. 7). Both optic discs were elevated, and retinal hemorrhage, neovascularization, and exudative retinopathy were noted. Atheromatous material was seen in the arterioles. Transantral orbital decompression was done on August 1, 1975. There was little change in vision, eye position, or papilledema. A transfrontal decompression was done, again with little change in vision. The eyes recessed by 3 mm. By May 1977 vision was 20/200 in the left eye and fingercount in the right.

Comment

It is my impression that in this patient visual loss resulted from a combination of venous congestion and radiation. The process started as Graves' ophthalmopathy, but the treatment with radiation led to radiation retinopathy. At neither the transfrontal operation nor the

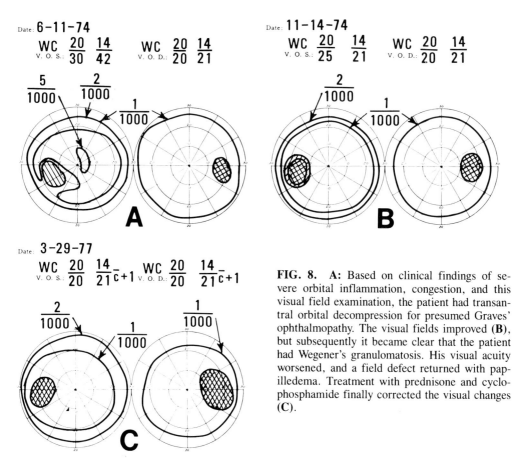

FIG. 8. **A:** Based on clinical findings of severe orbital inflammation, congestion, and this visual field examination, the patient had transantral orbital decompression for presumed Graves' ophthalmopathy. The visual fields improved (**B**), but subsequently it became clear that the patient had Wegener's granulomatosis. His visual acuity worsened, and a field defect returned with papilledema. Treatment with prednisone and cyclophosphamide finally corrected the visual changes (**C**).

transantral procedure did the orbital tissues look different than those seen with usual Graves' disease.

Case 10: Wegener's Granulomatosis

The second patient had clinical findings consistent with Graves' disease, but the process evolved into classic Wegener's granulomatosis with its first manifestation in the orbit.

In June 1974 a 52-year-old man experienced progressive exophthalmos and diplopia. Visual examination showed two diopters of papilledema on the left, a relative enlargement of the blind spot on visual field study, and a central scotoma on the left. The right eye was normal. There was no history of hyperthyroidism or thyroid disease. Prednisone, 60 to 80 mg/day, did not help. Decompression in June 1974 (Fig. 8A) revealed massively enlarged extrocular muscles and little orbital fat. The eyes did not recede. Vision improved, and the field defect cleared. By August 1974 severe periorbital edema, chemosis, and ocular congestion returned and double vision was troublesome. Orbital irradiation was used to 2,000 rads in 20 fractions, and steroids were continued. In November 1974 the congestive symptoms were worse, although vision was maintained and the visual fields were normal (Fig. 8B). Because of the possibility that another orbital process existed, the orbital fat was biopsied. Biopsy revealed acute and chronic inflammation with extensive acute necrotizing vasculitis and focal deposits of fibrinoid material. The diagnosis of orbital pseudotumor was considered.

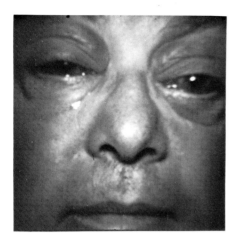

FIG. 9. Orbital lymphoma, as in this patient, can be a bilateral process which closely mimics Graves' ophthalmopathy in appearance.

Shortly after this, crusting and bleeding from the nose developed, and fluid was observed in the left ear. Nasal examination showed extensive crusting and a septal perforation. The anterior turbinates were gone. Multiple biopsy specimens showed subacute and chronic inflammatory changes, ulceration, plasmacytosis, and necrotizing vasculitis consistent with Wegener's granulomatosis. The sedimentation rate was 98 mm in 1 hr. Prednisone therapy, 60 mg every other day, was started. By January 1975 proteinuria was present, and the creatinine level was elevated. Prednisone therapy was continued, and the symptoms gradually improved. In October 1976 two diopters of papilledema was noted in the right eye. Cyclophosphamide, 100 mg/day, was added to the program. Within 3 months all systems were stable. Prednisone was discontinued in October 1977 and the cyclophosphamide in August 1978. At all subsequent follow-up visits the patient was well. His last visual field examination was normal, and vision was corrected to 20/20 in both eyes (Fig. 8).

Case 11: Chronic Sinusitis

The third patient seemed to have chronic sinusitis that presented with orbital symptoms only. This was the only patient we have seen with sinus disease as the basis for eye symptoms suggestive of Graves' disease. Roentgenograms of the sinus region are not a routine part of the preoperative evaluation.

Case 12: Orbital Lymphoma

The final patient had classic eye symptoms of Graves' disease, with proptosis, decreased vision, and bilateral field defects. There were no other symptoms. At decompression a bilateral process consistent with malignant lymphoma was uncovered and decompression was terminated (Fig. 9).

CONCLUSIONS

Until the biochemical process that produces the orbital pathology in Graves' ophthalmopathy is better understood and the process can be prevented or reversed, there will be a need for orbital decompression in some patients. Enlargement of the orbital space does not in itself directly attack the orbital process, and as such any operation can be considered only symptomatically palliative or rehabilitative therapy. Selection of appropriate patients is essential.

The predictability of recession following decompression depends on the patient's problem. The operation is most predictable in patients with congestive changes, visual field defects, and visual loss, in that order. The more unsuccessful is the treatment that precedes decompression, the less predictable the operation becomes. Because of the short hospital stay, few complications, and the high percentage of satisfied patients with these specific eye problems, the transantral orbital decompression seems to be a conservative form of treatment and not necessarily a treatment of last resort. For these specific problems, decompression seems more conservative than high-dose long-term corticosteroid therapy. We are less reluctant to decompress orbits early in the disease process today than when our experience began in 1969.

Assessment of the effectiveness of transantral decompression becomes more subjective as the indications expand to include cosmetic goals and when the operation is done as an adjunct to muscle surgery. In these circumstances decompression is only a part of a rehabilitative process that includes extraocular muscle surgery, upper and lower lid surgery, and at times lid and facial skin surgery.

EDITORS' COMMENT:

Advantages and Disadvantages of The Transantral Orbital Approach to Thyroid Decompression

The major disadvantage to the transantral orbital approach for management of thyroid exophthalmos may be that the surgical field is unfamiliar to the majority of ophthalmic surgeons who at times are primary care physicians for the patient. However, the expertise required to perform the transantral–ethmoidal decompression described by Walsh and Ogura can be obtained by the ophthalmologist if he or she is motivated to do so; if not, surgery performed by colleagues in otolaryngology is not an undesired alternative if the team approach to the complex problem of Graves' disease is compatible with the practice style of the community.

A second disadvantage to the transantral orbital approach for thyroid decompression, postoperative infection, may be more apparent than real. Decompressing the orbit through a contaminated field has not produced significant problems with orbital or sinus infection in a large series of cases. Postoperatively, orbital contents (because of multiple incisions placed into the periorbita to facilitate decompression) are in direct contact with sinus cavities with both the anterior orbital approach and the transantral approach. In point of fact, neither operation, perhaps surprisingly, is associated with a high incidence of postoperative sinusitis or orbital cellulitis.

Oral intubation does not preclude easy access to the antral-ethmoidal sinuses when approached via the Caldwell–Luc incision if the patient is properly positioned. The operating microscope should be employed to identify important landmarks during the course of the dissection. If worrisome bleeding occurs, one may be in a good, if not better, position to control hemorrhage from within the sinuses than from the "orbital" side.

Although the anterior orbital approach utilizes the incision and exposure familiar to ophthalmic orbital surgeons and allows for the same bony structures to be removed as in the transantral approach, there may be a tendency via the anterior approach to be timid with respect to removal of the posterior ethmoid air cells. Perhaps the issue cannot be easily settled, but our experience to date emphasizes that the secret to successful decompression of the orbital apex is removal of the ethmoid sinus, especially posteriorly; our clinical impression with regard to patients referred to our institution who require reoperation because of persistent signs and symptoms of Graves' disease is that the incidence of inadequate decompression via the anterior approach is higher than with the transantral approach. This tempers our enthusiasm for the anterior approach, and we select the transantral approach for most patients requiring decompression, especially those with optic neuropathy.

ADDITIONAL READING

1. DeSanto, L. W. (1972): Surgical palliation of ophthalmopathy of Graves' disease: transantral approach. *Mayo Clin. Proc.*, 47:989–992.
2. DeSanto, L. W. (1980): The total rehabilitation of Graves' ophthalmopathy. *Laryngoscope*, 90:1652–1678.
3. DeSanto, L. W., and Gorman, C. A. (1973): Selection of patients and choice of operation in Graves' ophthalmopathy. *Laryngoscope*, 83:945–959.
4. Gorman, C. A., DeSanto, L. W., MacCarty, C. S., and Riley, F. C. (1974): Optic neuropathy of Graves' disease: treatment by transantral or transfrontal orbital decompression. *N. Engl. J. Med.*, 290:70–75.
5. Ogura, J. H., and Pratt, L. L. (1971): Transantral orbital decompression for malignant exophthalmos. *Otolaryngol. Clin. North Am.*, 4:193–203.

The Eye and Orbit in Thyroid Disease, edited by
C. A. Gorman et al. Raven Press, New York 1984.

Ocular Muscle Surgery

John A. Dyer

Department of Ophthalmology, Mayo Clinic, Rochester, Minnesota 55905

The extraocular muscle abnormalities encountered in Graves' disease are dealt with in this chapter primarily in terms of the surgical experience resulting from treatment of some 287 patients operated on from 1968 to 1982. Many had prior orbital decompression with a surgical success rate in the order of 60% for one procedure, and those without decompression in the last group studied had a one-time surgical success of nearly 80%.

PATHOPHYSIOLOGY

In 1962 Brain (1) listed five conditions in which endocrine exophthalmos may be associated with ophthalmoplegia. The first of these, exophthalmic ophthalmoplegia, usually was bilateral and often severe in proportion to the ophthalmoplegia, and chemosis and lid retraction were often present. In mild or early cases the ophthalmoplegia often was unilateral or more severe on one side. Elevation and abduction usually were affected first with depression and adduction involved in the more severe cases only. In general, this thesis is still correct. In 1963 Grob (2) found ocular myopathy to be the most common myopathy associated with thyroid disease. He noted that eye signs may develop before there is any evidence of hyperthyroidism, and that a limitation of elevation occurs first and then a decrease in abduction. In the present discussion, Werner's class 4 (3) is of primary interest, i.e., extraocular muscle involvement.

Although some authors (1,2,4–6) believed that the hypotropia and reduced elevation of eyes was the result of "paralysis" of the superior rectus and possibly the inferior oblique muscles, other reports (7–12) confirmed that there is, in fact, fibrosis of the inferior rectus and often the medial rectus muscles which prevents elevation or abduction through a leash effect. This finding led Braley (13) in 1953 to record and report an increase in intraocular pressure on attempted upgaze with lowering of the pressure on downgaze. This is an additional and very positive indication of the restrictive nature of the ophthalmopathy. It behooves one to check the intraocular pressure with the affected eye in a relaxed position to avoid erroneous diagnosis and treatment for glaucoma.

DIAGNOSTIC AIDS

From the practical standpoint, restricted elevation, abduction, or both in the absence of a history of trauma or other obvious defect are indicative of Graves' ophthalmopathy. The clinical signs of elevated intraocular pressure on upgaze and a positive forced-duction test virtually clinch the diagnosis. Other examinations—e.g., computed tomography (CT) scans showing the enlarged muscles, electromyography, ultrasonography, and clinical tests which are discussed in detail in other chapters of this text—may add confirmatory evidence.

One must remember that the ophthalmologist frequently is the first to be consulted when vertical or horizontal diplopia occurs as the earliest manifestation of Graves' disease. One should consider myasthenia gravis as a possible cause of diplopia in these patients. Tensilon testing may help to establish the diagnosis. Moreover, ocular muscle involvement may occur without overt clinical or laboratory signs of the disease.

RESEARCH EXPERIENCE

The use of plastic implants as extensions of, or to, extraocular muscles or as a sleeve to surround them to prevent excessive scarring has been advocated for several years. Bowen and Dyer (14) used a Silastic strip in which Dacron mesh was embedded to act as a substitute tendon for the lateral rectus muscles in dogs. The material became enmeshed in a fibrous sleeve that adhered to the sclera beneath. Beisner (15) used medical-grade silicone elastomer and silicone-covered Dacron ribbons sutured under the tendons of rectus muscles in dogs. He concluded that these materials became firmly bound to the sclera and nullified any theoretical advantage as a tendon prosthesis.

On the other hand, Dunlap (16) considered Supramid Extra to be the most inert of the synthetic materials available. He believed that covering a muscle with a Supramid sleeve greatly reduced the postoperative scarring to the sclera or other nearby tissue. In my experience, these sleeves have a great tendency to extrude and must be sutured to the muscle with nonadsorbable suture material and be covered well by Tenon's capsule and conjunctiva.

Hiatt (17) used autogenous extraocular muscle to lengthen the action of another muscle and regarded this as a feasible procedure. He concluded that for a clinical and experimental procedure this tissue was as good as any synthetic material.

Because synthetic materials produce a greater inflammatory response and muscle tissue is difficult to manage as a transplant, the use of homologous sclera to serve as a substitute tendon seemed logical. Gamma-irradiated homologous sclera preserved by freezing was used experimentally in cats to extend the lateral rectus muscles (7). Because tissue reaction was negligible, human sclera prepared in a similar manner was used as an extension for medial and inferior rectus muscle surgery in humans with Graves' myopathy. The transplants were used in recession procedures only.

Although this proved to be a valid method of muscle extension, the tissues over the implants tended to melt away, and most patients complained of a thick mucoid discharge until the tissue was removed. I now find it totally satisfactory to use double-armed sutures from the recessed muscle passed through the original insertion site and tied, permitting the suture arms to act as an extension of the muscle which adheres to the sclera in the proper plane and angle of attachment. This technique may be used for adjustable sutures as well (Fig. 1).

SURGICAL CONSIDERATIONS

The taut fibrous ocular muscles found during a surgical procedure in patients with Graves' myopathy present a unique test of the surgeon's patience and skill. Because of the nature of the disease, postoperative scarring often is excessive, and a result that looks promising hours or days postoperatively may change to an overcorrection, a regression to the previous state, or the appearance of an entirely new muscle imbalance as weeks pass. Hence the patient must be apprised of the fact that a second, or a third, or even more procedures may be required. The primary goal is to achieve some degree of single binocular vision in the primary and reading positions; full rotations rarely are achieved.

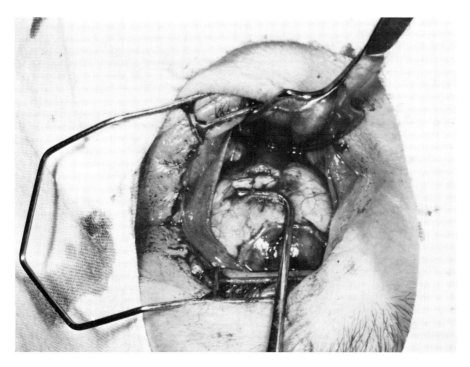

FIG. 1. Suture from muscle tied at the original insertion site, inferior rectus muscle.

Basically, the operation of choice is to relax the fibrous, restrictive ocular muscles—most frequently the inferior rectus muscles, secondly the medial recti, less often the superior muscles, and seldom the lateral recti. Some surgeons suggest complete severance of the scleral insertion (inferior muscles), whereas others recess 6 mm or more (18) as a standard procedure; others suggest a graded recession depending on the severity of restriction (7,12) or an adjustable suture technique so that a muscle can be advanced or recessed several hours postoperatively. This variety of opinions attests to the fact that there is still no panacea for surgical cure of the muscle imbalance. In my experience, reoperation is required in about 40% of patients.

Unless very careful and thorough dissection is done along the inferior rectus as far posteriorly as possible to relax or strip away the aponeurosis from the inferior rectus to the lower border of the tarsus, retraction of the lower eyelid may require later surgery. In my experience, any recession more than 5 to 6 mm results in this complication unless dissection is meticulous. A sharpened lid expressor (Weck) is an ideal instrument for separating these tissues in any muscle procedure. Figure 2 shows extensive fibrosis along the inferior rectus muscle and the tissue dissected away from the muscle. A large recession (i.e., more than 6 mm) was my choice formerly (7); however, although a complete myectomy or a large recession relieves the hypotropia or esotropia, it also creates an inability to depress the eyes into the reading position (inferior recti) or reduces convergence (medial recti) so that bifocals are rendered useless or the patient must hold objects upward in front of his eyes to read. This is particularly annoying when an operation is done on only one inferior muscle.

Other complications, e.g., exposure of the globes, may occur after the release of fibrotic ocular muscles with an increase in proptosis. In my opinion, if the proptosis is more than 22 to 23 mm (Hertel or Krahn exophthalmometer), serious consideration must be given to

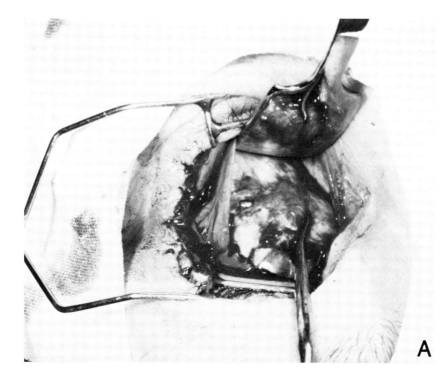

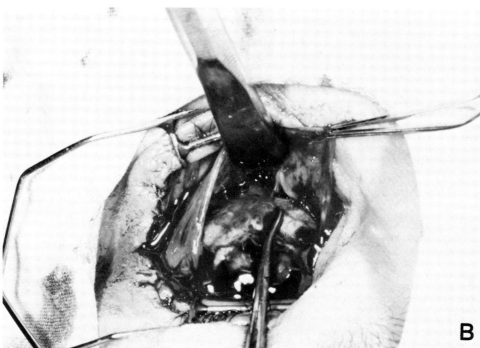

FIG. 2. A: Extensive fibrosis along the inferior rectus muscle. **B:** Tissue dissection away from the inferior rectus muscle.

orbital decompression before muscle surgery even if there is no threat to vision. The patient should be advised that about 40% of those with no ocular muscle imbalance before decompression have diplopia afterward, and that if an imbalance is present before decompression it will remain or be more severe after surgery.

The prime indications for orbital decompressions are diplopia with proptosis more than 22 to 23 mm, exposure of the globe, cosmesis, and progressive visual loss because of optic neuropathy. In any patient, a surgical procedure is not advised until the thyroid state is stable. Our otolaryngologists perform the transantral decompressions and anticipate 2 to 10 mm of regression in proptosis. A bilateral procedure usually is done to prevent asymmetry. Muscle surgery is delayed 2 to 4 months or longer to permit any ocular muscle change to occur and all tissue reaction to subside.

If only one inferior or medial rectus muscle is involved with minimal proptosis, a recession of the single muscle may suffice. After decompression, most patients require an operation on both inferior and medial muscles; this should be done as one procedure. From experience, I have found that a minimum recession usually suffices because the eye or eyes elevate or abduct more as time passes. To relax muscles further secondarily is much simpler than to repair an overcorrection. My results are best when recession of the medial rectus muscle is a standard 5 mm and recession of the inferior muscle varies from 2 to 6 mm so that the pupillary light reflexes from the operating room light are slightly above center in each eye while the patient is under anesthesia. This smaller recession permits the eyes to elevate adequately, yet depression is maintained for satisfactory reading.

The use of an adjustable suture is advocated by some surgeons; that is, once the muscle is released, the suture arms are passed through the original insertion close together (no scleral bite) and fastened with a slipknot or bow so that some hours later the suture may be tightened or relaxed to improve the eye position. Usually a maximum recession is performed and the muscle advanced if necessary. Because the postoperative course is so unpredictable in Graves' disease, I have found the variable recession technique best thus far. Vicryl or Dexon sutures of 5–0 or 6–0 caliber are preferred; the tensile strength is excellent and the tissue reaction minimal.

Many patients have a definite "A" pattern esotropia. Elevation and abduction of the eyes may be poor; the chin is tilted upward so that single vision can be obtained, and on upgaze the eyes converge excessively. In the past, I attributed this to the taut inferior muscles failing to relax (7); however, during surgery I noted that in many patients the upper half of the medial muscles often was very thick and swollen whereas the inferior portion was very fibrous and tight (Fig. 3), as are the inferior muscles. Subsequently, in these patients I have recessed the lower border of the muscle 2 to 3 mm more than the upper portion and displaced the muscles upward at least one muscle width (Fig. 3), as one would do in treating a child with "A" esotropia. Although my experience with these patients has been limited, my impression is that the results are definitely more satisfactory.

From experience I have learned also that a secondary hypertropia is best treated in most instances by a recession of the antagonist superior rectus muscle rather than an advancement of the previously recessed inferior muscle because the problem often is contracture of the superior muscle once the tight inferior muscle is relaxed. If the hyperdeviation is severe, the inferior muscle may require advancement also, but only after weakening of the superior muscle usually a maximum of 5 mm. Because of gradual secondary contracture of the antagonist superior or lateral rectus muscles in this disease, one should postpone further surgical intervention for several months. If the inferior muscle is permitted at surgery to retract freely with no measured recession, its secondary recovery is virtually impossible. In

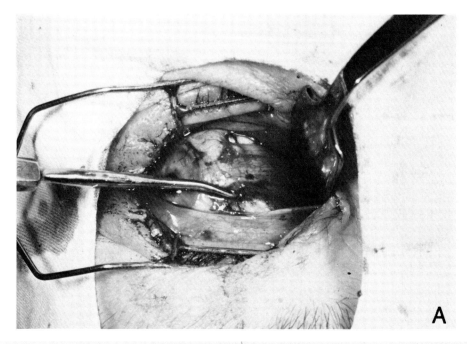

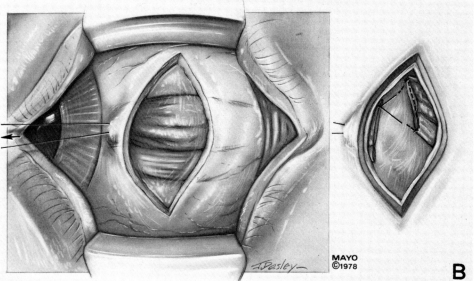

FIG. 3. Top: Surgical recession with upward placement of medial muscle, right eye. Note the thickened upper portion and fibrous lower portion of the muscle. This surgical photograph was taken above the left medial rectus muscle before recession. **Bottom:** Artist's conception.

severe cases in which a large recession is desired primarily, or in subsequent operations if further relaxation is desired, proper alignment of the muscles often is difficult.

If lower or upper eyelid retraction results in undue exposure of the eyes, surgery designed to correct these defects is in order. This always follows extraocular muscle surgery inasmuch as excessive upper eyelid retraction may result from the patient's thwarted effort to look up and is reduced when the fibrotic inferior muscles are relaxed.

At the Mayo Clinic a team approach has proved most satisfactory. This team includes an endocrinologist who certifies that the patient's disease is quiescent, an ophthalmologist, and an otolaryngologist who performs the transantral decompression on the advice of the ophthalmologist; at least two of these team members must examine the patient and suggest decompression for reasons previously discussed. Afterward, ocular muscle surgery and subsequent eyelid realignment are performed if needed.

CLINICAL EXPERIENCE

In previous papers (7,12) I reported on my surgical experience in 116 patients operated on from 1968 to 1975 and 83 patients who had muscle surgery from 1975 to 1978. An additional 91 patients were reviewed who had surgery from 1978 to 1982 with at least a year follow-up. All of these were primary surgical cases which I had performed and included those with or without prior orbital decompression. The overall results indicate that these are difficult patients in whom to achieve single binocular vision.

In each group the female/male ratio was 3:1. The average was 48 years for females and 49 years for males, with a range of 16 to 74 years. Orbital decompression was performed in 68 (59%) of group 1, 57 (69%) of group 2, and 46 (51%) of the last group. All of the patients had a transantral-ethmoidal type of decompression except for 7% of the first group.

Fifty-five percent of group 1 patients required one operation to obtain single binocular vision in the primary and reading positions, 63% of those in group 2, and 59% in group 3. A second procedure was required in 29% of group 1, 24% of group 2, and 35% of group 3, whereas three or more operations were necessary in 16% of group 1, 13% of group 2, and only 6% of the third group.

Time is on the side of the patient and the surgeon, as many of the patients who do not achieve single vision after multiple operations gradually suppress the second image or learn to cope with the situation. Patients with Graves' ophthalmopathy must be apprised that the progress is tedious and full of pitfalls.

Shorr et al. (19) reported on 50 consecutive patients who had ocular muscle surgery following orbital decompression. Of 32 patients who were orthotropic in the primary position prior to decompression, 11 (34%) developed strabismus postoperatively. In my experience, if no diplopia is present before decompression, 40 to 50% develop it postdecompression, whereas 100% of those with diplopia prior to decompression have it as severe or probably worse afterward. In Shorr's series of the 21 patients requiring muscle surgery, 14 (67%) required one operation, six (29%) needed two procedures, and one had three operations. It is obvious that more procedures may be required in patients with severe bilateral involvement than in those with a single muscle operated. In his discussion of this report, Rosenbaum postulated that the reduced abduction and the esotropia present in many of these patients resulted solely from tight inferior rectus muscles. In my opinion, reduced abduction always results from tight medial muscles, as does the "A" pattern esotropia (noted earlier in this chapter).

In an effort to reduce the number of procedures and exposures to anesthesia required for many of these patients, we performed muscle surgery immediately following the decompression in 13 patients, recessing those muscles that seemed constricted by forced-duction testing (hook beneath the muscle insertion). Whereas eight patients had diplopia preoperatively and five did not, eight had single vision postoperatively and five did not. Two of five patients without preoperative diplopia had it after surgery due to an overcorrection. In retrospect, this did not add to the success rate. Waiting a few weeks or months to perform muscle surgery probably is best, although it is obvious in many instances that the inferior or medial muscles may be entrapped in the decompressed sinuses.

Evans and Kennerdell (11) studied 45 patients who had ocular muscle surgery without prior decompression. Thirty (67%) achieved single vision in the primary position and 27 (60%) in the reading position. Thirteen underwent further surgery, with two requiring four operations. In my group 3, 45 of 91 patients did not have a prior decompression; 37 (82%) required one operation for single vision in the reading and primary positions, seven (16%) needed two procedures, and one had three to achieve single vision.

SUMMARY

When the thyroid state is stable and no further changes in ocular motility are occurring, surgical correction of diplopia is necessary to regain single vision in the primary and reading positions. Preliminary tests, including A-scan and A-scan ultrasonography, CT scan, saccadic velocity testing, and forced-duction tests, aid in excluding other causes of muscle abnormalities.

In the absence of proptosis and with minimal eyelid retraction, recession of the taut rectus muscles, most often the inferior and then the medial, is required. If proptosis is moderate (22 to 23 mm) and lid retraction is severe, preliminary orbital decompression is advised inasmuch as prior relaxation of the ocular muscles may cause increased proptosis and exposure of the eyes, which would necessitate emergency orbital decompression.

If severe proptosis creates a cosmetic blemish, or if exposure of the globes or optic neuropathy is a threat to vision, decompression should be done followed in 6 weeks or longer by ocular muscle surgery. After decompression, diplopia may occur in almost 50% of patients with no muscle imbalance preoperatively, whereas all patients with diplopia before decompression will have a more severe imbalance after decompression.

Although I previously advocated larger recessions of the fibrotic muscles (7), a smaller, graded recession of the inferior muscles after careful dissection is more accurate and prevents lower eyelid retraction (12). Transposition of the medial muscles upward with recession is helpful in many patients with an "A" pattern esotropia. With time, the antagonist superior rectus muscle contracts and must be recessed secondarily if a large inferior recession has resulted in overcorrection. Advancement of the inferior muscle(s) does not suffice. The use of scleral grafts to extend the ocular muscles and placement of Supramid sleeves or caps may be useful adjuncts in reoperations.

These findings have led to a decrease in the number of surgical procedures required to gain useful single vision for these patients. As a general rule, if the pupillary light reflexes from the operating room light are almost centered in each eye at the conclusion of surgery, the eyes will remain in this position when the patient awakens. Because of the fibrotic state of the muscles, full rotations seldom are regained.

When the thyroid state is stable, relieve the proptosis, straighten the eyes, and correct the eyelid retraction for most effective results.

REFERENCES

1. Brain, R. (1962): The diagnosis, prognosis, and treatment of endocrine exophthalmos. *Trans. Ophthalmol. Soc. U.K.*, 82:223–242.
2. Grob, D. (1963): Myopathies and their relation to thyroid disease. *N.Y. State J. Med.*, 63:218–228.
3. Werner, S. C. (1969): Classification of thyroid disease. *J. Clin. Endocrinol. Metab.*, 29:860–862 (letter to the editor).

4. Rundle, F. F., and Wilson, C. W. (1944): Ophthalmoplegia in Graves' disease. *Clin. Sci. Mol. Med.*, 5:17–29.

5. Goldstein, J. E. (1964): Paresis of superior rectus muscle: associated with thyroid dysfunction. *Arch. Ophthalmol.*, 72:5–8.

6. Woods, A. C. (1951): The ocular changes of hyperthyroidism. *West. J. Surg.*, 59:288–302.

7. Dyer, J. A. (1976): The oculorotary muscles in Graves' disease. *Trans. Am. Ophthalmol. Soc.*, 74:425.

8. Miller, J. E. (1961): Acquired strabismus in adults. *South. Med. J.*, 54:744–752.

9. Miller, J. E., van Heuven, W., and Ward, R. (1965): Surgical correction of hypotropias associated with thyroid dysfunction. *Arch. Ophthalmol.*, 74:509–515.

10. Smith, B., and Soll, D. B. (1960): Strabismus associated with thyroid disease. *Am. J. Ophthalmol.*, 50:473–478.

11. Evans, D. E., and Kennerdell, J. S. (1983): Extraocular muscle surgery for dysthyroid myopathy. *Am. J. Ophthalmol.*, 95:767–771.

12. Dyer, J. A. (1978): Ocular muscle surgery in Graves' disease. *Trans. Am. Ophthalmol. Soc.*, 76:125–139.

13. Braley, A. E. (1953): Malignant exophthalmos. *Am. J. Ophthalmol.*, 36:1286–1290.

14. Bowen, S. F., Jr., and Dyer, J. A. (1962): A silicone rubber tendon for extraocular muscle: an experimental study. *Invest. Ophthalmol.*, 1:579–585.

15. Beisner, D. H. (1970): Extraocular muscle recessions utilizing silicone tendon prostheses. *Arch. Ophthalmol.*, 83:195–204.

16. Dunlap, E. A. (1968): Plastic implants in muscle surgery: plastic materials in the management of extraocular motility restrictions. *Arch. Ophthalmol.*, 80:249–257.

17. Hiatt, R. L. (1973): Extraocular muscle transplantation. *Trans. Am. Ophthalmol. Soc.*, 71:426–458.

18. Schimek, R. A. (1972): Surgical management of ocular complications of Graves' disease. *Arch. Ophthalmol.*, 87:655–664.

19. Shorr, N., Neuhaus, R. W., and Baylis, H. I. (1982): Ocular motility problems after orbital decompression for dysthyroid ophthalmopathy. *Ophthalmology*, 89:323–328.

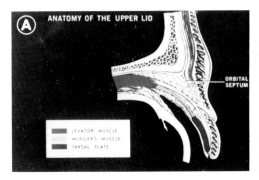

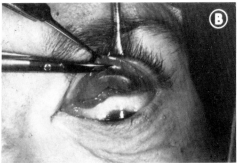

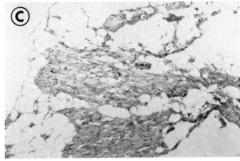

FIG. 2. A: Sagittal diagram depicting surgical anatomy of upper lid. **B:** Operative photograph showing attachments of levator aponeurosis to anterior tarsus. **C:** Photomicrograph of Müller's muscle layer and surrounding fat (hematoxylineosin, × 160).

that inserts onto the globe and a capsulopalpebral head that divides into three parts: an aponeurosis, a middle layer, and an inner capsular layer that forms the anterior portion of Tenon's capsule. In the upper lid of the human being, the capsulopalpebral head is analogous to the levator complex, which is composed of an aponeurosis and Müller's muscle. The lower lid has a retractor mechanism composed of two layers, a superficial layer inserting onto the lower border of the tarsus, the capsulopalpebral fascia (analogous to the levator aponeurosis of the upper lid), and Müller's muscle.

Some pertinent anatomic concepts about the upper lid can be understood from review of the sagittal diagram in Fig. 2A. The levator muscle originates in the periorbital tissues surrounding the lesser wing of the sphenoid bone, traverses the orbit (as a muscle) to Whitnall's ligament, and then becomes an aponeurosis. Six sites of attachment of the levator complex are important for the surgeon. The primary attachments include those fibers that pierce the orbicularis oculi at or near the junction of the pretarsal and preseptal muscle groups, insert in the skin, and thus create the lid fold. Additional attachments of the aponeurosis include those to the anterior tarsus. Some authors suggest that the anterior attachments are to the lower third of the tarsus. Our surgical dissections (Fig. 2B) confirm the findings of Anderson and Beard (5), who concluded that the fibers insert firmly to the lower two-thirds of the anterior tarsus with wispy attachments to the upper third. The levator aponeurosis has a strong lateral horn that divides the lacrimal gland into palpebral and orbital lobes and then attaches to the orbital tubercle and the lateral canthal tendon. The somewhat weaker medial horn inserts at the posterior lacrimal crest and periorbita of the medial orbital wall. Fibers extend from the undersurface of the levator muscle toward the conjunctival fornix and create the suspensory ligament of the fornix. Müller's muscle originates 12 to 14 mm above the tarsus, is situated posterior to the aponeurosis, and serves as yet another attachment of the levator complex. The levator muscle is innervated by the superior ramus of the third cranial nerve. In contrast, Müller's muscle is sympathetically innervated.

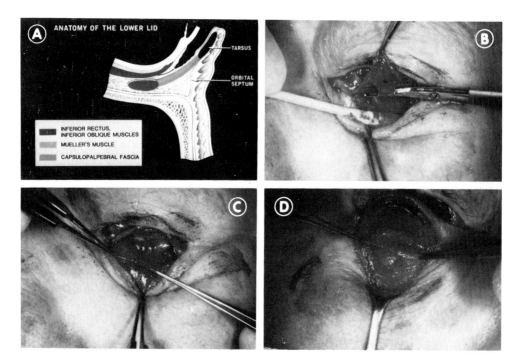

FIG. 3. **A:** Sagittal diagram depicting surgical anatomy of lower lid. **B:** Surgical photograph showing fornix attachments of conjunctiva. **C,D:** Lower lid retractor mechanism from the posterior and anterior approach.

The anatomy of the lower lid, similar to that of the upper lid, is shown in Fig. 3A. Both the upper and lower eyelids consist of the layers of skin, orbicularis muscle, tarsus, and conjunctiva. An aponeurosis, also termed the "capsulopalpebral fascia," can be identified in the lower lid. This fascia extends from the suspensory ligament of Lockwood to the lower border of the tarsus. It functions as a retractor in that the movement of the eye downward allows depression of the lower eyelid through this connection between the suspensory ligament and the tarsus. Although Jones (1) stated that the capsulopalpebral fascia inserts onto the inferior border of the tarsus, I am not certain that this is the case. To be completely analogous to the levator aponeurosis, the capsulopalpebral fascia should insert onto the anterior tarsus and also send fibers through the orbicularis to insert into the skin and create the lower lid fold.

As in the upper lid, Müller's muscle is readily identified in the lower lid posterior to the capsulopalpebral fascia. The most posterior extension of Müller's muscle and capsulopalpebral fascia surround the inferior oblique muscle and form part of the sheath (2). In the lower lid, one can readily identify fibrous bands that arise from the undersurface of Müller's muscle and insert into the conjunctiva; these bands form the inferior suspensory ligament of the fornix, as shown in Fig. 3B. Figures 3C,D illustrate that the capsulopalpebral fascia in the lower lid can be isolated surgically from either an anterior or a posterior approach.

The orbital septum is depicted in both sagittal diagrams (Figs. 2A and 3A). In the upper lid, the septum drapes onto the anterior surface of the levator muscle after it has become tendinous at approximately the level of Whitnall's ligament. The septum attaches to the aponeurosis at variable distances above the superior border of the tarsus. A central fat pad lies between the levator aponeurosis and the orbital septum. Incising the orbital septum from an anterior surgical approach exposes the preaponeurotic fat space. In the lower lid, the septum drapes over the anterior surface of the capsulopalpebral fascia and fuses with the fascia at variable distances from the inferior tarsal border. The orbital septum encloses the preaponeurotic fat space inferiorly. A strong bond of fascia between the orbital septum and the deeper capsulopalpebral fascia separates the larger nasal fat pad from the smaller temporal fat pad. We do not believe that there are three separate fat pockets in the lower eyelid, as mentioned in some reports.

Three further observations related to surgical anatomy are important. First, an unnamed space exists between the levator aponeurosis and Müller's muscle. This postaponeurotic space is important surgically because it must be identified during the conjunctival–Müller's muscle recession procedure. Second, the dictum that orbital fat always identifies the prea-poneurotic space in the upper and lower eyelids is not invariably true. Orbital fat can be present within the compartment of Müller's muscle, as shown in Fig. 2C. Finally, it should be emphasized that dissection and severance of the primary attachments of the levator aponeurosis to the skin alter the position of the lid fold. Such dissections increase the distance between the lid fold and the lash margin. Dissection of these attachments can alter the arch of the upper eyelid more than any other surgical maneuver.

DIFFERENTIAL DIAGNOSIS OF EYELID RETRACTION IN THYROID EYE DISEASE

The most common eyelid malposition in thyroid eye disease is lid retraction, the differential diagnosis of which is summarized as follows:

Graves' disease
Neurologic disease—Marcus Gunn phenomena; midbrain disease; hydrocephalus;
    parinaud's syndrome; trauma to cranial nerve III; aneurysm involving cranial nerve III
Sympathomimetic drugs
Cirrhosis
Congenital
Postsurgical retraction—ptosis surgery; lid reconstruction

Thyroid eye disease is by far the most common cause of eyelid retraction; however, upper eyelid retraction may be of neurologic importance. Paradoxical retraction may be noted in patients with the Marcus Gunn pupillary phenomenon. The most common neurologic cause of lid retraction is midbrain disease, especially involving the posterior commissure. For example, Collier's sign is lid retraction in the presence of midbrain disease. Eyelid retraction may be seen after trauma or with faulty regeneration of cranial nerve III after recovery from a bleeding intracranial aneurysm. This has been attributed to misdirection of cranial nerve III fibers. Walsh and Hoyt (6) observed lid retraction in patients with impending tentorial herniation. The instillation of sympathomimetic drugs into the conjunctival sac can be a cause of eyelid retraction. Summerskill and Molnar (7) have noted eyelid retraction more frequently in patients with hepatic cirrhosis than in the general population. Posey (8) has described retraction of the upper eyelids in a youngster presumed to have chorea.

Upper eyelid retraction can occur temporarily among infants whose mothers have thyroid dysfunction during pregnancy. Neonatal hyperthyroidism is rare (9), and most infants have lid retraction that has been attributed to long-acting thyroid stimulator (LATS) substances or other humoral substances that have crossed the placenta (10). We have observed one infant, approximately 1 year of age, with unilateral upper lid retraction that seemed to be a congenital abnormality. It is of interest that the mother had been treated for thyrotoxicosis when she was a child. Results of laboratory studies of her child have been normal to date.

Fascinating case studies have been reported by Johns et al. (11) and Givner (12). Johns et al. described the presence of bizarre involuntary movements of the eyelids and other eyelid muscles, including eyelid retraction, in a patient with thyrotoxicosis and myasthenia gravis. Givner reported on a myasthenic patient whose eyelids were "raised and lowered like marionettes." We have seen a similar patient with hyperthyroidism and no clinical or laboratory evidence of myasthenia. In this patient, severe eyelid retraction alternated with severe ptosis two to three times per minute. After several weeks this pattern was followed by permanent ptosis.

The common causes of lower eyelid retraction are the following:

Graves' disease
Postsurgical retraction—inferior rectus recession; blow out fracture repair
Posttraumatic
Postinflammatory
Congenital

The etiologic factors are similar to those in the upper lid. Thyroid disease is again the most frequent associated disorder. Iatrogenic complications related to surgical correction of strabismus are a cause of lower eyelid retraction. We have had to repair lower lid retraction after recession of the inferior rectus muscle because the capsulopalpebral fascia was displaced posterior to the original inferior rectus insertion. Upper eyelid retraction has been reported after recession of the superior rectus muscle for a similar reason (13). Repair of blow-out fractures can be followed by lower lid retraction if a subcilial incision is employed and scarring between the orbital septum and the lower eyelid retractors occurs. Posttraumatic causes of lower lid retraction include the more severe fractures with displacement of the inferior orbital rim, appreciable soft tissue injuries, and burns. Inflammatory orbital disease, e.g., Wegener's granulomatosis, can cause contracture of the lower lid tissues and resultant eyelid malposition. We have repaired congenital lower eyelid retraction that was associated with flattening of the malar eminence.

PATHOPHYSIOLOGICAL MECHANISMS OF EYELID MALPOSITION

In a classic report during the late 1930s, Pochin (14) was the first investigator to describe the mechanisms of eyelid retraction. The many factors that contribute to eyelid retraction are the following:

Thyrotoxicosis
Abnormal sympathetic tone
Inferior rectus contracture and fibrosis
Proptosis
Levator muscle contracture and fibrosis
Adnexal fibrosis
Overmedication

Abnormal sympathetic tone is thought to account for some element of upper lid retraction, producing excessive contraction of Müller's muscle (15). Evidence that increased sympathetic activity plays a role in lid retraction is found in the use of sympatholytic drugs, e.g., topical guanethidine sulfate: The 5% solution is less toxic to the cornea than the 10% solution, provides some relief of eyelid retraction, and causes miosis. Its use in the management of this disorder is limited because of the minimal relief of symptoms, lack of availability, and poor stability of the eyedrops (16).

Contracture and fibrosis of the inferior rectus muscle can stimulate overaction of the superior rectus muscle (in an attempt to maintain primary gaze position) and the levator muscle because of the common fascial sheaths and common embryologic origin of these two muscles. Evidence supporting this concept is found in the relief of upper lid retraction observed immediately after recession of the inferior rectus muscle.

Proptosis together with eyelid retraction, if both are of sufficient magnitude, can result in subluxation of the globe. The relief of proptosis rarely improves eyelid retraction completely, although the management of retraction becomes easier when proptosis is minimized.

Fibrosis of the levator muscle can be etiologically important in lid retraction. As with other extraocular muscles in thyroid disease, the levator muscle may be extremely large. Substantial enlargement is easily observed on coronal CT scans. The pathologic process is one of fibrosis and contracture leading to lid retraction. Adnexal fibrosis is important. Many patients with thyroid eye disease exhibit fibrosis and contracture of the soft tissues of the eyelid. The distal levator complex may be involved in an intense inflammatory process that diffusely involves the full thickness of the eyelid. The result can be eyelid malposition. Patients who are overmedicated with thyroid replacement or who are actively thyrotoxic exhibit eyelid retraction, at least some of which can be relieved with the adjustment of medical therapy or correction of hyperthyroidism.

The pathophysiological mechanisms in lower lid retraction are similar to those in upper lid retraction, although additional features are present. The mechanisms of lower eyelid retraction are summarized as follows:

Thyrotoxicosis
Abnormal sympathetic tone
Superior rectus contracture
Proptosis
Inferior rectus recession
Adnexal fibrosis
Overmedication

A normal sympathetic tone may play a role in lower lid as well as in upper lid retraction. Contracture of the superior rectus muscle and concomitant overactivity of the inferior rectus muscle can result in lower lid retraction because of the origin of the lower lid capsulopalpebral fascia. Proptosis complicates the correction of lower lid malposition. Recession of the inferior rectus muscle can be associated with lower lid retraction if the procedure is not accompanied by an attempt to free the insertion of the capsulopalpebral fascia from its origin at the suspensory ligament of Lockwood. Adnexal fibrosis, if present in the lower lid, can contribute to retraction. Overmedication with thyroid supplement can make lower lid retraction worse.

A less common eyelid malposition in thyroid eye disease is ptosis, which we have observed in five circumstances, as summarized here:

Myasthenia gravis
Levator aponeurosis disinsertion
Surgical repair of eyelid retraction

Transantral ethmoidal decompression
Idiopathically in association with eyelid retraction

Myasthenia gravis is associated with thyroid eye disease. Indeed, the patients with ptosis and thyroid disease should be assumed to have myasthenia gravis until proved otherwise. Improvement of ptosis with the use of intravenous Tensilon is the most useful single test. Antibodies to acetylcholine receptor are diagnostic of myasthenia gravis. In our experience, however, these antibodies are detected in only one-fourth to one-half of patients with ocular myasthenia.

Ptosis can result from disinsertion of the levator aponeurosis in the patient with thyroid-associated lid edema. One should be suspicious of an aponeurotic defect in the presence of severe ptosis, good levator function, a high lid fold, and thinning of the eyelid tissues allowing the color of the iris to be observed through the skin of the closed eyelid.

Ptosis may follow the surgical repair of eyelid retraction. We have observed profound bilateral ptosis in one patient immediately after transantral ethmoidal decompression. In 10 weeks, the ptosis completely cleared and was followed by lid retraction. Finally, we have noted rhythmic alternating ptosis and lid retraction in one patient, as noted earlier in this section.

Lower lid entropion in thyroid eye disease is almost exclusively a complication related to orbital decompression procedures, particularly transantral ethmoidal decompression. When it occurs, the lower lid is more entropic medially than temporally. The condition may resolve after a few months without treatment; however, we have found that most cases of entropion do not improve without surgical intervention. Tarsal fracturing procedures and other conventional entropion repairs are not helpful. The basic pathophysiological disturbance is oblique and downward traction of the lower lid retractors created by the decompression procedure. Recession of the lid retractors relieves this problem.

Lateral canthal obliquity sometimes follows decompression and is the result of malposition of the globe, not of the canthus. If the orbital floor is removed excessively during the decompression procedure, or if bony supports to the floor are insufficient, downward displacement of the globe results, and the lateral canthal angle has the appearance of being displaced upward. Such malposition can interfere with lid closure and can cause exposure keratitis as well as a cosmetic blemish.

MEASUREMENT OF EYELID RETRACTION

Our inability to quantify surgical procedures for relief of lid retraction may be related to our inability to measure lid retraction precisely. Measurement of the vertical height of the lid fissures is of no help in thyroid eye disease because the lower lids are often retracted, and thus the baseline from which vertical measurements are taken is variable. Moreover, measurements are dependent on the direction of gaze. The use of photography may be the best approach to evaluating lid retraction. One can project the image of the upper face and take measurements with a rule or a grid. Photography, however, does not capture the second-to-second variability in lid retraction that is so often present and that may be critical in assessing the magnitude of retraction. Measurement of lid retraction should be based on the clinical judgment of the trained observer as much as on taking a photograph under standardized lighting conditions or measurement with a millimeter rule.

As with ptosis, mild and severe degrees of upper lid retraction may be assessed more accurately than moderate degrees. The normal upper lid arch is approximately 1.5 to 2.0 mm below the 12 o'clock limbus. This position is usually midway between the upper border of the pupil, the size of which must be assessed, and the limbus. In mild lid retraction (1.0 to 2.0 mm), the lid is at or slightly above the 12 o'clock limbus. In severe lid retraction (5.0 to 8.0 mm), patients exhibit obvious stare. The sclera becomes glaringly prominent. In this situation, the millimeter rule can be used; the distance from the upper lid margin to the 12 o'clock limbus is measured and then 1.5 to 2.0 mm is added, which is the distance below the upper limbus at which most normal lids rest in primary gaze.

Moderate upper lid retraction (3.0 to 4.0 mm) is more difficult to measure and is often more variable than mild or severe retraction. The judgment of the observer is important in the assessment of the magnitude of retraction. It is helpful to assess the average amount of scleral baring in millimeters above the 12 o'clock limbus as one observes the patient in the office setting and then add 1.5 mm for the desired normal position. Once the patient knows that measurements are being taken, inaccuracies occur.

The lower lid margin normally is at the lower limbus. In contrast to the upper lid, lower lid retraction is relatively constant. Nonetheless, a variation of approximately 1 mm in normal lower lid position is associated with changes in facial expression—the lids move up with smiling. The use of the millimeter rule held vertically allows the examiner to determine whether retraction is mild, moderate, or severe (i.e., 2, 3, or 4 mm, respectively, between the limbus and the lower lid margin).

UPPER EYELID RETRACTION

Indications for Correction

Patients seeking correction of upper eyelid retraction may be grouped into four categories. Most patients, particularly those who have conspicuously asymmetrical lid retraction, seek correction for cosmetic reasons. A second group includes patients who complain of ocular discomfort and photophobia. In the third group, patients have objective evidence of keratitis, with or without corneal ulceration, and may urgently require a corrective procedure. Finally, a rare patient has a history of subluxation of the globe because of severe retraction of the eyelids and severe proptosis. Each patient may have one or more than one indication for operation.

Methods

Our current methods of repair evolved over the last 10 years, during which time more than 350 upper eyelid operations were performed in patients with thyroid eye disease. Early attempts at correction using well-tested methods were only partially successful.

Current Surgical Technique

Upper eyelid retraction should be corrected with the patient under local anesthesia and with the use of little or no sedation to allow cooperation between the patient and the surgeon. We prefer infiltrative anesthesia, achieved by injecting an agent just beneath the conjunctiva, followed by 10 to 15 min of massage. This method disturbs the tissue planes very little, makes them more visible because bleeding is minimized, and does not interfere appreciably with levator function or action of the protractors. Infiltrative anesthesia with added epinephrine prolongs the anesthetic time and achieves better hemostasis. The lid-elevating effect from epinephrine acting on Müller's muscle is of short duration and does not interfere with assessment of the lid arch or lid position.

Our technique is a staged procedure during which one, a combination of several, or all of five operative maneuvers may be chosen by the surgeon to correct the defect. The choices are made in a systematic and orderly manner. The decision to proceed with any of the surgical options is dependent on the intraoperative appearance of the lid arch and lid position. The list of options is as follows:

1. Recession of Müller's muscle and the conjunctiva
2. Transection of attachment of the levator aponeurosis to the anterior tarsus
3. Stretching of the levator aponeurosis
4. Transection of the primary attachments of the levator aponeurosis (the attachments that create the lid fold)
5. Temporal tarsorrhaphy

Figures 4A–Q depict an operative sequence on one patient in whom all five options were used. Figure 4A shows the patient's preoperative appearance in primary gaze. The upper lid is infiltrated with lidocaine hydrochloride (Xylocaine) and bupivacaine hydrochloride (Marcaine) with epinephrine, and the site is massaged for approximately 10 min. The eyelid is everted. A scalpel incision is then made through the conjunctiva and Müller's muscle for a distance of 3 to 4 mm in the central third of the eyelid, as shown in Fig. 4B. By using an iris spatula as a guide, the space between the levator aponeurosis and Müller's muscle is identified just above the tarsus, and Müller's muscle is severed from the upper tarsal border (Fig. 4C). In Fig. 4D the conjunctiva and Müller's muscle are maximally recessed. Care is taken to transect fully the fine attachments of Müller's muscle to its medial and lateral extents as well as centrally. The eyelid is then returned to its normal anatomic position, and the lid arch and the lid height are examined. In Fig. 4E Müller's muscle myotomy and recession have been completed on the right upper lid. Relief of lid retraction varies from patient to patient with this maneuver. Because only minimal change was noted in this case, we proceeded further. In Fig. 4F, the attachments of the levator aponeurosis are being severed from the anterior surface of the tarsal plate from canthus to canthus in order to weaken those attachments partially responsible for the malposition. This is the second of the five possible steps. Figure 4C shows the almost complete release of the attachments, allowing the tarsus to be rotated nearly 180°. Note that in Fig. 4H the right upper lid has been lowered slightly. This photograph shows the patient looking up slightly, a position that makes the right upper lid appear lower than it actually is. When assessing the eyelid, the surgeon must be aware of the gaze position of the patient. Further work is needed to achieve a satisfactory result.

In Fig. 4I the levator aponeurosis is being stretched vertically. As advocated by Tenzel, this maneuver is carried out along the entire width of the lid. Again, the lid arch and position are assessed after this third maneuver. As noted in Fig. 4J, some improvement has been achieved, but 1.5 mm of right upper lid retraction persists.

The fourth step is to transect the primary attachments of the levator aponeurosis to the skin. The surgeon may perform more or less dissection, depending on two factors: the concern of the patient regarding overcorrection and the unilateral or bilateral nature of the case. The dissection must be performed slowly; small groups of fibers are incised, and the lid position is assessed frequently. This caution is necessary because the release of small numbers of fibers can relieve large amounts of retraction. In Fig. 4K the aponeurosis is incised horizontally with a scissors along the upper tarsal edge. Figure 4L shows the surgeon severing those attachments of the aponeurosis that pass through orbicularis oculi to the skin.

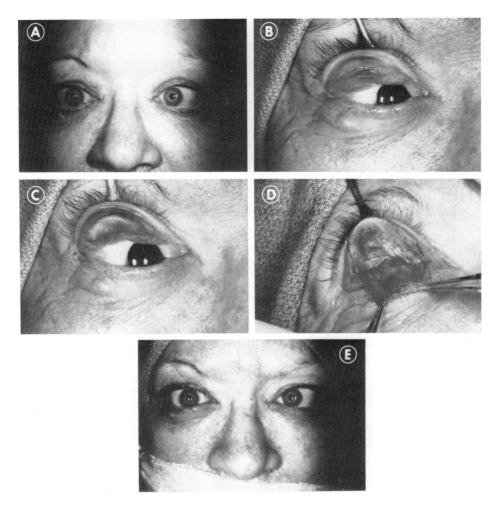

FIG. 4. A: Preoperative photograph. **B:** Müller's muscle myotomy. **C,D:** Müller's muscle recession. **E:** Intraoperative assessment of Müller's muscle surgical procedure on right upper lid. **F,G:** Transection of aponeurotic attachments to anterior tarsus. **H:** Intraoperative assessment of surgical procedure on right upper lid. **I:** Levator stretching. **J:** Intraoperative assessment after stretching of levator aponeurosis. **K,L:** Resection of primary attachments of levator aponeurosis. **M,N:** Tarsorrhaphy technique. **O:** Intraoperative assessment after tarsorrhaphy. **P,Q:** Preoperative and postoperative photographs of recession of both upper lid retractor mechanisms.

The final step that may be necessary is to add a temporal tarsorrhaphy. Figures 4M,N depict the salient features of the tarsorrhaphy, which we prefer to keep as simple as possible. The lid margins are abraded for a distance of 3 to 4 mm and then stitched together with 4-0 chronic catgut suture and a semicircular cutting needle. Figure 4O shows the patient who was still on the operating table after all five of the surgical options on the right upper eyelid had been completed. Figures 4P,Q are preoperative and immediately postoperative pictures, respectively, of the same patient after bilateral surgical procedures on the upper eyelid.

This photographic sequence illustrates our current approach to the management of upper eyelid retraction. Local anesthesia does not impede progress; rather, it allows cooperation between the patient and the surgeon. No one of these maneuvers provides the desired result,

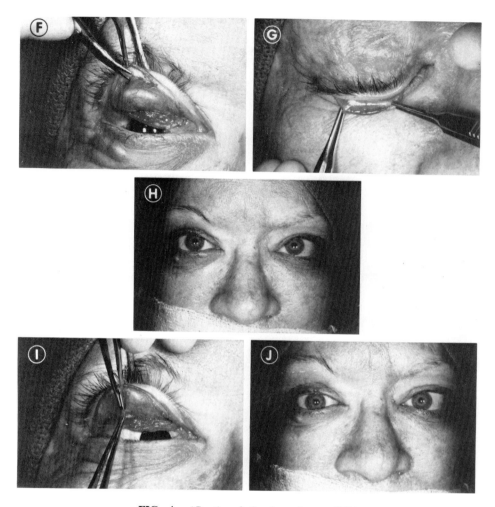

FIG. 4.   *(Continued. See legend on p. 273.)*

but a combination of several or all can achieve it in most instances with minimal operating time, less swelling than with the scleral grafting technique, and few complications. In our experience, this approach has allowed us to avoid setting rigid guidelines with respect to the quantity of surgical correction to be performed. Judgments are made intraoperatively on the basis of the response of the patient to a variety of manipulations, any one of which may have a broad range of effects.

Results

The pre- and postoperative photographs of selected patients from our series of eyelid operations are shown in Figs. 5A–N. Figures 5A,B are pre- and postoperative photographs of the repair of right upper lid retraction. No levator stretching or transection of levator attachments to the anterior tarsus were performed. Müller's muscle myotomy and recession were accomplished, followed first by transection of the primary levator attachments and then by tarsorrhaphy, which helped to suspend the right lower lid and minimize scleral baring inferiorly. The eyelids of the patient shown in Figs. 5C,D with moderate left upper

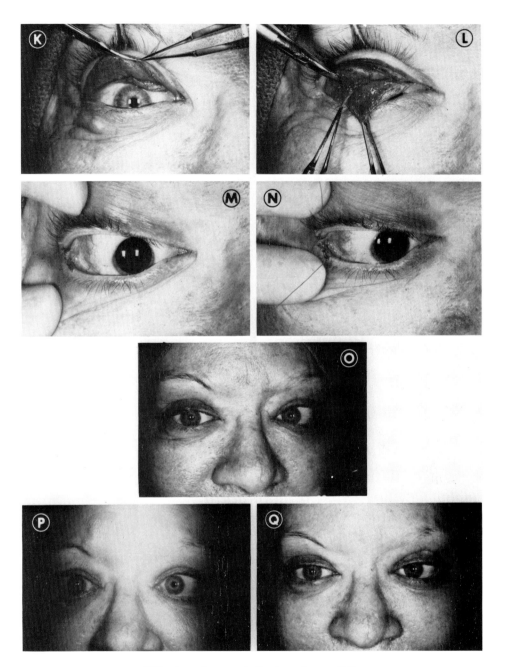

FIG. 4. *(Continued. See legend on p. 273.)*

lid retraction were repaired using all options except tarsorrhaphy. In the cases represented by Figs. 5E,F and 5G,H, tarsorrhaphy was performed in addition to all other options.

The patients depicted in Figs. 5I,J and 5K,L required all five operative maneuvers to correct, respectively, moderate and severe bilateral, symmetrical upper lid retraction. Even though the patient in Figs. 5M,N demonstrated equally severe bilateral upper lid retraction,

PREOPERATIVE   POSTOPERATIVE

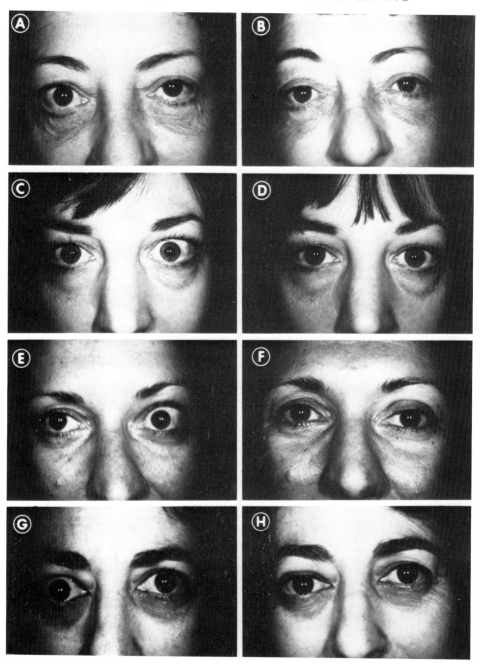

FIG. 5.   A–N: Preoperative and postoperative photographs of seven patients showing repair of upper lid retraction by current techniques.

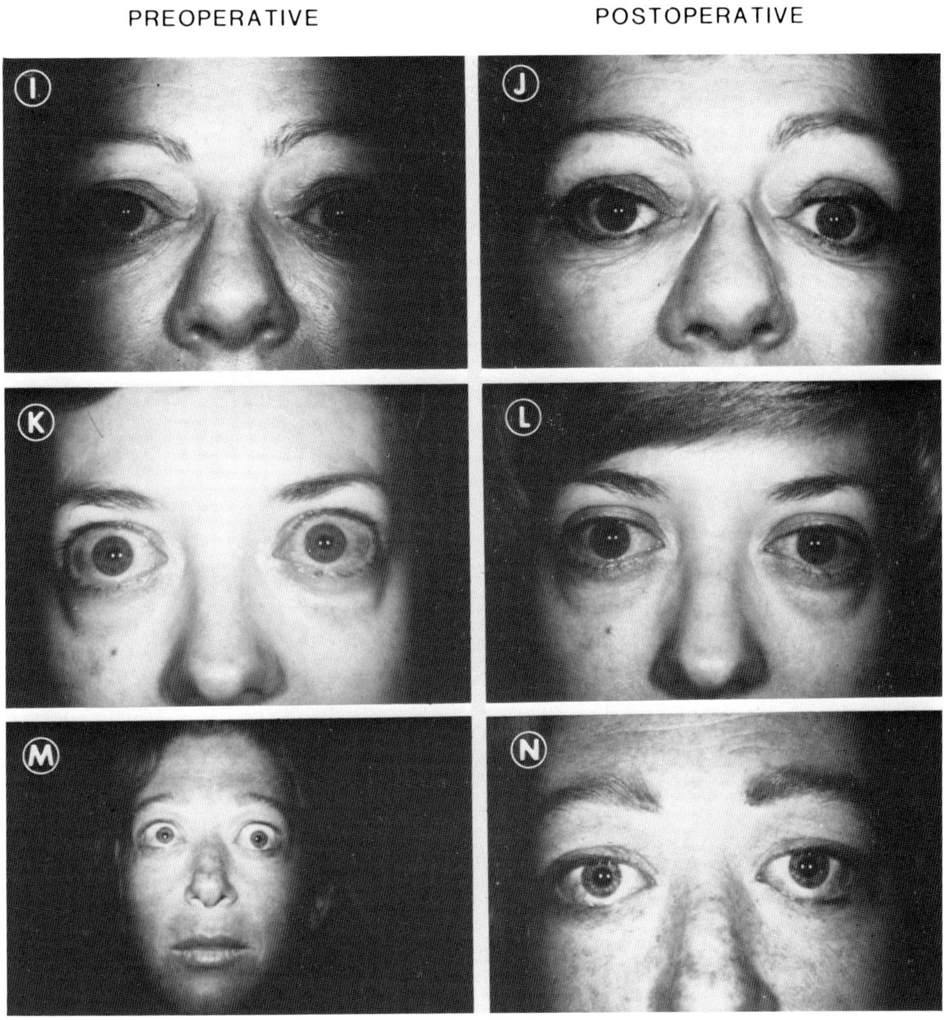

PREOPERATIVE   POSTOPERATIVE

FIG. 5. *(Continued)*

effective lid lowering was accomplished with only two maneuvers: (a) Müller's muscle myotomy; and (b) recession and transection of the levator attachments to the anterior tarsus. The case presentations in Fig. 5 illustrate the variability of response to individual surgical maneuvers and thus underscore the importance of the outlined approach.

Complications

The photographs in Figs. 6A–M depict the major complications that can be encountered. Figures 6A,B show pre- and postoperative photographs of a repair of upper lid retraction that resulted in undercorrection on the right and overcorrection on the left. Dissection was obviously inadequate on the right, perhaps because of faulty intraoperative assessment of lid position. Dissection on the left was too aggressive for similar reasons. The patient in Figs. 6C,D shows the temporal obliquity that can be observed when inadequate attention is given to the strong levator aponeurosis attachments. Further recession, perhaps with tarsor-

PREOPERATIVE   POSTOPERATIVE

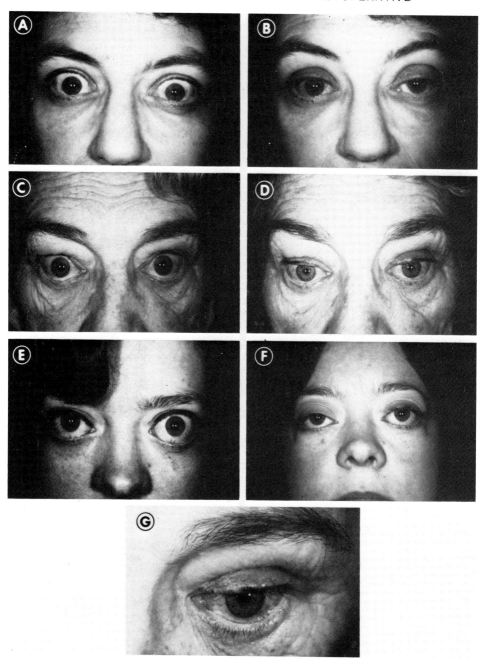

FIG. 6. **A,B:** Preoperative and postoperative photographs of patient with upper lid retraction; note undercorrection of right eyelid and overcorrection of left eyelid. **C,D:** Another patient before and after bilateral levator recessions; note temporal eyelid flare. **E,F:** Another patient who underwent levator recession of left upper eyelid; note apparent ptosis of right upper lid. **G:** Loss of lashes after damage to lash roots during resection of levator attachments to anterior tarsus. **H–K:** Postsurgical ptosis and repair with scleral graft. **L,M:** Concealment of upper lid retraction by redundant upper lid skin and brow droop.

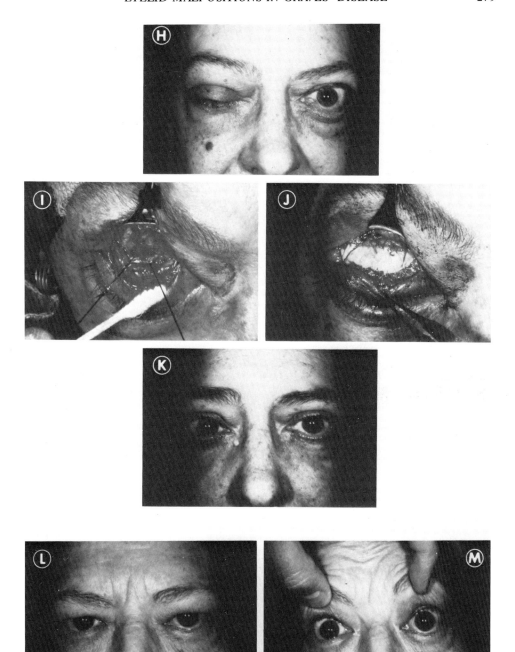

FIG. 6. *(Continued)*

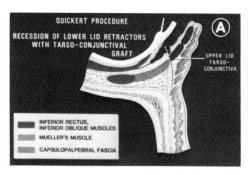

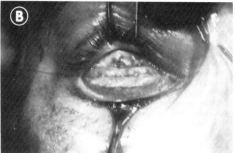

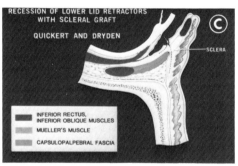

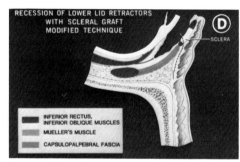

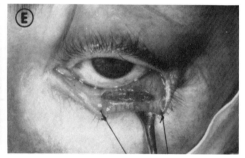

FIG. 7. A: Sagittal diagram depicting Quickert procedure. **B:** Surgical photograph of placement of upper lid tarsoconjunctiva after recession of lower lid retractors. **C:** Procedure first described for placement of scleral grafts into lower lid. **D,E:** Modified approach employing an intratarsal incision to facilitate retractor recession. **F,G:** Isolation of lower lid retractors. **H,I:** Scleral graft sutured in place. **J:** Examples of shapes of scleral grafts for placement into lower lids. **K:** Photograph one day postoperatively, showing mattress sutures through lower lid anchored to a cotton bolus. **L:** Scleral graft in place 6 weeks postoperatively.

rhaphy, is necessary to correct this malposition. Figures 6E,F show slight overcorrection of the left upper lid repair, and, surprisingly, the appearance of ptosis postoperatively of the right upper lid. In Fig. 6G there is a loss of cilia from the upper lid related to an overzealous resection of levator attachments to the anterior tarsus inferiorly.

Almost complete ptosis followed repair of upper eyelid retraction in the patient shown in Fig. 6H. Nine months later the right upper eyelid was explored anteriorly, the free levator aponeurosis was identified, and a large scleral graft was sutured to its distal end and then to the upper tarsus. This is shown in Figs. 6I,J. Figure 6K shows the result 1 year after repair of the ptosis.

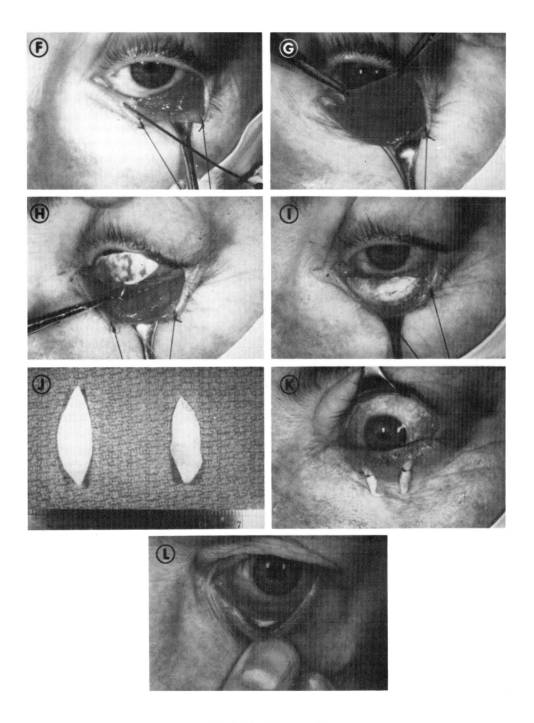

FIG. 7. *(Continued)*

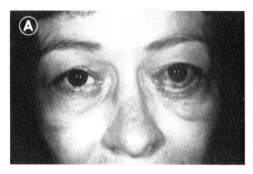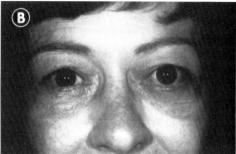

FIG. 8. **A:** Preoperative photograph of patient with left lower lid retraction. **B:** Photograph of same patient 1 year after placement of scleral graft in left lower lid.

The patient in Fig. 6L requested blepharoplasty. In this patient, dermatochalasis masked the presence of bilateral, moderately severe upper lid retraction, as shown in Fig. 6M. We have encountered patients who were dissatisfied with results of blepharoplasty because of the presence of eyelid retraction, which was not discussed with them preoperatively and which was masked by the redundant upper eyelid skin. This is not a complication of eyelid retraction repair, but it is important to mention as part of a discussion on complications.

LOWER EYELID RETRACTION AND ENTROPION

Indications for Correction

The indications for repair of lower eyelid retraction are similar to those for the upper eyelid and are also divided into four groups. Retraction repair is indicated for cosmetic reasons in properly motivated patients. The second group consists of patients who complain of ocular discomfort and photophobia with lower lid retraction alone or with involvement of the upper and lower eyelid. Keratitis with or without corneal ulceration prompts repair in a third group. Finally, a patient may suffer from subluxation of the globe because of excessive lid retraction and severe proptosis.

The indications for repair of entropion are the same. It is important to emphasize that lower lid retraction can coexist with lower lid entropion.

Methods

Measures to relieve malpositions of the lower eyelid were only recently developed. Techniques of repair were stimulated by the new anatomic concepts of Jones (1) and Beard and Quickert (2). Henderson (17) suggested recession of Müller's muscle of the lower lid as a means to correct lower eyelid malposition, but this method was only partially successful. Other procedures, e.g., Beard's tenotomy procedure, were advocated for repair of lower eyelid retraction (C. Beard, *oral communication*, January 1973). The most notable advance, however, began with Quickert and Dryden's report (18), which advocated the use of scleral transplantation as a means to correct lower eyelid retraction and to buttress the lower eyelid after recession of the lower lid retractors. Others followed with their modifications of this new procedure.

Figures 7A,B illustrate the original concept of repair of lower lid malposition, in which patients with upper lid ptosis and lower lid retraction were managed by upper lid tarso-myectomy, and the upper lid tarsus was preserved for the lower lid buttress after recession

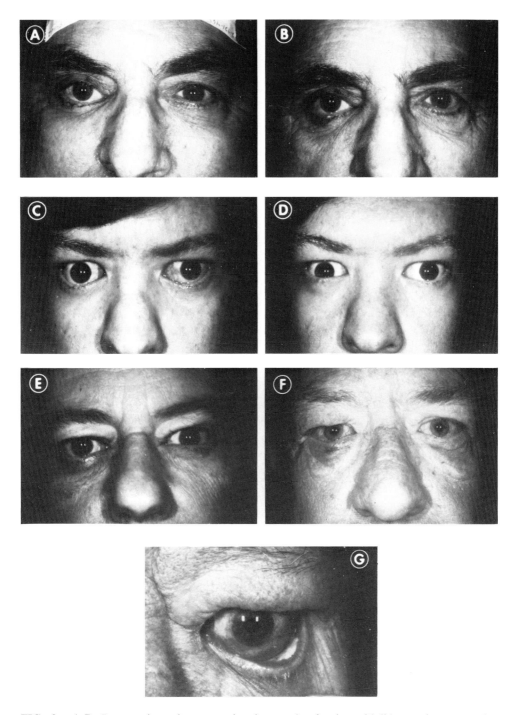

FIG. 9. **A,B:** Preoperative and postoperative photographs of patient with lid retraction; note undercorrection of right lower lid. **C,D:** Another patient before and after placement of scleral grafts in both lower lids; note overcorrection of right lower lid. **E:** Postoperative obliquity of left lower lid arch. **F:** Suture abscess of right lower lid. **G:** Migration of scleral graft.

of the lower lid retractor mechanism. The concept of scleral transplantation soon followed and is diagrammed in Fig. 7C. A previously reported modification of the recession procedure is diagrammed in Fig. 7D (19). The point of emphasis is with the placement of an intratarsal incision, as shown in Fig. 7E. This allows for the block resection of conjunctiva, Müller's muscle, and capsulopalpebral fascia attached to a tarsal remnant (Figs. 7F,G). This approach facilitates dissection, minimizes bleeding, and makes suturing of the scleral graft easier, as shown in Figs. 7H,I. The scleral graft is spindle-shaped (Fig. 7J). The height of the graft is 2.5 to 3 times the amount of vertical correction desired. Figure 7K shows an immediate postoperative result, with mattress sutures in place to tamponade the graft. Figure 7L depicts epithelialization of the graft 6 weeks postoperatively.

Results

Figures 8A,B show preoperative and 1-year postoperative results after recession of the left lower lid retractors and placement of a scleral graft. This patient had previously undergone a 4-mm recession of the left inferior rectus muscle for correction of vertical strabismus related to thyroid myopathy.

Complications

To our knowledge, detailed descriptions of the incidence and types of complications associated with this operation have not been reported. The most common complication is undercorrection of lid retraction, as shown in Figs. 9A,B. This result is related, in part, to our inability to quantitate preoperatively the size of the graft that is required; it is also partially related to graft contraction over time. Dryden and Soll (20) expressed the opinion that an immunologic rejection process probably accounts for scleral shrinkage. Their conclusions were based, in part, on a histologic study reviewed in written communication with Yanoff (1977).

Although overcorrection is unusual in our experience, it does occur. Figures 9C,D show pre- and postoperative photographs of lower lid repairs with scleral grafts. The left lower lid repair is satisfactory; the right lower lid repair shows overcorrection several months postoperatively. An additional complication is obliquity of the lid arch, as shown in the left lower lid in Fig. 9E. This complication occurs when the graft is too small or is sutured too far nasally. Suture abscess, such as that shown in Fig. 9F, and pressure necrosis with graft exposure on the skin surface can occur, but they can be minimized with the use of a less-reactive suture, e.g., nylon, and the avoidance of trauma to the orbicularis during the procedure so that a muscular cushion is present between the scleral graft and the lower eyelid skin. Graft migration, as shown in Fig. 9G, is related to poor suturing technique. Transient lid edema subsides within a few weeks. Corneal abrasions from the suture line can be avoided by suturing with fine plain catgut, with knots buried in the nasal and temporal fornices. Constant attention to the lacrimal excretory system during the medial dissection prevents transection of the inferior canaliculus.

As mentioned previously, lower lid entropion, especially medially, seems to be a problem unique to the patient who has undergone transantral ethmoidal decompression. It may occur independently or with eyelid retraction. When entropion exists alone, repair can usually be achieved by recessing the lower lid retractor mechanism without placing a scleral graft. The patient shown in Fig. 10A–F illustrates our approach to entropion when it exists alone or in association with mild lower eyelid retraction. The right lower eyelid was entropic, as shown in Figs. 10A,B. Recession of the lid retractor mechanism is accomplished with special

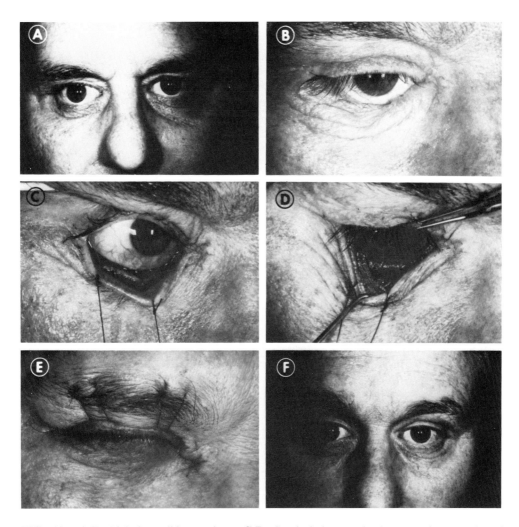

FIG. 10. A,B: Right lower lid entropion. **C,D:** Surgical photographs demonstrating recession of lower lid retractor mechanism. **E:** Photograph on first postoperative day with traction sutures in place. **F:** Photograph 3 months postoperatively.

attention given to the medial half of the eyelid where the entropion is usually the most prominent, as noted in Figs. 10C,D. The lower lid is sutured upward to the brow for 1 week, as depicted in Fig. 10E. The postoperative result, 3 months later, is shown in Fig. 10F.

STATISTICAL ANALYSIS OF SURGICAL RESULTS

No published studies have analyzed statistically the types of eyelid repair in a large number of patients with Graves' disease. Such studies may be beneficial because they can help to determine which procedure or combination of procedures is most efficacious. It has been our impression that results have improved during a 10-year experience, during which time a total of more than 350 operations have been done.

Caution must be used in retrospective studies of this kind, as they can yield only a limited amount of useful information. Our patients were not participants in a randomized or controlled study. In our approach to the study, however, we posed several important questions. What were the common factors in the signs and symptoms of patients with eyelid retraction related to Graves' disease? Which of these factors could be attributed to retraction only, and which could be attributed to a more dynamic loss of muscle function that could not be simply measured in terms of static lid retraction? What were the effects of using sutures in recession techniques, particularly in the upper lid? What were the effects of using scleral grafting materials in the relief of eyelid retraction? What was the efficacy of a combination of surgical procedures as they related to the repair of upper lid retraction?

Methods

The records of patients who underwent their first surgical procedure for lid retraction caused by Graves' disease between January 1, 1977, and December 30, 1980, were reviewed. This process yielded a total of 77 patients. Patients who had coexistent lid disease from other causes were excluded from this study. Data were collected on a procedure-by-procedure basis; and associated ocular findings of Graves' ophthalmopathy, the amount of preoperative eyelid retraction, the nature of the operation, the amount of postoperative eyelid retraction, and the complications of surgical procedures were encoded. The amount of eyelid retraction was determined not only from measurements in the patient's chart but also from photographs analyzed by an observer who had no prior knowledge of the patient or the surgical procedure. Most of the patients had pre- and postoperative photographs taken in the primary position gaze.

With respect to rotational involvement, we considered our patients to have abnormalities in extraocular movements if any restriction in the cardinal fields of gaze was recorded for one or more extraocular muscles. Proptosis was considered to be present if >20 mm was measured with the Krahn exophthalmometer in either eye or if there was a >3 mm difference between the two eyes. In most of our patients, we used the presence of positive rose bengal staining as the indicator of corneal involvement. Definite chemosis and injection had to be present for signs of congestive ophthalmopathy to be recorded. We defined optic nerve involvement as loss of visual acuity and visual field in the absence of other ocular disease. All patients with optic neuropathy had field loss established at least by a tangent screen examination.

The encoded data were subjected to standard statistical tests, including determination of the mean, median, and standard deviation (SD) for each of the variables as well as the determination of significance by using the chi-square test and Pearson's correlation coefficient. When analyzing ocular findings associated with lid retraction, we grouped patients into three categories—those with 1 to 2 mm of lid retraction (mild), those with 3 to 4 mm of lid retraction (moderate), and those with 5 mm or more of lid retraction (severe)—to minimize small differences among these patients and to minimize the effect of variability among observers.

Seventy-seven patients underwent a total of 104 operations that included 139 upper eyelid procedures and 50 lower eyelid procedures for a total of 189 separate eyelid procedures. This information is summarized in Table 1. We excluded the third and fourth procedures of three patients from subsequent statistical analysis. This resulted in 185 eyelid procedures for study.

Results

Population Characteristics

The population characteristics of our patients are summarized in Table 1. The mean age of the group was 47 years, and the range was 17 to 78 years. A substantial preponderance

TABLE 1. *Lid retraction in Graves' disease: 77 patients (1977–1980)*

General information:
  154 Eyes in patients with Graves' ophthalmopathy with eyelid retraction ranging
      from 0 to 8 mm
  104 Operations
      135 Upper lid procedures—114 first procedures; 21 repeat procedures
      50 Lower lid procedures—46 first procedures; 4 repeat procedures
      185 Separate eyelid procedures
Population characteristics:
  Age
      Mean, 47 years
      Median, 49 years
      Range, 17–78 years
      Five highest—65, 67, 67, 67, 78
      Five lowest—17, 18, 20, 25, 25
  Sex—9 male; 68 female
Clinical status at time of first operation:
  Supplemental thyroid—71% on; 29% off
  Clinical status—1% hypothyroid; 99% euthyroid
  Serum T_4—8% > normal; 81% normal; 11% < normal
Decompression prior to surgery:
  Transantral decompression—bilateral, 44; unilateral, 0; none, 33
  Elapsed time between decompression and eyelid surgery (first operation)—mean,
      18 months; median, 13 months; range, 3–77 months
Muscle surgery prior to surgery for lid retraction:
  Muscle surgery
      Vertical procedure   13
      Horizontal procedure   8
      Both procedures   59
      No procedure   74
      Total   154 eyes
  Elapsed time between muscle surgery and eyelid surgery (first operation)—
      mean, 12 months; median, 7 months; range, 0–66 months

---

of women was noted. At the time of the first operation, 71% of patients were taking supplemental thyroid medication, 99% were considered to be euthyroid preoperatively as evaluated by an internist, and 81% had a normal level of total serum thyroxine.

Relationship to Other Procedures

As noted in Table 1, transantral orbital decompression was performed in more than half of our patients before their eyelid operations. In every instance, the transantral decompression was bilateral. The mean elapsed time between transantral orbital decompression and the first eyelid operation was 18 months, with a range of 3 to 77 months.

Table 1 also provides data relative to the performance of surgical correction of strabismus in our patient population. In most instances, correction of squint was done before operation for lid retraction.

Five patients had concomitant strabismus and eyelid retraction operations, one of whom had had such concomitant procedures on two occasions. The mean elapsed time between muscle operation and the first eyelid operation was 12 months, and the range was 0 to 66 months.

Eye Findings

We analyzed our patients with eyelid retraction to determine the relationship between eyelid abnormalities and other findings of Graves' disease according to the American Thyroid

TABLE 2. *Presenting findings in 77 patients with eyelid retraction due to Graves' disease at the time of first operation*

ATA classification	Not present	Unilateral	Bilateral
Class I: eyelid retraction	1	12	64
Class II: chemosis, injection	44	4	29
Class III: proptosis (20/3)	35	8	34
Class IV: rotational involvement	23	4	50
Class V: corneal involvement	51	4	22
Class VI: optic neuropathy	70	4	3

TABLE 3. *ATA classification findings versus eyelid retraction in 154 eyes[a]*

Retraction (mm)	Class II +	Class II −	Class III +	Class III −	Class IV +	Class IV −	Class V +	Class V −	Class VI +	Class VI −	No.
None	2	25	6	21	11	16	5	22	2	25	27
1	3	0	2	1	2	1	1	2	1	2	3
2	14	24	11	27	23	15	11	27	4	34	38
3	15	22	20	17	31	6	15	22	1	36	37
4	8	16	18	6	15	9	7	17	1	23	24
5	6	3	5	4	8	1	0	9	0	9	9
6	5	2	5	2	6	1	3	4	0	7	7
7	8	0	8	0	7	1	5	3	2	6	8
8	1	0	1	0	1	0	1	0	0	1	1
χ_3^2	28.72		29.06		16.15		3.04		χ_2^1 177		
	<0.001		<0.001		<0.1		0.39		18		

[a]Data taken from first encounter with 77 patients who eventually had eyelid retraction surgery.

Association (ATA) classification. Table 2 depicts the relationship between eyelid retraction and the other classes of involvement in Graves' disease at the time we initially saw our patients. Rotational involvement (class IV) was the most common associated finding, followed by the presence of proptosis (class III) and then chemosis and injection (class II). When class V findings were present (corneal involvement), most patients had bilateral involvement of the corneas; in contrast, when the class VI finding of optic neuropathy was noted, an equal number of patients had unilateral and bilateral involvement. Review of our class I findings of eyelid retraction revealed that most patients (64) had bilateral eyelid retraction, whereas in 12 patients it was unilateral. Eyelid retraction was not considered to be present in one patient. This patient did have Graves' disease with obliquity of the lid arch, however, and this was repaired at the patient's request.

Table 3 illustrates the correlation between the classes of eye involvement and the degree of eyelid retraction. The findings of chemosis and injection (class II), proptosis (class III), and extraocular rotation involvement (class IV) were significantly related to the degree of lid retraction, but corneal involvement (class V) and optic neuropathy (class VI) were not. From the statistical standpoint, these data represent 77 observations, as 77 pairs of eyes were analyzed. Patients with findings in one eye, in our opinion, tend to have similar findings in the other eye. Because of this, we compiled similar data for all right eyes as

TABLE 4. *Indications for first surgical repair of eyelids[a]*

Indication	None	Unilateral	Bilateral
Pain	34	12	31
Photophobia	58	2	17
Cosmetic	12	18	47
Corneal involvement	51	5	21
Subluxation	76	0	1

[a]Some patients had more than one indication.

TABLE 5. *Indications at time of first procedure on an eyelid as a function of lid retraction (upper lids only)*

Retraction (mm)	Pain		Photophobia		Cosmetic		Corneal staining	
	+	−	+	−	+	−	+	−
0–2	8	23	2	29	12	19	3	28
3–4	15	45	8	52	27	33	12	48
5–7	6	17	6	17	10	13	4	19

compared with all left eyes, and the findings were the same as the findings noted in Table 3 with respect to statistical significance.

We analyzed the multifactorial relationships among corneal changes, rotational abnormalities, and degree of retraction. As retraction increased, there was an increased incidence of corneal involvement combined with rotational involvement. When retraction was 0 to 2 mm, 11 (16%) of 68 patients had both corneal and rotational involvement. When retraction was from 3 to 4 mm, 17 (28%) of 61 patients had both. When retraction was 5 mm or more, nine (36%) of 25 patients had both. This trend was not quite statistically significant ($p = 0.09$). Patients who had involvement of the extraocular muscles showed no increase in corneal involvement as retraction increased. In patients with corneal involvement, there was a trend toward increased involvement of the extraocular muscles with greater degrees of retraction, but this trend also was not statistically significant ($p = 0.13$).

Indications for Operation

The data in Table 4 depict the indications for surgical repair at the time each of our 77 patients had the first operation. Some patients had more than one indication. Of importance is the fact that the major indication for eyelid operation was cosmetic. In only one of our cases was subluxation of the eyelids behind the globe an indication. Analysis of these data also revealed that cosmesis was the sole indication for surgery in 54 eyelids, the presence of pain and cosmesis were indications in 47 instances, and pain alone prompted surgery in 13 instances.

We analyzed the four indications for which sufficient data were available to determine if an association existed between the degree of lid retraction and any one or more indications for surgery. These data are depicted in Table 5. We found that there was no statistically significant association between any of the indications for operation and the degree of eyelid

TABLE 6. *Use of anesthesia*

Procedure	Local with i.v.	General	Local without i.v.
First operation			
Upper lids only	50	1	—
Both lids	12	3	1
Lower lids only	7	3	—
All operations			
Upper lids only	58	1	—
Both lids	24	6	2
Lower lids only	9	4	—

retraction ($p > 0.10$ for each group when lid retraction was grouped into 2 mm or less, 3 to 4 mm, and 5 to 7 mm).

Anesthesia

Table 6 depicts the use of anesthesia at first operation and at all operations. At first operation, general anesthesia was selected for 10% of our patients. These seven patients received general anesthesia because they were anxious and because we anticipated a prolonged operating time. Similarly, for all operations, general anesthesia was used in about 10% of patients. A few patients in whom local infiltrative anesthesia was used did not require intravenous sedation.

Surgical Procedures

Surgical procedures performed on the upper lids were analyzed according to frequency in Table 7. This table shows only the first and second procedures performed on upper eyelids. The most frequently performed combination of procedures was Müller's muscle myotomy and recession and transection of the primary attachments of the levator aponeurosis at the upper border of the tarsus. Thirty-eight patients (28% of our patient population) underwent this combination of surgical procedures. The next most frequent approach to upper eyelid retraction was Müller's muscle myotomy and recession combined with the transection of the levator attachments to the anterior tarsus, which was performed in 25 patients (19% of the population). Of the 135 upper eyelids operated on, 90 eyelids required transection of the primary attachments of the levator aponeurosis to accomplish an effective repair.

The efficacy of the six most common procedures performed for upper eyelid retraction is analyzed in Table 8. In terms of producing change, the data show that Müller's muscle myotomy and recession combined with transection of the attachments of the levator aponeurosis to the anterior tarsal plate and transection of the primary attachments of the levator aponeurosis was the most effective procedure, producing a mean change in eyelid retraction of 3.4 mm (group C). This was followed closely by the group of patients in whom Müller's muscle myotomy and recession was performed, followed by transection of the primary attachments of the levator aponeurosis combined with a tarsorrhaphy (group D). The third group of patients in whom there was a large mean change between pre- and postoperative measurements was the group that underwent Müller's muscle myotomy and recession and transection of the primary attachments only (group A).

The range of change which each of these combinations of procedures produced in pre- and postoperative measurements of lid retraction is striking. For example, patients undergo-

TABLE 7. *Methods used (all upper lid procedures) by frequency*

	Müller's Myotomy	Transection of Levat Attach to Ant Tarsus	Levator Stretching	Transection 1° Attachments	Tarsorraphy
38	●			●	
25	●	●			
19	●	●		●	
16	●			●	●
12	*			●	
11	●				
5	●	●	●		
3					●
2	●	●	●	●	
2	●	●		●	●
1	●		●		
1	*			●	●

*Already done on previous operation

TABLE 8. *Efficacy of the six most common procedures for eyelid retraction: A comparison*

	Müller's Myotomy	Transect Anterior	Levator Stretch	Transect Primary	Tarsorph	N	Mean Pre	Mean Post	Mean change	Range of Change
A	▬			▬		38	3.8	0.6	3.2	0-7
B	▬	▬				25	2.6	0.7	1.9	0-2
C	▬	▬		▬		19	4.3	0.9	3.4	0-7
D	▬			▬	▬	16	4.4	1.2	·3.2	1-7
E	▬			▬		12	1.7	0.9	0.8	0-3
F	▬					11	2.3	0.7	1.6	0-3

ing Müller's muscle myotomy and recession, transection of the anterior attachments to the tarsal plate, and transection of the primary attachments of the levator aponeurosis (group C) had a range of change of 0 to 7 mm.

We analyzed the data to determine if an association existed between the amount of eyelid retraction present when the patient was first seen and the number of procedures ultimately

TABLE 9. *Amount of retraction at presentation is not a predictor of how many procedures will be required to fix the retraction (upper lids)*

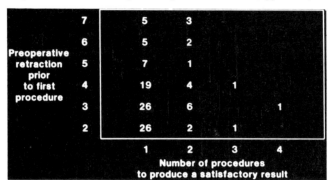

		1	2	3	4
Preoperative retraction prior to first procedure	7	5	3		
	6	5	2		
	5	7	1		
	4	19	4	1	
	3	26	6		1
	2	26	2	1	

Number of procedures to produce a satisfactory result

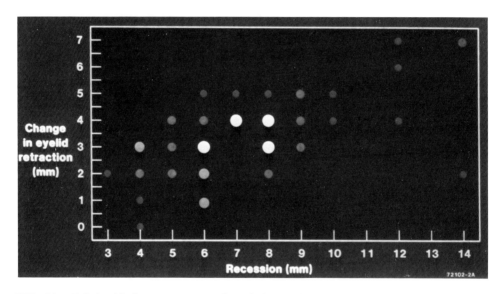

FIG. 11. Relationship between amount of surgical recession and amount of correction at time of first operation on each upper eyelid. Smallest dot represents single patient; the next larger dot represents two patients; each large gray dot represents three patients; and each large white dot represents four patients.

required to correct upper eyelid retraction. The data (Table 9) show that the amount of upper eyelid retraction seen initially was not a predictor of how many procedures would be required to achieve a satisfactory result. Sufficient data did not exist to report this analysis for repair of lower lid retraction because we had only four repeat procedures on lower eyelids during this 4-year period.

Figure 11 illustrates that a direct relationship does exist, however, between the millimeters of retractor recession performed at the first operation for repair of upper eyelid retraction and the change in the amount of eyelid retraction that was achieved. For each 1 mm of retraction that was corrected, 2 mm of recession was accomplished. Pearson's coefficient of 0.62888 is significant ($p < 0.0001$).

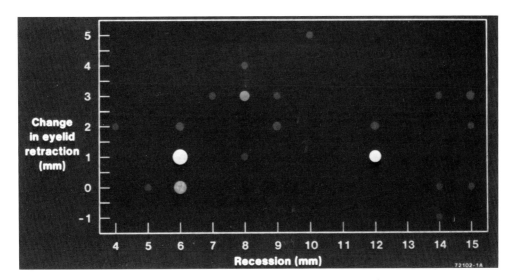

FIG. 12. Relationship between amount of surgical recession and amount of correction at time of first operation on each lower eyelid. Size conversion is identical to that of Fig. 11. Large gray dot represents seven patients; large white dot represents eight patients.

Figure 12 depicts the result of 50 procedures for lower eyelid retraction. The mean preoperative lid retraction was 2.2 mm, the mean postoperative lid retraction was 0.7 mm, and the mean change produced in 46 lids was 1.5 mm. Producing relief of lid retraction in repeat lower eyelid operations was more difficult; we achieved a mean change of 0.3 mm. The data in Fig. 12 show that for the lower lid no relationship exists between the millimeters of retractor recession that are performed and the degree of change in the eyelid retraction.

Special Considerations: Effect of Sutures on Retractor Recession of the Upper Lid

We have been uncertain about the efficacy of placing a running plain catgut suture between the underbelly of the orbicularis muscle and the recessed levator aponeurosis, Müller's muscle, and conjunctiva. To assess the effects of such sutures during repair of upper eyelid retraction, we compared those who were repaired with sutures with those repaired without any suture material. There was no statistical difference between the two groups preoperatively; however, a statistically significant difference did exist postoperatively (Table 10). Patients undergoing a repair with sutures had a mean change in lid retraction of 4.23 mm compared with a mean change of 3.26 mm in those patients who were repaired without sutures. For procedures that were performed identically except for the addition of suture placement to the recessed upper eyelid retractor mechanisms, a mean difference of 1.1 mm was found.

Efficacy of Scleral Grafts

Before this 4-year series, the use of upper lid scleral grafts had been abandoned. We do, however, have experience with a large number of lower eyelid operations in which scleral grafts were used in an attempt to correct retraction. In addition, we had the opportunity to compare the efficacy of scleral grafts in the treatment of lower eyelid retraction with lower eyelid retractor recession alone.

TABLE 10. *Effect of sutures on retractor recession*

Retraction	mm
With sutures (13 lids)	
Mean preoperative retraction	4.46
Mean postoperative retraction	0.23
Mean change	4.23
Without sutures (49 lids)	
Mean preoperative retraction	4.20
Mean postoperative retraction	0.94
Mean change	3.26

Sutures significantly enhance the amount of recession achieved ($p = 0.027$ for mean change).

TABLE 11. *Efficacy of scleral grafts in lower eyelid procedures*

Eyelids	Mean	SD	Median	Range
Eyelids with scleral grafts ($N = 18$)				
Preop retraction	3.4	1.0	3.5	2 to 5
Postop retraction	1.1	1.0	1	0 to 3
Difference	2.3	1.1	2	0 to 5
Patients without scleral grafts ($N = 32$)				
Preop retraction	1.5	1.1	2	0 to 3
Postop retraction	0.6	0.9	0	0 to 3
Difference	0.9	1.2	1	−1 to 3

Table 11 depicts the data comparing all lower eyelid procedures done with and without scleral grafts. Eighteen eyelids underwent scleral grafting. These eyelids had a mean preoperative retraction of 3.4 mm and a mean postoperative retraction of 1.1 mm. Patients who had recession of lower eyelid retractors without placement of scleral grafts had a mean preoperative retraction of 1.5 mm and a mean postoperative retraction of 0.6 mm. Statistical analysis showed that these two groups were quite different preoperatively. Patients who had scleral grafts had more preoperative retraction than did patients who did not receive grafts. Of nine patients who had more than 3 mm of preoperative lid retraction, all had scleral grafts. Preoperative versus postoperative retraction for these patients is plotted in Fig. 13. Forty-nine of 50 eyelids were either unchanged or improved by surgical intervention. A single eyelid showed more retraction postoperatively. Of five patients who began the operation with eyelid retraction and who were unchanged by the procedure, four did not have scleral grafts. The eight patients who had preoperative retraction of zero underwent operative repair of medial entropion. Excluding these eight patients, 11 (46%) of 24 procedures without grafts failed to correct to zero. Eleven (61%) of 18 procedures with scleral grafts did not correct to zero. This difference, which suggested that it is difficult to attain "zero retraction" results with a scleral graft, was almost statistically significant ($\chi = 3.34$; $p = 0.07$).

Complications

Table 12 depicts the complications tabulated for lower and upper eyelid first procedures. The most common complication of upper eyelid surgery was ptosis. Of seven eyelids, six

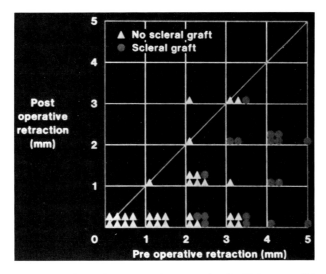

FIG. 13. Graph of preoperative and postoperative retraction in 50 lower eyelids with and without scleral grafts.

had ptosis of 1 mm or less, and one had ptosis of 2 mm. Three eyelids had obliquity of the lid arch. Two had a lid fold disturbance (which was regarded as separate from an obliquity of the lid arch). Two eyelids had persistent lid edema. Other complications were isolated.

In the first procedures for the lower eyelid, two eyelids had cyst formation within a scleral graft, two had worsening of preexisting keratitis, one had a lid arch obliquity, and one had a migration of the scleral graft. Of the six complications for the first lower lid procedure, half were associated with a scleral graft, although scleral grafts were done in only one-third of all first lower eyelid procedures.

The complications encountered in performing repeat (second) procedures are also listed in Table 12. The complication rate for 21 reoperations in the upper lid was 19%, and in the lower lid it was 50%. The total number of repeat operations, however, was small.

Complications of upper and lower eyelid operations not encountered by us within the framework of this series are also given in Table 12. We have encountered these complications outside of the period of this study. Among the 160 first eyelid procedures, there were 24 complications—a complication rate of 15%.

Discussion

Population Characteristics

Our population characteristics were consistent with those reported in other series of patients with Graves' ophthalmopathy (21). The female/male ratio was about 7:1. As we have previously stated, the metabolic status did not correlate with the signs and symptoms of Graves' ophthalmopathy. The total serum thyroxine level at the time that our patients were first seen was recorded as normal, above normal, or below normal. More detailed serologic testing was occasionally necessary to delineate the specific thyroid abnormality, but not all of our patients had these studies. However, 99% were judged to be clinically euthyroid by an internist.

TABLE 12. *Complications*

Complication	No.
First procedures:	
Upper eyelids	
Ptosis	7
1 mm or less	6
2 mm	1
Obliquity of lid arch	3
Lid fold disturbance	2
Persistent lid edema	2
Lid fold disturbance with lid edema and corneal erosion	1
Obliquity of lid arch with lid edema	1
Leaking of tarsorrhaphy	1
Hematoma	1
Lower eyelids	
Preexisting keratitis made worse than before	2
Granulomatous cyst	2
Obliquity of lid arch	1
Graft migration	1
Second procedures:	
Upper eyelids	
Obliquity of lid arch	1
Ptosis	1
Preexisting obliquity not corrected	2
Lower eyelids	1
Preexisting keratitis worse than before	1
Lower lid granuloma	1
Not encountered in this series:	
Upper eyelids	
Loss of cilia	
Infection	
Lower eyelids	
Graft exposure	
Infection	
Persistent lid edema	
Transection of canaliculus	
Keratitis	
Graft shrinkage	

Relationship to Other Procedures

Early in our experience, and for convenience for our patients, surgical correction of strabismus was performed concomitantly with eyelid procedures. This approach was abandoned because of the complexities involved in attempting to quantitate the amount of lid retraction during alteration of the vertical muscles. In addition, general anesthesia was required for most strabismus operations, which placed us at a disadvantage in eyelid repair.

With regard to the relationship to other procedures, the surgical rehabilitation of the patient with Graves' ophthalmopathy begins with decompression, followed by a strabismus operation; it ends with procedures on the eyelids. In some cases, surgical correction of strabismus antecedent to decompression can cause acute corneal decompensation if proptosis is borderline. The release of tight rectus muscles allows the globe to come forward and makes exposure more likely, particularly in the presence of impaired motility. Generally, in those patients whose measurements are 22 mm or greater on Krahn exophthalmometry, and who require surgical correction of strabismus, decompression should be considered in order to avoid corneal complications (22). Eyelid operations should be performed when orbital procedures have been completed, when extraocular muscles have been rearranged, and when the clinical picture is stable.

Eye Findings: ATA Classification

In the absence of control data, statements about our patients in comparison with all patients with Graves' disease cannot be made. Of the six main classes of involvement of the eye common to Graves' disease, eyelid retraction was obviously the most prevalent in these patients. The second most common finding was rotational involvement, followed by proptosis, injection, and chemosis. In the presence of retraction, these patients had a tendency to have keratitis when the rotations were involved. This is not seen in Table 3 because the data are not displayed in a multifactorial fashion. Before this study, it was our clinical impression that patients exhibiting severe eyelid retraction often had no corneal involvement when rotational disturbances were minimal. In contrast, severe corneal involvement was noted in patients with mild eyelid retraction if motility disturbance was severe. The frequency of rotational involvement with corneal involvement does, in fact, increase as retraction increases. In our patients who had involvement of the rotations, an increase in retraction was not accompanied by a significant increase in corneal involvement. None of our measurements reflected the disturbance in eyelid movement and the blink in patients with Graves' disease. Indeed, these data call attention to the need to evaluate these factors.

Indications for Operation

The most common indication for operation in our series was cosmetic; however, in a substantial number of patients, pain was a major factor in arriving at a decision for surgical intervention. The pain was usually of corneal origin. The amount of lid retraction was not helpful with respect to which indications for operation were present.

Anesthesia

Early in our experience, general anesthesia was commonly used when lower eyelid surgical procedures were performed. However, local anesthesia became the preferred approach to the repair of lower eyelid retraction when our operating time became shorter and thus patients were able to tolerate the procedure better. For upper eyelid procedures, local anesthesia is mandatory for assessment of changes in the relief of eyelid retraction on a minute-to-minute basis, as the retractor mechanism is released. Currently, virtually all patients are managed with local, infiltrative anesthesia, rather than regional or general anesthesia.

Surgical Procedures

Müller's muscle myotomy and recession were performed on most patients because we chose to approach the eyelid retractors from the conjunctival side. Patients not having Müller's muscle myotomy and recession were those who underwent tarsorrhaphy only or those who had had a previous procedure. When the muscle was maximally recessed at the time of the first operation, it usually did not reattach. Review of Table 8 shows that the common denominator among the most effective procedures was transection of the primary attachments of the levator aponeurosis at the upper border of the tarsal plate as they pierce the orbicularis oculi to create the lid fold. Although transection of the primary attachments was the most efficacious, a compromise had to be made in terms of alteration of the lid fold. If lid retraction is to be relieved, the lid fold must be raised. Patients must be made aware preoperatively that the lid fold will be altered even when the surgical result is satisfactory.

The data show that Müller's muscle myotomy and recession alone produce an average of 1.5 mm of a lid-lowering effect. Transection of the primary attachments is usually responsible for an additional 2 mm of lid lowering. When transection of the levator attachments to the anterior tarsus is added to the operative procedure, another 0.5 mm of relief of eyelid retraction seems to be obtained. These impressions are not only from mean observations from our statistics but also from individual observations of our patients.

The range of change in relief of eyelid retraction within each group of patients varied considerably. For example, Müller's muscle myotomy and recession, transection of levator attachments to anterior tarsus, and transection of primary attachments resulted in a range of change from 0 to 7 mm. Müller's muscle myotomy and recession alone resulted in a range of change from 0 to 3 mm. This variability underscores the difficulty in the repair of these patients and the imperfections in our technique.

The data in Table 9 show that one cannot predict how many procedures will be necessary on the basis of the degree of eyelid retraction. Before this study, we would have assumed that greater degrees of eyelid retraction would necessitate more operations than mild retraction, but the data do not support that assumption. Patients must be informed in advance of the potential need for repeat procedures.

In Fig. 11, a relationship, though variable, is demonstrated between millimeters of recession and relief of eyelid retraction in the upper lid. This permits some guidelines for the surgeon when the recession is being performed. For example, 4 mm of recession may be required for 2 mm of eyelid retraction, or 14 mm of recession may be required for 7 mm of eyelid retraction. No such relationship exists for the lower lid.

Special Considerations: Effect of Sutures on Retractor Recession of the Upper Lid

The use of sutures in levator recession can enhance an effective repair. For the same amount of surgical correction, sutures may increase the effect by about 1 mm. We prefer to use a running 6-0 plain catgut suture with knots tied in the nasal and temporal fornices to anchor the recessed eyelid retractor mechanism to the underbelly of the orbicularis oculi.

Efficacy of Scleral Grafts

For our 50 lower lid procedures, those patients having scleral grafts had substantially more preoperative lid retraction than those not having scleral grafts; thus the two populations were not comparable. The data suggest that repair of lower eyelid retraction both with and without grafts may be successful in completely relieving retraction about 50% of the time. Although they were not significant, the data indicate that it may be more difficult to obtain a perfect result when a graft is used. Alternative graft materials may be useful in obtaining a more reliable result in correcting lower lid retraction.

Complications

The most frequent complication associated with first procedures on upper eyelids in our series was ptosis. We were encouraged by the finding, however, that six of seven eyelids with this complication had only 1 mm or less of ptosis and that a seventh had 2 mm of ptosis. We believe that ptosis is difficult to induce in patients who have Graves' disease. To the contrary, our major difficulty has been with undercorrection. Obliquity of the lid arch was characterized most commonly by temporal flare. This abnormality was a result of failure to adequately recess the stronger temporal horn of the levator complex. Later in this series, this complication became less frequent as we became more aggressive in recessing the temporal horn. We noted more complications associated with scleral grafting than without scleral grafting in the lower lid.

CONCLUSIONS

On the basis of our presentations in this chapter, the following conclusions can be made:

1. Chemosis and injection, proptosis, and extraocular muscle involvement are all associated with increasing degrees of eyelid retraction. Optic nerve involvement is not.

2. Corneal involvement in Graves' ophthalmopathy is more frequent if motility is affected.

3. The most common indications for repair of eyelid retraction are cosmesis, pain, and photophobia.

4. Local infiltrative anesthesia is necessary so that the patient's cooperation may be elicited, as surgical manipulations are assessed on a minute-to-minute basis. General anesthesia is best reserved for the rare, difficult procedure.

5. Once the patient's cooperation has been obtained, the choice of surgical procedure should depend on the known efficacy of the various components. The most frequent combination of procedures in our study was the performance of Müller's muscle myotomy and recession and transection of the primary attachments of the levator aponeurosis. The latter is the common denominator of all the most effective procedures.

6. It may be deduced that approximately 1.5 mm of a lid-lowering effect is produced by Müller's muscle myotomy and recession alone. On the average, transection of the primary attachments may be responsible for an additional 2.0 mm of lid lowering. Transection of levator attachments to the anterior tarsus results in about 0.5 mm of lid lowering. The placement of sutures may produce another 1.0 mm of effect.

7. The amount of eyelid retraction present is not helpful in determining how many procedures will be necessary to produce a satisfactory result.

8. The amount of surgical recession results in a somewhat predictable relief of retraction in the upper lid but not in the lower lid.

9. Scleral grafts are effective in producing some relief in lower lid retraction when the disorder is severe. The solution is not ideal, however, because use of scleral grafts is associated with more complications.

10. The complication rate for first procedures was 15% in this series. The complication rate increased when subsequent procedures were necessary.

REFERENCES

1. Jones, L. T. (1968): A new concept of the orbital fascia and rectus muscle sheaths and its surgical implications. *Trans. Am. Acad. Ophthalmol. Otolaryngol.*, 72:755–764.
2. Beard, C., and Quickert, M. H. (1969): *Anatomy of the Orbit: A Dissection Manual.* Aesculapius, Birmingham, AL.
3. Callahan, A. (1966): *Reconstructive Surgery of the Eyelids and Ocular Adnexa.* Aesculapius, Birmingham, AL.
4. Berke, R. N., and Wadsworth, J. A. C. (1955): Histology of levator muscle in congenital and acquired ptosis. *Arch. Ophthalmol.*, 53:413–428.

5. Anderson, R. L., and Beard, C. (1977): The levator aponeurosis: attachments and their clinical significance. *Arch. Ophthalmol.*, 95:1437–1441.
6. Walsh, F. B., and Hoyt, W. F. (1969): *Clinical Neuro-Ophthalmology*, Vol. 1, 3rd ed. Williams & Wilkins, Baltimore.
7. Summerskill, W. H. J., and Wolnar, G. D. (1962): Eye signs in hepatic cirrhosis. *N. Engl. J. Med.*, 266:1244–1248.
8. Posey, W. C. (1902): Unusual choreiform alterations in the width of the palpebral fissure of both eyes, occasioned by spasm of the levator palpebrae muscles. *J. Nerv. Ment. Dis.*, 29:419–421.
9. Ainslie, M. B. (1980): Thyroid disorders in children. *Bull. St. Louis Park Med. Clin.*, 24:233–246.
10. Lewis, I. C., and MacGregor, A. G. (1957): Congenital hyperthyroidism. *Lancet*, 1:14–16.
11. Johns, R. J., Knox, D. L., Walsh, F. B., and Renken, H. J. (1962): Involuntary eye movements in a patient with myasthenia and hyperthyroidism. *Arch. Ophthalmol.*, 67:35–41.
12. Givner, I. (1964): Abnormal movements of the lids. *Int. Ophthalmol. Clin.*, 4:45–53.
13. Schimek, R. A. (1972): Surgical management of ocular complications of Graves' disease. *Arch. Ophthalmol.*, 87:655–664.
14. Pochin, E. E. (1939): The mechanism of lid retraction in Graves' disease. *Clin. Sci.*, 4:91–101.
15. Gay, A. J., and Wolkstein, M. A. (1966): Topical guanethidine therapy for endocrine lid retraction. *Arch. Ophthalmol.*, 76:364–367.
16. Cartlidge, N. E. F., Crombie, A. L., Anderson, J., et al. (1969): Critical study of 5% guanethidine in ocular manifestations of Graves' disease. *Br. Med. J.*, 4:645–647.
17. Henderson, J. W. (1965): Relief of eyelid retraction: a surgical procedure. *Arch. Ophthalmol.*, 74:205–216.
18. Quickert, M. H., and Dryden, R. M. (1971): Lower eyelid advancement. Read before the American Society of Ophthalmic Plastic and Reconstructive Surgery, Las Vegas.
19. Waller, R. R. (1978): Lower eyelid retraction: management. *Ophthalmic Surg.*, 9:41–47.
20. Dryden, R. M., and Soll, D. B. (1977): The use of scleral transplantation in cicatricial entropion and eyelid retraction. *Trans. Am. Acad. Ophthalmol. Otolaryngol.*, 83:OP669–OP678.
21. Gorman, C. A. (1978): The presentation and management of endocrine ophthalmopathy. *Clin. Endocrinol. Metab.*, 7:67–96.
22. Dyer, J. A. (1976): The oculorotary muscles in Graves' disease. *Trans. Am. Ophthalmol. Soc.*, 74:425–456.

The Eye and Orbit in Thyroid Disease, edited by
C. A. Gorman et al. Raven Press, New York 1984.

Radiotherapy of Graves' Ophthalmopathy

*A. Pinchera, †L. Bartalena, *L. Chiovato, and *C. Marcocci

*Cattedra di Endocrinologia e Medicina Costituzionale and †Cattedra di Patologia Medica II,
University of Pisa, 56100 Pisa, Italy*

Orbital radiotherapy is currently used for the treatment of severe and progressive Graves' ophthalmopathy as an alternative to other major therapeutic measures, e.g., systemic corticosteroids and decompressive surgery. It may also be advantageously employed in combination with corticosteroids.

Radiotherapy of Graves' ophthalmopathy was introduced more than 50 years ago. Orthovoltage equipment delivering deep x-rays of relatively low energy were employed up to the early 1970s and have subsequently been replaced by supervoltage apparatus (linear accelerator, cobalt unit, or betatron) which provide high-energy x-rays with better collimation. In most of the early reports, the irradiation was primarily directed to the pituitary and the hypothalamus on the assumption that the eye changes were due to the hypersecretion of thyrotropin or a pituitary exophthalmogenic factor as a consequence of a hypothalamic dysfunction. As discussed elsewhere in this volume, the concept of a pathogenetic role of the pituitary in Graves' ophthalmopathy is no longer tenable, and several data indicate that this condition is related to autoimmune phenomena involving the retro-orbital tissues (8,12,20,45,46). Antibodies reacting with retro-orbital antigens (18), deposition of immune complexes (19), and/or cell-mediated immune reactions (22,30,41) have been implicated, but the precise mechanisms leading to the eye changes remain to be elucidated. Whatever the mechanisms, the most prominent histological changes are edema and a marked inflammatory infiltrate, consisting of lymphocytes and to a lesser extent plasma cells, mast cells, and macrophages (34). Gross enlargement of the extraocular muscles is the resulting macroscopic finding. The well-established radiosensitivity of lymphocytes provides the rationale for orbital radiotherapy of Graves' ophthalmopathy. The question of whether the effect of irradiation is due to suppression of a specific immune reaction or to a nonspecific anti-inflammatory effect remains to be clarified. An additional histological feature of Graves' ophthalmopathy is the increased content of hydrophilic intercellular mucopolysaccharides, which may contribute to the accumulation of local edema. Thus it is also conceivable that irradiation acts by reducing the secretion of hydrophilic glycosaminoglycans by retro-orbital fibroblasts.

The procedures, risks, and indications of radiotherapy of Graves' ophthalmopathy are discussed in the present review, and the results obtained in different series are analyzed with particular reference to our own experience. The role of orbital irradiation in relation to other forms of treatment is also considered.

RADIOTHERAPY PROCEDURES

Deep x-ray delivered by orthovoltage equipment (170 to 250 kV) has been used for several years. Methods of irradiation, dosimetry, and size and location of fields have varied considerably in different series. Irradiation was aimed to the pituitary (3,4,11,16), the orbits (11,16,17), or both regions (14,33,39). The hypothalamus was explicitly used as a primary target only in some instances (14,39), but it is conceivable that this region was encompassed by irradiation to the pituitary or the orbits due to the poor collimation of the x-rays delivered by orthovoltage equipment. Similarly, the orbits were also involved by x-rays directed to the pituitary and vice versa. It has been calculated that irradiation of the pituitary via a lateral field delivers roughly the same dose of x-rays to the posterior aspect of the orbits as to the pituitary (11). On the other hand, irradiation of the orbit via an anterior field may deliver up to 43% of the skin dose to the pituitary (17).

Two to four fields of variable size have been employed in different studies. Daily doses ranging from 50 to 400 rads were delivered per each field, and the total dose received by each patient over a period of 4 to 6 weeks ranged from 800 to 9,000 rads. These doses were calculated at the skin level. Owing to the low energy of the orthovoltage radiation, the actual dose delivered to the target tissues was considerably lower. A further drawback of this irradiation technique is the occurrence of substantial side scatter of x-rays, which may expose the lens and the anterior chamber of the eye to unnecessary radiation.

Many of these problems have been overcome by the availability of supervoltage apparatus, delivering well-collimated, high-energy x-rays. Kriss and his group (7,20) first applied supervoltage radiotherapy to the treatment of Graves' ophthalmopathy using a 4- to 6-meV linear accelerator. In this technique the x-ray beam was directed to the orbit, sparing the lens, cornea, pituitary, and hypothalamus. A lateral irradiation field was individualized to each patient and shaped to fit three anatomical landmarks: the lateral canthus of the eye (marked by a small lead piece), the anterior border of the sella turcica, and the upper limit of the maxillary antrum. The x-ray beam directed to this 4×5 cm triangular field was angled 5° posteriorly in order to avoid the contralateral lens. The correctness of the beam alignment was verified by a double-exposure film, in which the first exposure was limited to the treatment field and the second was made after opening the collimators. Particular care was taken to ensure a good collimation of the beam, keeping the edge of the field which slices posterior to the lens as sharp as possible. A total dose of 2,000 rads, divided in 10 equal daily fractions alternating left and right lateral fields, was delivered during a 2-week period. Similar procedures were adopted by other authors (5,6,42,44,48), using 4- to 6-meV linear accelerators. A modification of the technique for x-ray beam direction to protect the lens from irradiation was suggested by Covington et al. (6), who located the anterior margin of the radiation field 12 mm backward from the corneal plane marked by a fine pinpoint light. Kriss et al. (21) modified their original procedure, which employed a posterior angulation of the beam to protect the cornea and the lens. To this purpose, a beam-splitting technique with the central axis of the beam corresponding to the anterior border of the treatment field was used. This resulted in a more satisfactory distribution of orbital muscle irradiation while protecting the cornea and lens.

A betatron delivering 42-meV x-rays has been used for orbital radiotherapy by Fritsch et al. (10). Field sizes varied between 4×4 cm and 5×8 cm. In the latter case, the pituitary was encompassed by the radiation. A 3° posterior angulation of the x-ray beam was used to spare the lens. A total orbital dose of 1,600 rads, divided in eight equal daily fractions, was delivered over a 2-week period.

Cobalt units for supervoltage orbital radiotherapy of Graves' ophthalmopathy have been employed by several workers (5,10,13), including ourselves (2). We have been using cobalt equipment with a 50-cm source-to-skin distance. The radiation field (4×4 cm) had the anterior border located just behind the lateral canthus and the posterior border located just

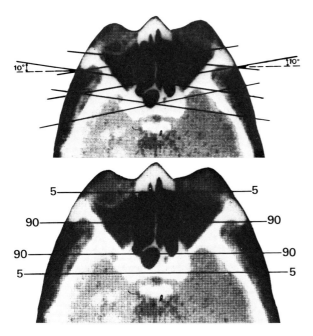

FIG. 1. Orbital cobalt radiotherapy. Radiation field superimposed on computerized transaxial scans of the orbits. **Top:** Left and right 4×4 cm fields are angled 10° posteriorly. **Bottom:** Typical isodose distribution. Values are expressed as a percentage of the midline dose. Doses delivered to the hypothalamus, pituitary, contralateral lens, and cornea are less than 5%. (From ref. 2.)

anterior to the sella turcica. The floor and the roof of the orbit represented the lower and upper limit of the radiation area. The field was angled 10° posteriorly in order to avoid irradiation of the contralateral cornea and lens. The head of the patient was stabilized by a head holder. The isodose distribution, analyzed by computer assisted tomography (CT), showed that the dose delivered to the lens, cornea, pituitary and hypothalamus was less than 5% (Fig. 1), with very low penumbra and side scatter. Ten daily doses of 200 rads were given in 2 weeks, up to a total dose of 2,000 rads to each eye calculated at midline. Essentially the same technique was used by Brennan et al. (5) and Grauthoff et al. (13), but a lower total dose (1,000 rads per eye) was given by the latter group of workers. The conditions adopted by Fritsch et al. (10) were similar to those described above for betatron irradiation. These included a total orbital dose of 1,600 rads and the use of two field sizes, one of which encompassed the pituitary.

Admittedly, the cobalt unit may not achieve the same degree of x-ray collimation with minimal penumbra provided by the linear accelerator. Due to the greater posterior angulation of the beam, generally required by cobalt radiotherapy units to spare the cornea and lens, the dose distribution to the extraocular muscles is not uniform. According to our calculation, variations in the medial rectus ranged from 5% at its anterior extremity to 90% at about midpoint.

Orbital irradiation may be combined with simultaneous systemic corticosteroid treatment. Any supervoltage unit may be used in association with prednisone or other steroids in this class in equivalent doses. Treatment schedules adopted in different centers have been variable (13,48). In our own institution (2), cobalt radiotherapy was combined with 6α-methylprednisolone. Corticosteroid treatment was started with 70 to 80 mg methylprednisolone daily for about 3 weeks. The dose was gradually tapered by 5 mg weekly until a daily dosage of 20 mg was reached, and thereafter by 2.5 to 5 mg every 2 to 3 weeks. Treatment was discontinued after 5 to 6 months. Large doses were administered parenterally by intramuscular injection, and small doses were given orally.

RISKS AND COMPLICATIONS OF ORBITAL RADIOTHERAPY

Orbital irradiation may carry the risk of unwanted damage to ocular and extraocular structures encompassed in the radiation field. Particular care should be used when planning the radiation procedure in order to spare the lens, cornea, pituitary, and hypothalamus. This may be achieved by the use of supervoltage apparatus delivering well-collimated high-energy x-rays and should be checked by an accurate evaluation of the isodose distribution. Untoward side effects are much more likely to occur with orthovoltage equipment because it is impossible to prevent the large penumbra and the considerable side scatter of the radiation. For this reason, the use of such equipment for the treatment of Graves' ophthalmopathy is no longer recommended. Although most of the complications listed below have been observed after radiotherapy of eye diseases other than Graves' ophthalmopathy, e.g., malignant tumors (15,25), they should be taken into consideration in any treatment involving the orbital region.

Transient Manifestations

Minor and transient side effects have been rather frequently observed in patients submitted to orthovoltage radiotherapy for Graves' ophthalmopathy. These included skin erythema, local epilation, headache, serous otitis, abnormal taste sensation, conjunctivitis, and an increase in periorbital edema (3,4,11,16,17,39). In patients submitted to supervoltage radiotherapy side effects have been much less frequent, the more common manifestations being a transient increase in periorbital and conjunctival edema (6,7). In our experience, this did not occur when cobalt orbital radiotherapy was combined with systemic corticosteroids. Mild headache, maculopapular facial rash, and eyelid erythema have occasionally been observed by some workers (5,42).

Lid, Conjunctiva, and Lacrimal Apparatus

Inflammatory changes of the eyelids and conjunctiva due to radiation may be followed by sequelae including lid deformities (entropion or ectropion), epiphora, keratinization of the palpebral conjunctiva, atrophy and telangiectasia of the skin and conjunctiva. Exposure of the lacrimal glands to radiation may result in qualitative and quantitative changes of the tears, leading to dry and irritable eyes and keratitis. These complications have not been reported in patients submitted to orbital radiotherapy for Graves' ophthalmopathy.

Cornea

The normal cornea is said to be radioresistant, but this may not be the case when sepsis and trauma or other predisposing conditions, e.g., exposure keratitis associated with proptosis and chemosis, are present. Direct irradiation of the cornea without special protection may induce pericorneal injection, heralded by the appearance at the limbus of the normally invisible pericorneal blood vessels. Corneal edema involving the superficial layers can subsequently occur, and this is associated with a decreased corneal reflex. The edema may lead to superficial or deep keratitis, which may ultimately result in corneal ulceration (25). To our knowledge, corneal lesions following radiotherapy for Graves' ophthalmopathy have not been reported in the literature.

Lens

Cataract is a well-known complication of irradiation of the lens. It is due to damage of the epithelial cells, resulting in lens fiber disorganization. Characteristically, the initial changes of radiation cataract are located at the posterior pole of the lens with the appearance of a gradually enlarging dot opacity. Granular opacities and vacuoles surround the central opacity and may then extend to the anterior subcapsular region, producing changes which may not be distinguished from other types of cataract (29). The severity and the rate of progression of radiation cataract are dose-dependent. It has been reported that a total dose of 1,150 rads causes cataract in all cases, whereas the minimum effective dose in a single administration is 200 rads (29). Fractionation of radiation doses tends to reduce their cataractogenic effects and delays the onset of cataract changes (29). The mean latent period for the development of cataract is 2 years, with a range of 6 months to 35 years. Age is an important factor, as lenses of children appear to be more sensitive to radiation (32). Radiation cataract has been frequently observed in patients submitted to direct radiation to the lens for orbit malignancies, but only one doubtful case has been reported after orthovoltage radiotherapy for Graves' ophthalmopathy (17). Although the development of radiation cataract has been carefully sought in several series using supervoltage orbital radiotherapy, no case has been detected.

Retina

In contrast to the maturing retina (26,37,38), the adult retina is known to tolerate relatively large doses of radiation (25). In exceptional cases, excessive irradiation may produce damage to the retinal vasculature, leading to retinal hemorrhages. Radiation retinopathy after radiotherapy for Graves' ophthalmopathy at high doses has been reported in a single patient by one group of workers (1). Details on the source, dose, and duration of radiotherapy were not given. Conversely, no retinal damage was observed in several series in which irradiation doses up to 2,000 rads were used. In children submitted to supervoltage orbital radiotherapy for retinoblastoma, some deleterious effects on the retina have been observed using high doses up to 6,000 rads, but no significant damage occurred in children receiving 3,000 rads or less (21). Because the retina is necessarily included in the treatment field of orbital radiotherapy for Graves' ophthalmopathy, the limit of 3,000 rads should not be exceeded.

Pituitary and Hypothalamus

Multiple endocrine deficiencies have been observed after radiotherapy of pituitary tumors (24) and may also occur after radiation to the head and neck for extrapituitary neoplasms, e.g., carcinomas of the nasopharynx or paranasal sinuses (36). This may result from lesions to the pituitary itself, the hypothalamus, or both (35). Nontumorous adenohypophyseal tissue seems to be relatively radioresistant. This may explain the absence of clinical hypopituitarism in patients submitted to pituitary irradiation for Graves' ophthalmopathy.

Carcinogenic Effect

The potential risk of radiation-induced tumors should also be considered. An increased frequency of thyroid and salivary gland tumor has been observed in subjects given radiation to the head and neck for benign conditions during childhood (15). Severe Graves' ophthalmopathy is mostly observed in adults. Radiation-induced tumors have not been so far reported in patients submitted to radiotherapy for Graves' ophthalmopathy.

SELECTION OF PATIENTS AND INDICATIONS FOR ORBITAL RADIOTHERAPY

Orbital radiotherapy is an aggressive and vigorous treatment for Graves' ophthalmopathy and requires appropriate selection of patients. Factors to be taken into major consideration

TABLE 1. *Categories of eye involvement in Graves' ophthalmopathy[a]*

Soft tissue	Proptosis (mm over upper normal limit)	Eye muscle	Cornea	Acuity	Score
Slight redness, chemosis, periorbital edema, minimal symptoms	3–4	Infrequent diplopia at extremes of gaze	Slight stippling	20/25–20/40	1
Moderately severe redness, chemosis, periorbital swelling and symptoms	5–7	Frequent diplopia, moderate limitation of movement	Marked stippling and symptoms	20/45–20/100	2
Conjunctival redundancy, marked edema, severe symptoms	8	Severe, constant muscle dysfunction	Ulceration	<20/100	3

Modified from Kriss et al. (21).
[a]Ophthalmopathy index = sum of scores for all five categories.

include severity, duration, and progression of the eye disease. Contraindications and unresponsiveness to systemic corticosteroids should also be considered. The extent of eye involvement should be carefully evaluated by physical examination, exophthalmometry, tests for extraocular muscle function, retinoscopy, tests of visual field and acuity, tonometry, and corneal examination. Orbital ultrasonography and computerized tomography are helpful diagnostic techniques and are especially useful in doubtful cases, e.g., patients with ophthalmopathy but no evidence of present or past thyroid disease. The thyroid status should be assessed by appropriate clinical and laboratory criteria.

Severity of Ophthalmopathy

Patients with mild ophthalmopathy do not require major forms of treatment and can be managed by simple conservative measures. Radiotherapy should be considered when the eye manifestations are severe and result in significant impairment of customary daily activity. This may be produced by severe inflammatory changes of soft tissues, marked proptosis leading to corneal exposure, extraocular muscle dysfunction resulting in limitation of movements and/or diplopia, corneal lesions, and loss of visual acuity. A useful tool for assessing the degree of ophthalmopathy and evaluating the results of treatment is the ophthalmopathy index proposed by Donaldson et al. (7) and based on the American Thyroid Association classification of the eye changes of Graves' disease (47). To calculate this index, a numerical score graded from 0 to 3 according to severity is assigned to each category of eye involvement (soft tissues, proptosis, extraocular muscle, cornea, sight loss) and their sum is then determined (Table 1). In agreement with others (21), we consider orbital radiotherapy only in patients with an ophthalmopathy index of 4 or more.

Duration and Progression of Ophthalmopathy

An inverse relationship between duration of eye changes and efficacy of treatment has been observed by several workers, more favorable results usually being obtained when symptoms have been present for less than 2 years (2,3,7). A poor response to radiotherapy is expected in long-lasting, stable ophthalmopathy, and especially in the case of fixed ophthalmoplegia, presumably in relation to the presence of irreversible fibrotic changes. The time elapsed from the onset of the opthalmopathy should not be considered an absolute criterion for the selection of patients, as recent exacerbations occurring in long-lasting ophthalmopathy may also respond favorably to radiotherapy. In this regard, the rate of progression has been suggested as the main factor predicting the outcome of therapy (21). Progression of the disease should be evaluated by repeated ophthalmological examinations over a period of weeks or months, if it is not clearly apparent on the basis of historical data.

Contraindications and Unresponsiveness to Corticosteroids

Although the choice between orbital radiotherapy and systemic corticosteroids depends largely on the experience of the various centers, the former is clearly indicated in patients with contraindications to corticosteroid usage, e.g., the presence of diabetes mellitus, peptic ulcer, hypertension, osteoporosis, acute psychosis, tuberculosis, or other infectious diseases. Radiotherapy should also be considered in patients developing major side effects from corticosteroids and in those who failed to respond to an adequate trial with these drugs.

Thyroid Status

Graves' ophthalmopathy is most often associated with a history of hyperthyroidism. The severity and the course of the eye conditions are largely independent of the evolution of the thyroid disease. The selection of patients for orbital radiotherapy may be made irrespective of the thyroid status, but any thyroid dysfunction needs to be corrected by appropriate measures.

The majority of the patients referred for treatment of ophthalmopathy had their hyperthyroidism controlled by previous therapy. Patients with hypothyroidism following surgical or radioactive thyroid ablation should be maintained euthyroid with thyroxine replacement therapy. Patients with active thyrotoxicosis and those who are euthyroid under antithyroid drug therapy raise the question of the type and the timing of treatment of hyperthyroidism. Thyroid ablative therapy, and especially radioiodine treatment, may be followed by worsening of the eye changes (23). Although no controlled studies are available, some clinicians believe that this occurs less frequently after institution of antithyroid drug therapy. A transient increase of circulating thyroid-stimulating antibodies and other thyroid antibodies is observed after radioiodine therapy of Graves' disease (31), whereas a reduction is found during antithyroid drug treatment (9,27,28,31). It remains to be established whether these phenomena have any bearing on the course of eye changes of Graves' disease. In the absence of more precise information, we favor the use of antithyroid drugs as the treatment of hyperthyroidism. When a more definitive form of treatment is desired, we recommend the use of combined therapy with ^{131}I and antithyroid drugs. Admittedly, this is a controversial problem, and ^{131}I therapy combined with systemic corticosteroids (prednisone 20 to 40 mg/day for 3 months) to prevent any exacerbation of eye changes has been advocated by others (21).

Graves' ophthalmopathy occasionally occurs in the absence or presence of a history of thyrotoxicosis (euthyroid or hypothyroid Graves' disease) (40). It has been reported that orbital radiotherapy is less effective in this group of patients (21), but available data are not sufficient to draw any conclusion.

ROLE OF ORBITAL RADIOTHERAPY IN RELATION TO OTHER FORMS OF TREATMENT

Orbital radiotherapy and other forms of treatment for Graves' ophthalmopathy do not necessarily represent alternative therapeutic measures, as they may be useful in combination or in sequence.

During and after the course of irradiation some palliative and simple measures may help to reduce symptoms. Dark glasses may be beneficial in reducing photophobia. Eyedrops containing methylcellulose act as a lubricating agent and may alleviate the transient worsening of conjunctival irritation, which may be induced by radiation. Treatment with eyedrops containing 5% guanethidine or, preferably, the β-blocking agent timolol (0.25 to 0.5%) may be effective in controlling lid lag.

The choice among orbital radiotherapy, systemic corticosteroids, or a combination of these two methods of treatment is a matter of controversy. Corticosteroids are probably more effective than radiotherapy in providing prompt control of soft tissue manifestations but have the disadvantage of producing cushingoid features and possibly other relevant untoward effects. No major side effects of orbital irradiation have been reported when appropriate techniques were used, except for a transient exacerbation of irritative changes and periorbital edema. In our experience the latter phenomena do not occur when orbital radiotherapy is combined with systemic corticosteroids. The final selection of the therapeutic method ultimately depends on the experience of the individual centers. Among those using orbital radiotherapy, Kriss et al. (7,21) advocated this procedure as the treatment of choice. According to other workers (5,6), systemic corticosteroids should be given as a fair trial for several weeks, and orbital radiotherapy should be reserved to the patients who fail to respond or experience major side effects. We favor the use of orbital radiotherapy combined with high doses of systemic corticosteroids in all patients with severe Graves' ophthalmopathy and no contraindications to corticosteroid treatment, whereas others recommend low doses of corticosteroids only in patients receiving ^{131}I therapy for coexisting thyrotoxicosis (21). As discussed in a preceding section, orbital radiotherapy alone is indicated when contraindications to systemic corticosteroids are present. As an alternative, retrobulbar injection of corticosteroids may be used in such patients in combination with orbital radiotherapy in order to potentiate the effect of the latter and avoid the risks of systemic corticosteroids. We are currently evaluating the effectiveness and the advantages of this form of treatment.

Irreversible eye muscle dysfunction and/or eyelid retraction may require appropriate corrective surgical procedures. Eyelid and eye muscle surgery are best performed when the inflammatory changes are quiescent and other signs are stable. This process can be accelerated by orbital irradiation, thus permitting earlier surgical correction. A period of 1 to 2 years should elapse after radiotherapy before considering eye surgery.

RESULTS OF RADIOTHERAPY OF GRAVES' OPHTHALMOPATHY

There are several reports on orthovoltage radiotherapy for Graves' ophthalmopathy since its beneficial effects were first described by Thomas and Woods in 1936 (43). A precise evaluation of the results obtained in many of these studies is hampered by the limited number of patients, the variability in dosimetry, the different irradiation targets (pituitary, hypothalamus, orbits), the wide range of the severity of eye changes, and the lack of definite and uniform criteria to quantitate the degree of ophthalmopathy before and after therapy. The results obtained in some of the larger and better documented studies are now briefly analyzed.

In 1951 Jones (17) described 29 patients with Graves' ophthalmopathy submitted to radiotherapy directed to the orbits using both lateral and anterior radiation fields. Amelioration or disappearance of soft tissue changes was obtained in most cases, whereas proptosis and ophthalmoplegia responded poorly. By irradiating the pituitary, Beierwaltes (3) observed a reduction of at least 2 mm in proptosis with a parallel improvement in the edema and inflammatory changes in 13 of 28 patients. Silvestrini and Pasargiklian (39) irradiated the hypothalamus, the pituitary, and the orbits in a series of 23 patients and reported improvement of variable degree in about 50% of the patients with soft tissue changes and/or proptosis and in 40% of those with ophthalmoplegia. By irradiating the same targets using different ports of entry, Guinet and Mornex (14) described an overall positive effect in more than 50% of 23 patients. In a large series of 112 patients submitted to irradiation to the pituitary, the orbits, or both, a general improvement of ophthalmopathy was observed by Horst et al. (16) regardless of the irradiated region. Corneal lesions, proptosis of recent onset and optic neuropathy showed the most favorable responses, whereas only scanty effects were noted on extraocular muscle involvement. Ravin et al. (33) described the results obtained in a series of 37 patients using the same technique as Beierwaltes. Improvement of soft tissue changes was observed in many patients, a reduction of proptosis of at least 3 mm in more than one-third of cases, whereas only one of 33 patients with extraocular muscle involvement responded favorably. Interestingly, a marked amelioration or resolution of optic nerve involvement occurred in eight of nine patients with this complication.

In view of the current concepts excluding a pathogenetic role of the pituitary and the hypothalamus in Graves' ophthalmopathy, the beneficial effects reported in patients submitted to direct irradiation of these regions might be regarded as surprising. However, as discussed in a preceding section, it is reasonable to assume that the orbits were inevitably encompassed in the radiation field directed to the pituitary and the hypothalamus when orthovoltage equipments were used. Thus it seems that orbital rather than hypothalamic–pituitary irradiation accounted for the positive results described above.

In 1973 Donaldson et al. (7) at the Stanford University School of Medicine reported the first study on the effects of orbital radiotherapy for the treatment of Graves' ophthalmopathy using a linear accelerator. In addition to the technical advantages offered by the well-collimated high-energy x-ray beam generated by the supervoltage apparatus, the authors employed an ophthalmopathy index to attempt a quantitative assessment of the degree of ocular involvement both before and after therapy. The treatment group comprised 23 patients with severe and progressive ophthalmopathy, with an index score ranging from 4 to 12. Excellent or good results, as assessed by variations in the ophthalmopathy index and by clinical criteria, were observed in 65% of patients, and none was made worse. Initial responses were apparent during the second week of treatment, and further improvement occurred during subsequent weeks or months. Beneficial effects were also obtained in several patients who had previously responded poorly to systemic corticosteroid therapy. Among the various classes of eye change, severe asymmetrical extraocular muscle paresis was found to be the least susceptible to orbital radiotherapy. Results were generally less satisfactory in patients with longstanding ophthalmopathy, but the main factor determining the outcome of treatment seemed to be the rate of progression of the disease. Patients with rapidly progressive eye changes experienced the most favorable responses. Since their original report, these authors have enlarged their series to 121 patients (21). Eighty patients were treated by radiotherapy alone, and an overall excellent or good response was obtained in 67% of cases. When the various categories of eye involvement were analyzed, the percentages of improvement were 95% for soft tissue changes, 60% for both proptosis and extraocular muscle involvement, 50% for corneal lesions, and 85% for sight loss. Among the 41 patients who required eyelid or eye muscle surgery following radiotherapy, the final percentage of favorable results reached 81%. Interestingly, of the 12 patients with no history of hyperthyroidism included in the present series, only four responded favorably to orbital irradiation.

Results of other studies using linear accelerator for orbital irradiation have been satisfactory to a variable degree. Covington et al. (6) reported good responses in five of seven patients with severe ophthalmopathy. Improvement occurred within 3 months and was most impressive in the case of optic neuropathy. Varying degrees of amelioration were also noted in soft tissue changes and, to a lesser extent, in proptosis. Trobe et al. (44) submitted to orbital irradiation six patients with bilateral ophthalmopathy associated with optic neuropathy, five of whom had failed to respond to oral corticosteroids. Significant improvement of visual acuity occurred in six of the 12 eyes involved. Yamamoto et al. (48) described the effects of orbital irradiation in nine patients, including five who did not respond to corticosteroids and two with relapses following plasmapheresis. Good responses were obtained in four, fair or no responses being observed in the remaining five. Improvement of soft tissue changes was apparent within 3 to 4 weeks, whereas a period of 3 to 7 months was required for the effect on proptosis. Of the 14 patients submitted to orbital radiotherapy by Brennan et al. (5), 10 were irradiated by linear accelerator. Six of them had failed to respond to previous corticosteroids. With one exception, a reduction in soft tissue inflammation and proptosis was observed in all cases, and improvement of myopathy occurred only in three of the six cases involved. Much less satisfactory results were reported by Teng et al. (42) in a series of 20 patients with moderately severe ophthalmopathy. About one-third of the patients showed some improvement, but the benefit was not impressive and was mainly confined to soft tissue changes. Proptosis improved in 25% of cases, and longstanding ophthalmoplegia only rarely responded favorably.

To our knowledge, the betatron as a source of supervoltage x-rays for the treatment of ophthalmopathy has been used only by Fritsch et al. (10) in a series of 68 patients. In about half of the cases the irradiation field also encompassed the pituitary. An objective improvement was achieved in only 30% of patients regardless of the radiation field.

Orbital cobalt radiotherapy for Graves' ophthalmopathy has been used by several groups. Eight of the 10 patients treated by Grauthoff et al. (13) experienced significant improvement of eye changes, and the mean ophthalmopathy index of the whole group decreased from 6.7 to 3.0. Soft tissue changes, proptosis, and corneal lesions accounted for most beneficial effects, whereas myopathy remained unchanged. Most of the patients had had variable unsuccessful courses with systemic corticosteroids, and four of them received 20 to 60 mg of prednisolone after the initiation of radiotherapy. The results were apparently unaffected by the concomitant corticosteroid administration. Favorable results were also reported by Brennan et al. (5) in their four patients treated by orbital cobalt radiotherapy, which included three cases of unresponsiveness to systemic corticosteroids. Similar to other studies, amelioration occurred in soft tissue changes, proptosis, and corneal lesions, but little effect was noted in extraocular muscle paresis. The overall results did not differ from those obtained by the same workers using a linear accelerator. At variance with these data, only 20% of the 15 patients submitted to orbital cobalt radiotherapy by Fritsch et al. (10) showed an objective improvement.

In our institution orbital cobalt radiotherapy has been mostly used in combination with high doses of systemic corticosteroids. Methylprednisolone was started simultaneously with radiotherapy, using 70 to 80 mg/day for the first 3 weeks and progressively reduced doses thereafter. Treatment was discontinued after 5 to 6 months. The results obtained in a series of 36 patients with severe ophthalmopathy have been previously reported (2). Assessment of the results of therapy by clinical criteria and determination of the ophthalmopathy index at least 12 months after discontinuation of corticosteroids showed an excellent or good response in 26 patients (72%) and no case of worsening (Table 2). In several cases, the

TABLE 2. *Overall responses to combined treatment with systemic methylprednisolone and orbital cobalt radiotherapy in 36 patients with Graves' ophthalmopathy*

| Clinical assessment | No. of patients | Mean ophthalmopathy index ($\pm$ SE) | | Mean duration of symptoms (months) |
		Initial	Final	
Excellent response	12	6.2 $\pm$ 2.1	0.5 $\pm$ 0.5[a]	10
Good response	14	6.2 $\pm$ 1.3	1.8 $\pm$ 0.7[a]	31
Slight response	9	7.3 $\pm$ 1.6	3.9 $\pm$ 1.1[a]	35
No response	1	6	6	108

[a]$p < 0.001$ versus initial value.

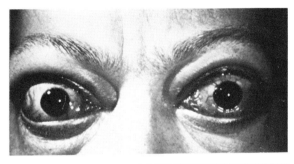

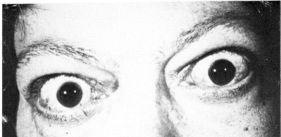

FIG. 2. Responses to orbital cobalt radiotherapy combined with systemic corticosteroids in a patient with severe Graves' ophthalmopathy. **Top panel:** Before treatment (ophthalmopathy index = 10). **Middle panel:** Two months after initiation of treatment (ophthalmopathy index = 4). **Bottom panel:** Twelve months after initiation of treatment, 6 months after discontinuation of corticosteroids (ophthalmopathy index = 1).

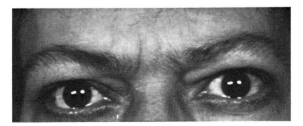

effect of treatment was dramatic, as exemplified by the patient reported in Fig. 2. The mean ophthalmopathy index was reduced from 6.5 to 2.1, with a net change of −4.4. There was an inverse relationship between the efficacy of treatment and the duration of ophthalmopathy, less favorable results being obtained when eye symptoms had been present for more than 2 years. Among the categories of eye involvement, soft tissue changes were most favorably influenced by the treatment, regression or significant improvement being observed in 97% of the cases involved (Table 2). Variable degrees of amelioration of

TABLE 3. *Overall results of orbital supervoltage radiotherapy in various series*

Radiation apparatus	No. of patients	Percent of favorable results	Ref.	Radiation apparatus	No. of patients	Percent of favorable results	Ref.
Linear accelerator	23	65	7[a]	Linear accelerator[b]	41	81	21[a]
	7	71	6	Betatron	68	30	10
	6	50	44	Cobalt unit	10	80	13[a]
	20	35	42[a]		15	20	10
	9	45	48[a]		4	75	5
	10	70	5	Cobalt unit[c]	36	72	2[a]
	80	67	21[a]				

[a]Data based on changes of the ophthalmopathy index.
[b]Followed by eye muscle or eyelid surgery.
[c]Combined with systemic corticosteroids.

extraocular muscle dysfunction were found in 93% of cases, but complete remission was mostly observed in patients with newly developed ophthalmoplegia; the response of long-standing muscle involvement in general was only partial. Reduction of proptosis of 2 to 7 mm occurred in 19 of 34 patients (56%). Both patients with severe sight loss showed complete restoration of visual acuity within the first few weeks of treatment. A prompt response was also observed in the inflammatory manifestations, whereas proptosis and ophthalmoplegia responded more slowly. Ocular symptoms recurred in four patients at variable times after the end of treatment, but in only one case was orbital decompression required. Since this study was completed, 26 additional patients have been submitted to the same therapeutic schedule, and similarly favorable results have been obtained. When considering the combined therapy, one should take into account the well-known risks of high-dose corticosteroids. During the past 10 years, we have treated a total of 88 patients with systemic methylprednisolone either alone or in combination with orbital cobalt radiotherapy. Cushingoid features occurred in most cases but subsided after discontinuation of treatment. The development of a moderate increase in intraocular tension, transient depressive psychosis, and diabetic syndrome requiring insulin was observed in three instances. An additional patient developed an acute febrile illness within the first month of corticosteroid treatment, which was diagnosed elsewhere as infectious encephalitis, possibly due to the herpes simplex virus. Whether this illness was related to the corticosteroid administration remains conjectural. These complications raise the question of to what extent the addition of systemic corticosteroids to orbital supervoltage radiotherapy is justified. To our knowledge, there is no controlled study comparing combined therapy with orbital radiotherapy alone. In the absence of this information and in view of the overall satisfactory results so far obtained, we regard systemic corticosteroids as a valuable adjunctive measure to orbital cobalt radiotherapy. The added benefit from combined therapy might be less relevant when a linear accelerator rather than a cobalt unit is used.

In most of the studies reviewed above, orbital radiotherapy by supervoltage equipment, regardless of whether it is associated with systemic corticosteroids, has resulted in a significant improvement of Graves' ophthalmopathy in the majority of cases (Table 3). In general, the most favorable responses have been observed in patients with recent onset of the disease, emphasizing the need for early treatment of Graves' ophthalmopathy. This is in keeping with the concept that radiotherapy may reverse phlogistic infiltration of retro-orbital tissue but is not effective when the infiltrate has been replaced by fibrotic tissue. Soft tissue changes and optic neuropathy have been almost uniformly found to respond more promptly and dramatically. Proptosis, newly developed ophthalmoplegia, and corneal lesions also showed beneficial effects. It is worth noting that virtually no case of worsening has been observed after orbital irradiation, that the number of patients requiring subsequent orbital decompression has been very limited, and that favorable results have also been obtained in patients with unresponsiveness to corticosteroids.

On the other hand, rather disappointing results have been reported by some workers using the linear accelerator (42), betatron (10), or cobalt unit (10). The reasons for such discrepancies are unclear, but differences in the radiation technique and in the selection of patients may account for some of these negative results. The experience with the use of the betatron for the treatment of Graves' ophthalmopathy is limited to a single study, which requires further confirmation. Detailed information on the patients submitted to orbital cobalt radiotherapy by Fritsch et al. (10) is lacking. The series of 20 subjects treated by Teng et al. (42) using a linear accelerator included nine who had rather mild ophthalmopathy with an index score of less than 4, and 13 who had symptoms of ophthalmopathy lasting for more than 2 years. The limited beneficial effects reported by these authors were mainly confined to the patients with recent onset of the disease. In view of the data discussed above, the unresponsiveness of the remaining patients may be explained by the indurative changes associated with longstanding ophthalmopathy. Of the eight patients submitted by us to cobalt radiotherapy alone, favorable results have been obtained only in the two cases with less than 1 year duration of the ophthalmopathy, whereas the mean duration of eye disease in the six unresponsive patients was more than 5 years.

Support for the concept that radiotherapy has a favorable influence on Graves' ophthalmopathy derived from the controlled trial carried out in our institution, in which the effects of systemic corticosteroids alone were compared with those of the combined treatment with orbital cobalt radiotherapy and systemic corticosteroids (2). The study was carried out in a series of 24 consecutive patients with severe ophthalmopathy randomly assigned to either of these methods of treatment. Mean initial ophthalmopathy indices did not differ in the two groups. Amelioration of eye changes with a significant reduction of the index score was observed in both groups. However, the results obtained in the patients submitted to combined therapy were moderately, but significantly, more satisfactory than those observed in the 12 patients given systemic methylprednisolone alone (Fig. 3). These data clearly indicate that the favorable response to the combined therapy is not solely due to the action of methylprednisolone and that orbital cobalt radiotherapy has an intrinsic beneficial effect.

CONCLUSIONS

Radiotherapy is an established method for the treatment of severe Graves' ophthalmopathy. In view of the current concepts on the pathogenesis of the disease, the irradiation should be confined to the orbits, using appropriate conditions to avoid exposure of the lens, cornea, pituitary, and hypothalamus. Although some favorable results have been obtained with orthovoltage equipment, the use of this type of irradiation is discouraged because of poor collimation, wide penumbra, and considerable side scatter. Supervoltage apparatus generating well-collimated high-energy x-rays are recommended. In this regard, the linear accelerator offers some advantage with respect to a cobalt unit, but both are effective. Experience with betatron radiotherapy for Graves' ophthalmopathy is still limited. Orbital radiotherapy is an aggressive and vigorous treatment for Graves' ophthalmopathy and should be reserved to patients with severe eye manifestations resulting in significant impairment of customary daily activity. It may be used as an alternative to systemic corticosteroids, and the choice

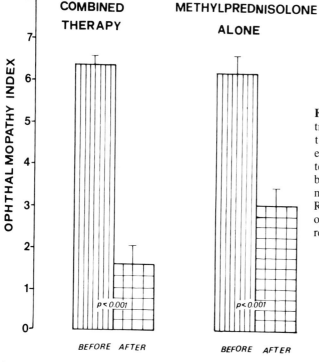

FIG. 3. Comparison of results of treatment in two groups of 12 patients each randomly assigned to either combined therapy with systemic methylprednisolone and orbital cobalt radiotherapy or systemic methylprednisolone treatment alone. Results are expressed as the mean ophthalmopathy index + SE. (From ref. 2.)

between these two methods largely depends on the experience of the individual center. Unresponsiveness to corticosteroids does not contraindicate orbital radiotherapy, as beneficial effects have been observed in several patients who failed to improve after previous corticosteroid trials. Duration and progression of the disease are important factors in the outcome of radiotherapy, as stable and longstanding eye changes are less likely to respond favorably. Satisfactory and even dramatic responses to supervoltage orbital radiotherapy have been reported in several studies. Each of the five categories of eye involvement may be favorably influenced, usually with a greater and more rapid improvement of soft tissue changes and optic neuropathy. Newly developed ophthalmoplegia, proptosis, and corneal lesions are also susceptible to varying degrees of amelioration. It is worth noting that no worsening of eye changes after radiotherapy has been observed, and side effects have so far been limited to transient manifestations. The results of orbital radiotherapy may be further improved by subsequent eyelid or eye muscle surgery. Orbital radiotherapy has been successfully used in combination with systemic corticosteroids, and the combined therapy has proved more satisfactory than systemic corticosteroids alone. The question of whether combined therapy is more advantageous than orbital radiotherapy alone remains to be clarified. Results of orbital radiotherapy as discussed in this chapter can be compared to those following orbital decompression as described in Chapter 17.

ACKNOWLEDGMENTS

The authors are grateful to Dr. M. Laddaga, Istituto di Radiologia; Drs. G. Lepri, G. Cavallacci, and C. Marconcini, Clinica Oculistica; and Dr. D. Andreani, Clinica Neurologica of the University of Pisa for helpful cooperation and valuable suggestions; to Dr. L. Baschieri, Patologia Medica II of the University of Pisa for continuous advice and encouragement; and to Miss A. Pisani for skillful secretarial assistance.

This study was supported by research grants from the Consiglio Nazionale delle Ricerche and the Ministero della Pubblica Istruzione, Rome, Italy.

REFERENCES

1. Bagan, S. M., and Hollenhorst, R. W. (1976): Radiation retinopathy after irradiation of intracranial lesions. *Am. J. Ophthalmol.*, 88:694–699.
2. Bartalena, L., Marcocci, C., Chiovato, L., Laddaga, M., Lepri, G., Andreani, D., Cavallacci, G., Baschieri, L., and Pinchera, A. (1983): Orbital cobalt irradiation combined with systemic corticosteroids for Graves' ophthalmopathy: comparison with systemic corticosteroids alone. *J. Clin. Endocrinol. Metab.*, 56:1139–1144.
3. Beierwaltes, W. H. (1953): X-ray treatment of malignant exophthalmos: a report on 28 patients. *J. Clin. Endocrinol. Metab.*, 15:1090–1100.
4. Blahut, R. J., Beierwaltes, W. H., and Lampe, I. (1963): Exophthalmos response during roentgen therapy. *AJR*, 90:261–268.
5. Brennan, M. W., Leone, C. R., Jr., and Janaki, L. (1983): Radiation therapy for Graves' disease. *Am. J. Ophthalmol.*, 96:195–199.
6. Covington, E. E., Lobes, L., and Sudarsanam, A. (1976): Radiation therapy of exophthalmos: report of seven cases. *Radiology*, 122:797–799.
7. Donaldson, S. S., Bagshaw, M. A., and Kriss, J. P. (1973): Supervoltage orbital radiotherapy for Graves' ophthalmopathy. *J. Clin. Endocrinol. Metab.*, 37:276–285.
8. Doniach, D., and Florin-Christensen, A. (1975): Autoimmunity in the pathogenesis of endocrine exophthalmos. *Clin. Endocrinol. Metab.*, 4:341–350.
9. Fenzi, G. F., Hashizume, K., Roudebush, C. P., and DeGroot, L. J. (1979): Changes in thyroid-stimulating immunoglobulins during antithyroid therapy. *J. Clin. Endocrinol. Metab.*, 48:572–576.
10. Fritsch, R., Hassenstein, E., and Dausch, D. (1981): Ergebnisse der Retrobulbärbestrahlung bei beginner endokriner ophthalmopathie. *Strahlentherapie*, 157:305–309.
11. Gedda, O., and Lindgren, M. (1954): Pituitary and orbital roentgen therapy in the hyperophthalmopathic type of Graves' disease. *Acta Radiol. (Stockh.)*, 42:211–220.
12. Gorman, C. A. (1978): The presentation and management of endocrine ophthalmopathy. *Clin. Endocrinol. Metab.*, 7:67–96.
13. Grauthoff, H., Wuttke, H., and Frommhold, H. (1980): Zur Strahlentherapie der endokrinen orbitopathie. *Strahlentherapie*, 156:469–474.
14. Guinet, M. M. P., and Mornex, R. (1956): Les manifestations oculaires au cours de l'hyperthyroidie. *Rev. Lyon Med.*, 5:933–982.
15. Hazen, R. W., Pifer, J. W., Toyooka, E. T., Livingood, J., and Hempelmann, H. (1966): Neoplasms following irradiation of the head. *Cancer Res.*, 26:305–311.
16. Horst, V. W., Sautter, H., and Ullerich, K. (1960): Radiojodiagnostik und strahlentherapie der endokrinen ophthalmopathie. *Dtsch. Med. Wochenschr.*, 85:794–798.
17. Jones, A. (1951): Orbital x-ray therapy of progressive exophthalmos. *Br. J. Radiol.*, 24:637–646.
18. Kodama, K., Sikorska, H., Bandy-Dafoe, P., Bayly, R., and Wall, J. R. (1982): Demonstration of a circulating autoantibody against a soluble eye-muscle antigen in Graves' ophthalmopathy. *Lancet*, 2:1353–1356.
19. Konishi, J., Herman, M. M., and Kriss, J. P. (1974): Binding of thyroglobulin and thyroglobulin-antithyroglobulin immune complex to extraocular muscle membrane. *Endocrinology*, 95:434–446.
20. Kriss, J. P., Konishi, J. H., and Herman, M. (1975): Studies on the pathogenesis of Graves' ophthalmopathy (with some related observation regarding therapy). *Recent Prog. Horm. Res.*, 31:533–561.
21. Kriss, J. P., McDougall, I. R., and Donaldson, S. S. (1983): Graves' ophthalmopathy. In: *Current Therapy in Endocrinology 1983–1984*, edited by D. T. Krieger and W. Bardin, pp. 104–109. Decker, New York.
22. Kriss, J. P., and Mehdi, S. Q. (1980): Pathogenesis of Graves' ophthalmopathy. In: *Autoimmune Aspects of Endocrine Disorders*, edited by A. Pinchera, D. Doniach, G. F. Fenzi, and L. Baschieri, pp. 127–141. Academic Press, New York.
23. Kriss, J. P., Pleshakov, V., Rosenblum, A. L., Holderness, M., Sharp, G., and Utiger, R. (1967): Studies on the pathogenesis of the ophthalmopathy of Graves' disease. *J. Clin. Endocrinol. Metab.*, 27:582–593.
24. Lawrence, A. W., Pinsky, S. M., and Goldfine, I. D. (1971): Conventional radiation therapy in acromegaly: a review and reassessment. *Arch. Intern. Med.*, 128:369–373.
25. Lederman, M., Jones, C. H., and Mould, R. F. (1973): Radiotherapy in eye disease. In: *Textbook of Radiotherapy*, edited by G. H. Fletcher, pp. 440–456. Lea & Febiger, Philadelphia.
26. Lucas, D. R. (1961): The effect of x-radiation on the mouse retina at different stages of development. *Int. J. Radiat. Biol.*, 3:105–124.
27. Marcocci, C., Chiovato, L., Mariotti, S., and Pinchera, A. (1982): Changes of circulating thyroid autoantibody levels during and after therapy with methimazole in patients with Graves' disease. *J. Endocrinol. Invest.*, 5:13–19.
28. McGregor, A. M., Petersen, M. M., McLachlan, S. M., Rooke, P., Smith, B. R., and Hall, R. (1980): Carbimazole and the autoimmune response in Graves' disease. *N. Engl. J. Med.*, 303:302–307.

29. Merriam, G. R., and Focht, E. F. (1957): A clinical study of radiation cataracts and the relationship to dose. *AJR*, 77:759–785.
30. Munro, R. E., Lamki, L., Row, V. V., and Volpé, R. (1973): Cell-mediated immunity in the exophthalmos of Graves' disease as demonstrated by the migration inhibition factor (MIF) test. *J. Clin. Endocrinol. Metab.*, 37:286–292.
31. Pinchera, A., Liberti, P., Martino, E., Fenzi, G. F., Grasso, L., Rovis, L., Baschieri, L., and Doria, G. (1969): Effects of antithyroid therapy on the long-acting thyroid stimulator and the antithyroglobulin antibodies. *J. Clin. Endocrinol. Metab.*, 29:231–238.
32. Prasad, K. N. (1974): *Radiation Biology*. Harper & Row, New York.
33. Ravin, J. G., Sisson, J. C., and William, T. K. (1974): Orbital radiation for the ocular changes of Graves' disease. *Am. J. Ophthalmol.*, 79:285–288.
34. Riley, F. C. (1972): Orbital pathology in Graves' disease. *Mayo Clin. Proc.*, 47:975–979.
35. Samaan, N. A., Bakdasm, M. M., Caderao, J. B., Cangir, A., Jesse, R. H., and Ballantyne, A. J. (1975): Hypopituitarism after external irradiation: evidence for both hypothalamic and pituitary origin. *Ann. Intern. Med.*, 83:771–777.
36. Samaan, N. A., Cangir, A., Maor, M. H., Sampiere, V. A., and Jesse, R. H. (1979): Effect of irradiation on the hypothalamic pituitary and thyroid function in patients with tumors of the head and neck. In: *Recent Advances in the Diagnosis and Treatment of Pituitary Tumors*, edited by J. A. Linfoot, p. 148. Raven Press, New York.
37. Shively, J. N., Phemister, R. D., and Epling, G. P. (1967): Alterations in the fine structure of the mature retina of dogs irradiated as neonates. *Exp. Eye Res.*, 6:278–282.
38. Shively, J. N., Phemister, R. D., Epling, G. P., and Jensen, R. (1976): Pathogenesis of radiation-induced retinal dysplasia. *Invest. Ophthalmol.*, 9:888–900.
39. Silvestrini, F., and Pasargiklian, E. (1955): *L'Esoftalmo endocrino*. Stabilimento Poligrafico Belforte, Livorno.
40. Solomon, D. H., Chopra, I. J., Chopra, U., and Smith, F. J. (1977): Identification of subgroups of euthyroid ophthalmic Graves' ophthalmopathy. *N. Engl. J. Med.*, 296:181–185.
41. Tao, T. W., Gatenby, P., and Kriss, J. (1982): Production and regulation of antithyroglobulin (anti-Tg) in vitro by B and T cells subsets from human peripheral blood. In: *Proceedings of the 58th Annual Meeting of the American Thyroid Association, Quebec*, abstract T-20.
42. Teng, C. S., Crombie, A. L., Hall, R., and Ross, W. M. (1980): An evaluation of supervoltage orbital irradiation for Graves' ophthalmopathy. *Clin. Endocrinol. (Oxf.)*, 13:545–551.
43. Thomas, H. M., and Woods, A. C. (1936): Progressive exophthalmos after thyroidectomy. *Bull. Johns Hopkins Hosp.*, 59:99–113.
44. Trobe, J. D., Glaser, J. S., and Laflamme, P. (1978): Dysthyroid optic neuropathy. *Arch. Ophthalmol.*, 96:1199–1209.
45. Volpé, R. (1981): *Auto-immunity in the Endocrine System*. Springer-Verlag, New York.
46. Wall, J. R., Henderson, J., Strakosh, C. R., and Joyner, D. M. (1981): Graves' ophthalmopathy—a review. *Can. Med. Assoc. J.*, 124:855–866.
47. Werner, S. C. (1976): Modification of the classification of the eye changes of Graves' disease: recommendation of the Ad Hoc Committee of the American Thyroid Association. *J. Clin. Endocrinol. Metab.*, 44:203–204.
48. Yamamoto, K., Saito, K., Takai, T., and Yoshida, S. (1982): Treatment of Graves' ophthalmopathy by steroid therapy, orbital radiation therapy, plasmapheresis and thyroxine replacement. *Endocrinol. Jpn.*, 29:495–501.

The Eye and Orbit in Thyroid Disease, edited by
C. A. Gorman et al. Raven Press, New York 1984.

Medical Therapy

William M. McConahey

*Division of Endocrinology and Department of Internal Medicine, Mayo Clinic,
Rochester, Minnesota 55905*

A number of medical treatments have been advocated for ophthalmopathy of Graves' disease. Although none has proved to be ideal, some do have a definite place in the treatment of certain types of ophthalmopathy. In this chapter we discuss these modalities and see how they fit into the therapeutic picture.

THYROID ABLATION WITH RADIOIODINE

Soon after Adams and Purvis (1–4) reported finding a long-acting thyroid stimulator (LATS) in the serum of some patients who had Graves' disease, it was found that LATS is usually detectable and sometimes quite elevated in the serum of those who have ophthalmopathy of Graves' disease (34,36,39). This led to the conjecture that LATS might have a causative role in ophthalmopathy, in that perhaps the thyroid cells produced LATS, which then acted on the eye tissues. The finding that LATS is a thyroid-specific antibody (23,32) supported the hypothesis that removal or destruction of all thyroid tissue in patients with severe ophthalmopathy might lead to a reduction in LATS levels and result in improvement in the eye signs. Catz and Perzik (17,18,38) reported that total ablation of the thyroid by surgery brought about a disappearance of LATS from the serum or a great decrease in its level along with a marked improvement in the infiltrative changes of ophthalmopathy and some regression of the proptosis, and Bauer and Catz (7) reported the same observations if the thyroid ablation was done with radioiodine. These workers believe that the aim in the treatment of ophthalmopathy should be total ablation of all thyroid tissue and that to determine if this has been achieved a neck scan using 5 to 25 mCi of ^{131}I should be done, preceded by the intramuscular injection of 10 units of thyrotropin daily for 3 days (7,16). Bauer and Catz (7) reported on 18 patients with progressive malignant exophthalmos whom they treated with radioiodine in an effort to ablate the thyroid glands. In the patients in whom these studies were done, LATS could no longer be detected following the radioiodine treatments except in one patient in whom the titer decreased but did not disappear. The total dose of ^{131}I used ranged from 8 to 303 mCi with a mean of 76.4 mCi. In four of the patients no functioning thyroid tissue could be detected, but in all the others thyroid tissue could still be demonstrated using a scanning dose of 5 mCi of ^{131}I preceded by thyrotropin. They reported marked improvement in the infiltrative changes of ophthalmopathy in all 18 patients and some improvement in proptosis.

Other workers have not found such good results from attempts to ablate thyroid tissue with radioiodine. Werner et al. (48) saw no effect on the eye disease in one patient so treated. Pequegnat et al. (37) studied 57 patients who had active and generally progressive ophthalmopathy of Graves' disease and who had ^{131}I treatment in an effort to ablate all thyroid tissue. The individual doses of ^{131}I ranged from 20 to 100 mCi. Radioiodine scans utilizing 1 mCi of ^{131}I were done on 46 patients after their therapeutic dose or doses of radioiodine, in 23 of whom no evidence of any residual thyroid tissue could be demonstrated. LATS assays were performed on the serum of 40 patients before and after the radioiodine treatment; moderate to high levels were found in 19 before treatment and in 16 after treatment. There was no significant correlation between LATS level and thyroid uptake of radioiodine after treatment. Of the 57 patients so treated, 40% improved after treatment, 35% were unchanged, and 25% became worse. There were six patients who after treatment had no thyroid localization of radioiodine and whose LATS titers turned from positive to negative. Of these six patients the ophthalmopathy improved in one, was unchanged in one, and became worse in four. The authors concluded that it had not been established that ophthalmopathy of Graves' disease could be altered by treatment with large doses of radioiodine.

Volpé et al. (45) administered large doses (60 to 100 mCi) of ^{131}I to 13 patients who had ophthalmopathy. Two of these patients had no residual thyroid tissue demonstrated with the use of thyrotropin followed by a 5-mCi dose of ^{131}I, and two others had negative neck scans using a 1-mCi dose. In none of the patients was there improvement in the eye signs and symptoms, nor was there a consistent significant decrease in LATS titers.

Boyle et al. (10) gave to two patients with severe ophthalmopathy ablation doses of up to 100 mCi of ^{131}I at 6-month intervals until a 5-day uptake of less than 0.2% of a 5 mCi dose of ^{131}I (preceded by thyrotropin) was achieved without seeing any improvement in the eye disease. Two other patients with severe ophthalmopathy served as controls. The authors concluded that thyroid ablation was not, at least in the short term, useful therapy for ophthalmopathy of Graves' disease.

GUANETHIDINE EYEDROPS

Although guanethidine eyedrops are not commercially available in the United States, it has been shown that lid retraction (which usually is a part of the ophthalmopathy) can be decreased by local instillation of the adrenergic blocking agent guanethidine. The strength of the guanethidine drops used has been 2, 5, 10, and 20%, with the 5% strength being found preferable. Two percent drops are much less effective, and 10 and 20% drops commonly cause eye pain and punctate keratitis. However, 5% guanethidine eyedrops administered one to four times per day have seldom caused side effects and may be expected to decrease lid retraction but not to affect proptosis, ophthalmoplegia, or conjunctival or periorbital edema. Gay and Wolkstein (25) treated nine patients with 10% eyedrops and found improvement in the lagophthalmos, lid lag, or lid retraction on upward gaze. The effect began within 6 to 8 hr after the instillation of one drop and lasted 32 to 38 hr. Cant et al. (14) treated 81 patients with upper eyelid retraction for an average of 54 weeks with either 10, 5, or 2% guanethidine eyedrops. They found the treatment effective in almost all cases. For the reasons already stated, they advised the use of 5% drops instilled into the eyes three times a day. They found that when treatment was stopped the eyes of most of the patients returned to their former position. Crombie and Lawson (19) and Bowden and Rose (9) reported that in addition to decreasing lid retraction the instillation of 5% guanethidine eyedrops decreased the proptosis, although others (14,25,28) have not found any effect on proptosis. A decrease in the intraocular pressure in patients so treated has been noted by Crombie and Lawson (19) and Cartlidge et al. (15).

β-ADRENERGIC BLOCKADE

As might be expected, the oral administration of a β-adrenergic blocking agent has an effect on the lid retraction of Graves' disease. Grossman et al. (27) studied the effects of sotalol on the peripheral manifestations of thyrotoxicosis in a double-masked controlled study on 10 patients. They found a decrease in stare, lid lag, and globe lag in the patients but no decrease in proptosis.

ORAL CORTICOSTEROIDS

The most frequently used medical treatment of severe ophthalmopathy of Graves' disease is the oral administration of corticosteroids. In 1953 Kinsell et al. (31) reported improvement in nine such patients who received large doses of both cortisone and ACTH. In 1955 a study from England (11) reported moderate to marked improvement in eight of 28 patients treated with either cortisone or ACTH, usually in relatively small doses. In 1958 McCullaugh et al. (33) treated 10 patients with both hydrocortisone by mouth and ACTH by intravenous injection; all 10 patients had improvement of conjunctival irritation and edema, lacrimation, ocular pain, and lid edema, but only two had any decrease in proptosis.

In 1966 Werner (47) reported remarkable immediate improvement following the sustained administration of unusually large doses of prednisone (120 to 140 mg/day) to two patients with far-advanced eye changes of Graves' disease, but he pointed out that this treatment could not be relied on to induce a permanent remission.

Many reports have now appeared (5,12,22,30,35,42) to document the immediate beneficial effects of giving large doses of corticosteroids to patients who have severe ophthalmopathy of Graves' disease. Daily doses of prednisone, in the vicinity of 60 mg or more, must be given. With this treatment most observers report the prompt improvement in the inflammatory components of the disease (i.e., chemosis, injection, lid edema, and lacrimation). If visual impairment due to optic neuropathy is also present, the visual acuity is frequently improved dramatically by large-dose steroid therapy. Improvement in ophthalmoplegia or in proptosis is usually not found to occur to any significant degree with the use of steroids. Because of the well-known and potentially serious side effects of high-dose steroid therapy, the dose must be gradually decreased in step-wise fashion as rapidly as is practical.

Steroid therapy is far from ideal treatment for the ophthalmopathy of Graves' disease. It does not cure the disease but only arrests the symptoms until a spontaneous remission may occur. High-dose or even medium-dose steroid therapy should not be given for more than a short period, and often when the dose is decreased or stopped the disease exacerbates in all its severity. However, for the patient with extremely severe infiltrative ophthalmopathy or with rapidly decreasing vision due to optic neuropathy, treatment with high doses of prednisone can be expected to give impressive immediate improvement. All investigators agree that better results with steroid therapy can be expected for patients whose symptoms have been present for a short period of time than for those with more chronic disease. Once the fibrosis which occurs with chronic exophthalmos has developed, no decrease in proptosis can be expected with the use of high-dose steroid therapy. In this situation surgery offers the best rehabilitative approach.

An interesting report by Bartalena et al. (6) compared methylprednisolone alone with methylprednisolone combined with orbital cobalt irradiation in the treatment of ophthalmopathy of Graves' disease. Of 12 patients treated with only methylprednisolone 33% had a good response, whereas 72% of 36 patients treated with both methylprednisolone and cobalt irradiation to the orbits had either an excellent or a good response.

SUBCONJUNCTIVAL INJECTION OF CORTICOSTEROIDS

Several workers have reported success with the subconjunctival or retrobulbar injection of corticosteroids for treatment of ophthalmopathy. Garber (24) treated 15 patients with such injections using 10 to 15 mg of methylprednisolone acetate and reported that all patients obtained relief from the symptoms of ocular discomfort, ranging from moderate to dramatic, after the first injection. The number of injections varied from two to 18 over time periods ranging from 2 to 24 months. The intervals between injections were lengthened progressively as indicated. The aim of treatment was to maintain improvement until a spontaneous remission of the disease occurred.

Other workers have been less enthusiastic about such injections. Riley (40) treated 27 patients, most of whom had relatively mild disease. Initially he injected methylprednisolone acetate once every 2 weeks. Later he injected Celestone Soluspan every 3 or 4 days and finally a mixture of both of these agents into the eyes every 7 to 10 days. He reported minor improvement in most patients. Because of the possibility that such subconjunctival or retrobulbar injections may cause glaucoma, Riley *(personal communication)* cautioned that they should not be used for a prolonged period.

However, Trobe et al. (44) saw no perceptible change in five eyes treated with repeated retrobulbar injections of 60 mg of triamcinolone acetonide (Kenalog). Haddad (28) advocated the injection of steroids into the retrobulbar or subtenon space as a test for the effectiveness of oral steroid therapy. If there was massive proptosis or orbital edema, he injected dexamethasone or hydrocortisone sodium succinate (and not methylprednisolone acetate) retrobulbarly; if there was muscle involvement with limitation of eye motion, he injected the material into the subtenon space in the intermuscular quadrants. If improvement was noted within 24 to 48 hr, he believed that oral steroid therapy would probably be effective and therefore instituted treatment with large doses of prednisone. If steroid injection produced little or no improvement, no oral prednisone therapy was given.

IMMUNOSUPPRESSION

Because of the suggested autoimmune pathogenesis of the ophthalmopathy of Graves' disease, treatment with immunosuppressive agents has been tried. In 1970 Burrow et al. (13) treated five patients with azathioprine 2 mg/kg/day for periods of 8 to 11 weeks for three patients and for more than 36 weeks for one. These four patients had no evidence of drug toxicity, but the fifth patient had to stop treatment after 10 days because of nausea. In no patient did the authors see improvement in the ophthalmopathy.

In 1979 Bigos et al. (8) reported some success with the use of cyclophosphamide in three patients. One patient who had had the ophthalmopathy for 5 years was given 700 mg of cyclophosphamide intravenously per month for 12 months; she experienced resolution of diplopia and the feeling of tension and grittiness in her eyes, but proptosis was unchanged. A second patient, who was also being treated with prednisone, received oral cyclophosphamide 150 mg/day for 15 months. With this combined therapy the patient's diplopia improved and chemosis resolved. The third patient received cyclophosphamide 85 mg/day orally for 5 months with resolution of right papilledema, return of visual acuity in the right eye from 20/80 to 20/20, resolution of diplopia, and reduction of chemosis; proptosis was unchanged. The authors did not report any side effects from cyclophosphamide in the three patients treated.

Wall et al. (46) treated 24 patients who had active and progressive ophthalmopathy with cyclophosphamide in a dose of 50 to 150 mg/day (depending on the patient's age and weight) for up to 4 months. They noted improvement in the congestive changes in all 24 patients and improvement in eye muscle involvement in 11 of 20 who had this problem, but there was a significant decrease of proptosis in one or both eyes (of 2 mm or more) in only three of the 24 patients. Cyclophosphamide was generally well tolerated, although the drug had to be stopped in four patients because of persistent nausea in two and alopecia in two.

Winand and Mahieu (49,50) noted that of 433 patients with hyperthyroidism seen and treated in their clinic 50 developed malignant exophthalmos. They then performed the leukocyte migration test on 366 patients with hyperthyroidism and found it positive in 109 and negative in 254. They believe that those patients whose leukocyte migration test is positive are at risk of developing ophthalmopathy and those whose test is negative are not. They found that none of the 254 hyperthyroid patients with negative tests developed malignant ophthalmopathy. All of the 109 patients whose leukocyte migration tests were positive were being treated for the hyperthyroidism as well as with azathioprine in a dose of 1.5 mg/kg/day; none developed malignant ophthalmopathy. The authors advocate doing leukocyte migration tests on all patients who have hyperthyroidism and treating with azathioprine all those whose tests are positive. For patients who have developed severe ophthalmopathy, Winand (49) advocated the use of both high doses of corticosteroids and azathioprine 1.5 mg/kg/day.

PLASMAPHERESIS

Because it has been postulated that a specific immunoglobulin G (IgG) may be a causative factor in the ophthalmopathy of Graves' disease, and because plasmapheresis has been shown to be an effective form of treatment of myasthenia gravis and Goodpasture's syndrome, both of which are known to have tissue damage caused by a specific IgG, plasmapheresis has been tried in the treatment of ophthalmopathy. Dandona et al. (20,21) treated seven patients for ophthalmopathy with plasma exchange followed by prednisolone and azathioprine. Of these seven patients, four had acute exophthalmos of less than 5 months' duration and three had chronic exophthalmos of between 8 months' and 5 years' duration. All patients except one had a sequence of three or four sessions of plasmapheresis at each of which 2 to 3 liters of plasma were removed and replaced by plasma and/or human serum albumin and saline. One patient had a total of 6 liters of plasma removed in two sessions because of very severe thyrotoxicosis and schizophrenia. At the completion of the plasma exchange, the patients received azathioprine 2.5 mg/kg body weight and prednisolone in a dose of 80 mg/day for 2 days, 60 mg/day for 2 days, 40 mg/day for 1 week, 30 mg/day for 2 weeks, and 20 mg/day thereafter for at least 8 weeks. All four patients with acute exophthalmos had significant improvement in their exophthalmos within 48 to 72 hr of the first plasmapheresis session, prior to immunosuppression, and the improvement continued during the following period of immunosuppression. In the eight eyes of these four patients the proptosis decreased by a mean of 3.75 mm (1 mm in one eye and 3, 4, or 5 mm in the other seven eyes). In none of the three patients with chronic exophthalmos did plasmapheresis bring about any improvement in the eyes.

Sawers et al. (41) reported improvement in the ophthalmopathy of two patients treated with plasma exchange, prednisolone, and cyclophosphamide, and of one patient treated with plasma exchange and prednisolone. Glinoer et al. (26) treated a patient with malignant exophthalmos with four plasma exchanges of 2.5 liters each, prednisone 80 mg/day, and azathioprine 100 mg/day, with spectacular improvement in less than 2 weeks.

MISCELLANEOUS

Other therapeutic measures have been tried for ophthalmopathy of Graves' disease, all to no avail. These include metronidazole (Flagyl) (29) dextrothyroxine (43), and desiccated thyroid, L-thyroxine, and L-triiodothyronine (33).

CONCLUSION

There are no ideal medical treatments for ophthalmopathy of Graves' disease, but some do have limited value. No medical treatment can be expected to be of much help for chronic ophthalmopathy when fibrosis has developed. To have a chance for success, medical therapy should be applied early in the course of the disease.

Destruction of residual thyroid tissue by large doses of radioiodine, as advocated by Bauer and Catz (7), has not been found by most other workers to be of significant benefit to the affected eyes.

Five percent guanethidine drops instilled into the eyes of patients with relatively acute ophthalmopathy may be expected to decrease the degree of lid retraction, but the effect is temporary. When the drops are stopped, lid retraction recurs. In addition, guanethidine in a solution of greater than 5% commonly causes eye pain and punctate keratitis. Finally, guanethidine eyedrops are not commercially available in the United States.

Oral corticosteroids are of distinct benefit if used in large doses and in patients who have fairly acute and severe ophthalmopathy. The inflammatory components of the disease (i.e., chemosis, injection, lid edema, lacrimation, and irritation) frequently are greatly improved by steroid therapy, as is visual acuity when optic neuropathy is present. Proptosis and paresis usually are little benefited by such treatment. The problem with steroid therapy is that because of the development of serious side effects the drug cannot be administered for long periods in high doses; and when the dose is decreased or the drug is stopped, the ophthalmopathy often quickly worsens. The interesting report by Bartalena et al. (6) of the successful use of combining cobalt irradiation of the orbits with oral corticosteroid therapy needs confirmation. The results of orbital irradiation are reviewed in Chapter 21.

Although subconjunctival or retrobulbar injection of corticosteroids may be expected to be of moderate benefit to the inflammatory changes of ophthalmopathy, this treatment is hardly worth the risk involved and the nuisance of frequent injections.

Cyclophosphamide and azathioprine have been reported by some workers to be of help in the treatment of ophthalmopathy, but other reports have not been enthusiastic. The report by Winand and Mahieu (50) on the use of azathioprine to prevent ophthalmopathy during the treatment of hyperthyroidism in patients who have a positive leukocyte migration test is very interesting.

Plasmapheresis has not been used widely enough to enable us to assess its worth in the treatment of ophthalmopathy. It is expensive, difficult to do, and available only in fairly large medical centers. Certainly it is not the first line of treatment to consider. Because the patients whose ophthalmopathy was reported to improve after plasmapheresis were also treated with steroids and azathioprine or cyclophosphamide, it is difficult to determine the role of plasmapheresis in the improvement. Further studies are needed to assess its usefulness in the treatment of ophthalmopathy of Graves' disease.

REFERENCES

1. Adams, D. D. (1956): The clinical status of patients whose sera have given the abnormal response when assayed for thyrotrophin. *Proc. Univ. Otago Med. School*, 34:29–30.
2. Adams, D. D. (1958): The presence of an abnormal thyroid-stimulating hormone in the serum of some thyrotoxic patients. *J. Clin. Endocrinol. Metab.*, 18:699–712.
3. Adams, D. D. (1961): Bioassay of long-acting thyroid stimulator (L.A.T.S.); the dose-response relationship. *J. Clin. Endocrinol. Metab.*, 21:799–805.
4. Adams, D. D., and Purvis, H. D. (1956): Abnormal responses in the assay of thyrotrophin. *Proc. Univ. Otago Med. School*, 34:11–12.
5. Apers, R. C. L., Oosterhuis, J. A., Goslings, B. M., and Bierlagh, J. J. M. (1975): Prednisone treatment in endocrine ophthalmopathy. *Mod. Probl. Ophthalmol.*, 14:414–420.

6. Bartalena, L., Marcocci, C., Chiovato, L., Laddaga, M., Lepri, G., Adreani, D., Cavallacci, G., Baschieri, L., and Pinchera, A. (1983): Orbital cobalt irradiation combined with systemic corticosteroids for Graves' ophthalmopathy: comparison with systemic corticosteroids alone. *J. Clin. Endocrinol. Metab.*, 56:1139–1144.

7. Bauer, F. K., and Catz, B. (1966): Radioactive iodine therapy for progressive malignant exophthalmos. *Acta Endocrinol. (Copenh.)*, 51:15–22.

8. Bigos, S. T., Nisula, B. C., Daniels, G. H., Eastman, R. C., Johnston, H. H., and Kohler, P. O. (1979): Cyclophosphamide in the management of advanced Graves' ophthalmopathy. *Ann. Intern. Med.*, 90:921–923.

9. Bowden, A. N., and Rose, F. C. (1969): Dysthyroid eye disease: a trial of guanethidine eye drops. *Br. J. Ophthalmol.*, 53:246–251.

10. Boyle, I. T., Greig, W. R., Thomson, J. A., Winning, J., and McGirr, E. M. (1969): Effect of thyroid ablation on dysthyroid exophthalmos. *Proc. R. Soc. Med.*, 62:19–23.

11. Brain, R. (1955): Cortisone in exophthalmos: report on a therapeutic trial of cortisone and corticotrophin (A.C.T.H.) in exophthalmos and exophthalmic ophthalmoplegia by a panel appointed by the Medical Research Council. *Lancet*, 1:6–9.

12. Brown, J., Coburn, J. W., Wigod, R. A., Hiss, J. M., Jr., and Dowling, J. T. (1963): Adrenal steroid therapy of severe infiltrative ophthalmopathy of Graves' disease. *Am. J. Med.*, 34:786–795.

13. Burrow, G. N., Mitchell, M. S., Howard, R. O., and Morrow, L. B. (1970): Immunosuppressive therapy for the eye changes of Graves' disease. *J. Clin. Endocrinol. Metab.*, 31:307–311.

14. Cant, J. S., Lewis, D. R. H., and Harrison, M. T. (1969): Treatment of dysthyroid ophthalmopathy with local guanethidine. *Br. J. Ophthalmol.*, 53:233–238.

15. Cartlidge, N. E. F., Crombie, A. L., Anderson, J., and Hall, R. (1969): Critical study of 5% guanethidine in ocular manifestations of Graves' disease. *Br. Med. J.*, 4:645–647.

16. Catz, B. (1967): Remnant thyroid tissue. *N. Engl. J. Med.*, 276:985.

17. Catz, B., and Perzik, S. L. (1965): Subtotal vs. total surgical ablation of the thyroid: malignant exophthalmos and its relation to remnant thyroid. In: *Current Topics in Thyroid Research*, edited by C. Cassano and M. Andreoli, pp. 1183–1199. Academic Press, New York.

18. Catz, B., and Perzik, S. L. (1969): Total thyroidectomy in the management of thyrotoxic and euthyroid Graves' disease. *Am. J. Surg.*, 118:434–439.

19. Crombie, A. L., and Lawson, A. A. H. (1967): Long-term trial of local guanethidine in treatment of eye signs of thyroid dysfunction and idiopathic lid retraction. *Br. Med. J.*, 4:592–595.

20. Dandona, P., Marshall, N. J., Bidey, S. P., Nathan, A., and Havard, C. W. H. (1979): Successful treatment of exophthalmos and pretibial myxedema with plasmapheresis. *Br. Med. J.*, 1:374–376.

21. Dandona, P., Marshall, N., Bidey, S., Nathan, A. W., and Havard, C. W. H. (1980): Treatment of acute malignant exophthalmos with plasma exchange. In: *Proceedings of the 8th International Thyroid Conference*, pp. 583–586. *Australian Academy of Science*, Canberra.

22. Day, R. M., and Carroll, F. D. (1967): Corticosteroids in the treatment of optic nerve involvement associated with thyroid dysfunction. *Trans. Am. Ophthalmol. Soc.*, 65:41–51.

23. Dorrington, K. J., Carneiro, L., and Munro, D. S. (1966): Absorption of the long-acting thyroid stimulator by human thyroid microsomes. *J. Endocrinol.*, 34:133–134.

24. Garber, M. I. (1966): Methylprednisolone in the treatment of exophthalmos. *Lancet*, 1:958–960.

25. Gay, A. J., and Wolkstein, M. A. (1966): Topical guanethidine therapy for endocrine lid retraction. *Arch. Ophthalmol.*, 76:364–367.

26. Glinoer, D., Gaham, N., Sand, G., Libert, J., Grivegnee, A., Badjou, R., and Ermans, A. M. (1981): Exophthalmie maligne traitee par echange plasmatique. *Ann. Endocrinol. (Paris)*, 42:545–546.

27. Grossman, W., Robin, N. I., Johnson, L. W., Brooks, H., Selenkow, H. A., and Dexter, L. (1971): Effects of beta blockade on the peripheral manifestations of thyrotoxicosis. *Ann. Intern. Med.*, 74:875–879.

28. Haddad, H. M. (1973): Pathogenesis and treatment of endocrine exophthalmos. *Int. Surg.*, 58:482–484.

29. Harden, R. M., Chisholm, C. J. S., and Cant, J. S. (1967): The effect of metronidazole on thyroid function and exophthalmos in man. *Metabolism*, 16:890–898.

30. Hoffenberg, R., and Jackson, W. P. U. (1958): Adrenocortical steroids in malignant exophthalmos. *Lancet*, 1:693–695.

31. Kinsell, L. W., Partridge, J. W., and Foreman, N. (1953): The use of ACTH and cortisone in the treatment and in the differential diagnosis of malignant exophthalmos: a preliminary report. *Ann. Intern. Med.*, 38:913–917.

32. Kriss, J. P., Pleshakov, V., and Chien, J. R. (1964): Isolation and identification of the long-acting thyroid stimulator and its relation to hyperthyroidism and circumscribed pretibial myxedema. *J. Clin. Endocrinol.*, 24:1005–1028.

33. McCullaugh, E. P., Clamen, M., Gardner, W. J., Kennedy, R. J., and Lockhart, G., III (1958): Exophthalmos of Graves' disease: a summary of the present status of therapy. *Ann. Intern. Med.*, 48:445–469.

34. McKenzie, J. M. (1961): Studies on the thyroid activator of hyperthyroidism. *J. Clin. Endocrinol.*, 21:635–647.

35. Mulherin, J. L., Jr., Temple, T. E., Jr., and Cundey, D. W. (1972): Glucocorticoid treatment of progressive infiltrative ophthalmopathy. *South. Med. J.*, 65:77–80.

36. Noguchi, A., Kurihara, H., and Sato, S. (1964): Clinical studies on the long-acting thyroid stimulator. *J. Clin. Endocrinol.*, 24:160–165.

37. Pequegnat, E. P., Mayberry, W. E., McConahey, W. M., and Wyse, E. P. (1967): Large doses of radioiodine in Graves' disease: effect on ophthalmopathy and long-acting thyroid stimulator. *Mayo Clin. Proc.*, 42:802–811.

38. Perzik, S. L., and Catz, B. (1967): The place of total thyroidectomy in the management of thyroid disease. *Surgery*, 62:436–440.

39. Pinchera, A., Pinchera, M. G., and Stanbury, J. B. (1965): Thyrotropin and long-acting thyroid stimulator assays in the thyroid disease. *J. Clin. Endocrinol.*, 25:189–208.

40. Riley, F. C., discussion of paper by Ivy, H. K. (1972): Medical approach to ophthalmopathy of Graves' disease. *Mayo Clin. Proc.*, 47:992–992a.

41. Sawers, J. S. A., Irvine, W. J., Toft, A. D., Urbaniak, S. J., and Donaldson, A. A. (1981): Plasma exchange in conjunction with immunosuppressive drug therapy in the treatment of endocrine exophthalmos. *J. Clin. Lab. Immunol.*, 6:245–250.

42. Stewart, R. D. H. (1974): Thyroid eye disease. *Trans. Ophthalmol. Soc. Aust.*, 26:45–50.

43. Tengroth, B. (1964): D-Thyroxine in the treatment of patients with endocrine exophthalmos. *Acta Ophthalmol. (Copenh.)*, 42:859–863.

44. Trobe, J. D., Glaser, J. S., and Laflamme, P. (1978): Dysthyroid optic neuropathy. *Arch. Ophthalmol.*, 96:1199–1209.

45. Volpé, R., Desbarats-Schonbaum, M. L., Schonbaum, E., Row, V. V., and Ezrin, C. (1969): The effect of radioablation of the thyroid gland in Graves' disease with high levels of long-acting thyroid stimulator (LATS) *Am. J. Med.*, 46:217–226.

46. Wall, J. R., Strakosch, C. R., Fang, S. L., Ingbar, S. H., and Braverman, L. E. (1979): Thyroid binding antibodies and other immunological abnormalities in patients with Graves' ophthalmopathy: effect of treatment with cyclophosphamide. *Clin. Endocrinol. (Oxf.)*, 10:79–91.

47. Werner, S. C. (1966): Prednisone in emergency treatment of malignant exophthalmos. *Lancet*, 1:1004–1007.

48. Werner, S. C., Feind, C. R., and Aida, M. (1967): Graves' disease and total thyroidectomy: progression of severe eye changes and decrease in serum long acting thyroid stimulator after operation. *N. Engl. J. Med.*, 276:132–138.

49. Winand, R. (1976): La prevention et le traitement de l'exophthalmie endocrinienne. *Bull. Mem. Acad. R. Med. Belg.*, 131:226–234.

50. Winand, R., and Mahieu, P. (1973): Prevention of malignant exophthalmos after treatment of thyrotoxicosis. *Lancet*, 1:1196.

The Eye and Orbit in Thyroid Disease, edited by
C. A. Gorman et al. Raven Press, New York 1984.

Comprehensive Care

Colum A. Gorman

*Division of Endocrinology and Department of Internal Medicine, Mayo Clinic,
Rochester, Minnesota 55905*

Patients with severe Graves' ophthalmopathy frequently experience an illness which can last for months or years. During the illness they may encounter phases of hyper- and hypothyroidism and side effects from steroids or antithyroid drugs. Unfavorable changes in appearance may assault their body image and their personal relationships. They are often required to choose between no therapy and a variety of procedures (Table 1), all of which are unfamiliar and are more or less daunting. To make matters worse, at times they face these decisions and discomforts with a fragmented series of specialized physicians, each of whom may be expert in a narrow discipline but none of whom has a comprehensive overview of the whole person, of his or her disease, and of the risks and benefits connected with each therapeutic alternative. This chapter outlines the role that an informed internist/ endocrinologist may play in providing perspective, continuity, and structure in management of patients with Graves' ophthalmopathy.

PATIENT EVALUATION

Evaluation of the patient with Graves' ophthalmopathy should begin with a comprehensive general medical evaluation. The examiner seeks to determine the other medical conditions of the patient. How severe a threat do the medical disorders pose to life and well being? Are there contraindications to steroid therapy or to surgery? If the patient has been treated with systemic corticosteroids, what side effects are present? How significant are they? Skin bruising and weight gain are reversible. Peptic ulcers heal and weight gained can be lost again; but bone loss is irreversible, and compression fractures represent a permanent spinal deformity.

When the general medical status of the patient is clear, definition of thyroid status is the next priority. Periorbital edema is a consistent feature of hypothyroidism and is sometimes extreme. Hyperthyroidism may induce lid retraction and lid lag which can be normalized by restoring thyroid function to normal. Active untreated hyperthyroidism is a firm contraindication to surgery under general anesthesia. Hypothyroidism is a lesser surgical risk factor (3). What treatment has been directed toward the thyroid gland in the past? To what extent has it been successful. Can it be employed again?

When patients are hyperthyroid, it has been our consistent practice to treat them with radioiodine. In spite of the occasional literature references to exacerbations of ophthalmopathy after radioiodine therapy (1), we have had no such experience and the results of exophthalmometer measurements by Tamai et al. show that proptosis decreases when hypothyroid patients become euthyroid (2).

When the patient's general medical and thyroid status have been defined, the next step is to obtain a careful history of past therapy to the eyes, the success or lack of efficacy of that therapy, and the side effects resulting from it.

TABLE 1. *Treatment options for Graves' ophthalmopathy*

Indication	Treatment options[b]
Lid retraction and lid lag in conjunction with hyperthyroidism	Correct hyperthyroidism
Periorbital and lid edema	Do not sleep prone; elevate head of bed; use diuretics
Eyelids close normally but gritty, sandy sensation is present	1% Methylcellulose eye drops p.r.n.
Imperfect coverage of globe due to eyelid retraction; relatively slight proptosis	Systemic or retrobulbar steroids; supervoltage x-ray therapy; eyelid surgery
Intermittent diplopia	Await remission or progression; consider prisms
Persistent diplopia	Extraocular muscle surgery with or without preliminary decompression
Optic neuropathy; corneal ulceration; severe eye discomfort, particularly if unresponsive to steroids[a]	Orbital decompression; supervoltage x-ray therapy

[a]Combined with local measures to protect the cornea.
[b]It is assumed that thyroid over- or underactivity will be concurrently treated.

Then one can turn one's attention to an assessment of current eye status. How long is it since the first eye symptoms developed? Does the patient have eye pain, lacrimation, photophobia, visual blurring, or diplopia? Are the symptoms stable or progressive? Are they tolerable, or does the patient demand relief? If diplopia is present, is it intermittent or constant? Intermittent diplopia should not be treated surgically. It usually either becomes persistent, in which case surgical correction is feasible, or it clears spontaneously, in which case surgery is unnecessary. What is the status of the cornea, optic nerve, and extraocular muscles? Here the perception of patient and physician in regard to the severity of the problem are most likely to be at variance. To the patient, diplopia may be the most worrisome symptom because it is so dramatic an occurrence. In the physician's terms, diplopia, which can be readily corrected surgically or with prisms is of less concern than persistent blurring of vision, which may indicate optic neuropathy. Effective communication between patient and physician to reconcile their priorities helps to avoid later misunderstandings.

Patients with ophthalmopathy complain of three types of visual blurring which have different medical significance. Chemosis and lacrimation may cause momentary blurring which clears with blinking. This is the "wet windowpane effect." Blurring which is present only when both eyes are in use and which clears when either eye is closed is due to extraocular muscle imbalance. Persistently blurred vision in one or both eyes progressively worsening over a period of days or weeks is probably due to optic neuropathy.

PATIENT MANAGEMENT

An evaluation as just described allows the physician to assess treatment options for the eye condition in the context of the patient's general health and against the record of previous treatment successes, failures, and side effects. A series of important clinical decisions must be made:

1. Is this truly Graves' ophthalmopathy?
2. Is the patient euthyroid, hypothyroid, or thyrotoxic?
3. Is the condition stable or progressive?

4. What are the specific threats to function (corneal exposure, eye muscle involvement, optic nerve)?
5. Which symptom is most troublesome to the patient?
6. What treatment is best for vision, appearance, and comfort?

Advanced pulmonary disease or recent myocardial infarction may preclude surgical options. Severe osteoporosis or peptic ulcer disease contraindicate corticosteroid therapy. A patient who has had little improvement following lateral orbital decompression may be unwilling to consider transantral decompression even when the anticipated better results are outlined to the patient. The internist/endocrinologist is likely to see the patient with Graves' eyes at all stages of treatment. Ophthalmologists relatively rarely encounter the actively hyperthyroid or hypothyroid patient who has only slight lid retraction and stare, and ENT surgeons characteristically encounter the patient around the time of orbital decompression and seldom see early or mild forms of the disease.

The internist should accept as a specific responsibility the definition of the patient's general health, the ranking of medical problems, the control of thyroid function, and the identification of specific risks connected with anesthesia, surgery, or steroid therapy. The internist should explain to the patient why the eye condition may be progressing despite adequate therapy for the hyperthyroid state. This is a necessary step to defuse a patient's concern that in the face of progressing eye disease the therapy directed to the thyroid was somehow inadequate.

A flowchart for medical decision-making in patients with Graves' ophthalmopathy is shown in Fig. 1 and includes the following:

1. Does the patient have serious medical problems apart from the thyroid and eyes?
   No
   Yes—What are they? Define type and severity, risk to life, and well-being. Do they preclude anesthesia or steroid therapy?
2. Is the patient euthyroid?
   Yes
   No—Define thyroid abnormality and treat hyperthyroidism with ^{131}I or hypothyroidism with T_4.
3. Is the eye problem the highest priority for the patient and the physician?
   Yes
   No—Treat whatever is highest priority, then return to eyes.
4. Is the eye problem due to Graves' eyes?
   Yes
   No—treat the cause of eye problem; e.g., lymphoma, allergy, tumor.
5. How have the eyes been treated in the past? Success? Side effects?
6. Evaluate and establish priorities based on the eye examination.

These should be considered as general guides to our approach rather than as absolute imperatives which are invariably followed. Special circumstances may favor alternative modes of management.

Before discussing the plan of therapy with the patient by telephone or in person, the ophthalmologist, ENT surgeon, and endocrinologist should confer. Specifically, the overall treatment plan and the sequence of each step should be reviewed. This ensures that during subsequent consultation a consistent management theme is presented to the patient. If surgery is recommended to the patient, we explain the reason for the surgery, the potential side

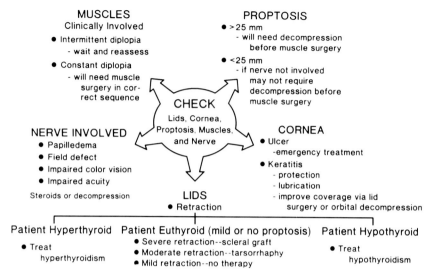

FIG. 1. Flowchart for medical decision-making in patients with Graves' ophthalmopathy: eye exam.

TABLE 2. *Discussion preceding transantral orbital decompression*

1. Why this procedure at this time?
    Discuss alternatives
2. How is the operation performed?
    Explain relevant anatomy
    Site of incision—sublabial—no external incision
    Stay in hospital
    Duration of disability
    Will eyes be bandaged postoperatively? Not usually
3. General surgery risks and complications:
    Risks of general anesthesia
    In steroid-treated patients, need for supplemental steroids during surgery
4. Specific risks and potential complications:
    Diplopia[a]; numb upper lip[b]; possibility of visual loss[c]; CSF leak[c]; limited
        improvement[d]; nasoantral fistula especially in steroid-treated patients[d]
5. Duration of stay in hospital and disability:
    3–4 days, duration of disability determined by outcome
    No work with dangerous machinery until any diplopia corrected
    Even if diplopia present, office work is feasible with eye patch
6. Postoperative plans:
    Taper and stop steroids within 1–2 weeks
    Probable need for muscle surgery in 6 weeks
    Possible need for lid surgery

[a]High probability, 30%.
[b]Inevitable, 100%.
[c]Very low probability, 1–2%.
[d]Medium probability, ±10%.

effects, complications of the specific operation, and the staging of surgical procedures. Discussion with the patient before transantral orbital decompression should cover all the points in Table 2. Numbness of the upper lip is an almost inevitable consequence of the procedure. Diplopia is frequent, but the risks of cerebrospinal fluid (CSF) leakage or visual loss are very slight. Similar discussions should precede surgery on extraocular muscles and on eyelids. The discussion preceding eye muscle surgery, where the patient has already had or does not need orbital decompression, includes the following:

1. How eye muscles work to move globe and maintain single vision.
2. Explanation of the problem—restricted eye motion due to tethering.
3. Proposed solution—advance or recession of one or more muscles.
4. Local or general anesthesia. General anesthesia is preferred.
5. Why we must wait until condition is stable, off steroids, before surgery is undertaken.
6. Possibility of a need for a second or third operation if first is not successful.
7. Possibility of a need for eyelid surgery (particularly following recession of inferior recti).
8. General surgical risks (bleeding, infection, etc.)
9. Stay in hospital—1 to 2 days.

The discussion preceding eyelid surgery, where the patient has already had or does not need orbital decompression or eye muscle surgery, is as follows:

1. Nature of the problem—retraction with consequent exposure of cornea.
2. Which lid surgical procedures were selected to solve the problem and why.
3. Perfection is not attainable—what degree of improvement is acceptable to patient and is attainable by physician.
4. Local anesthesia.
5. General risks—bleeding, infection.
6. Specific risks—overcorrection, ptosis; undercorrection, persistent retraction; alteration of upper lid fold position.

In summary, the elements of comprehensive care as we try to practice it are (a) continuity of care by an informed physician; (b) breadth of perspective in viewing the patient's eye condition relative to other medical problems; (c) a balanced assessment of relative risks from various forms of treatment; (d) a correctly staged, skillfully executed, and clearly communicated treatment plan; (e) and the development of concordance between the priorities of patient and physician.

REFERENCES

1. Gwinup, G., Elias, A. N., and Ascher, M. S. (1982): Effect on exophthalmos of various methods of treatment of Graves' disease. *JAMA*, 247:2135–2138.
2. Tamai, H., Nakagawa, T., Ohsako, N., Fukino, O., Takahashi, H., Matsuzuka, F., Kuma, K., and Nagataki, S. (1980): Changes in thyroid function in patients with euthyroid Graves' disease. *J. Clin. Endocrinol. Metab.*, 50:108–112.
3. Weinberg, A. D., Brennan, M. D., Gorman, C. A., Marsh, H. M., and O'Fallon, W. M. (1983): Outcome of anesthesia in surgery and hypothyroid patients. *Arch. Intern. Med.*, 143:893–897.

Subject Index